THE HOSPITAL RESEARCH AND EDUCATIONAL TRUST

Being a Health Unit Coordinator

Fifth Edition

Kay Cox-Stevens, R.N., M.A.
Health Careers Specialist
Professor, Saddleback College
Mission Viejo, California

D1605073

Prentice Hall

Prentice Hall
Upper Saddle River, New Jersey 07458

Notice

The procedures described in this textbook are based on consultation with medical authorities. The author and publisher have taken care to make certain that these procedures reflect currently accepted clinical practice; however, they cannot be considered absolute recommendations.

The material in this textbook contains the most current information available at the time of publication. However, federal, state, and local guidelines concerning medical clerical practices can change rapidly. The reader should note, therefore, that new regulations may require changes in some procedures.

It is the responsibility of the reader to familiarize himself or herself with the policies and procedures set by federal, state, and local agencies, as well as the institution or agency where the reader is employed. The authors and the publishers of this textbook, and the supplements written to accompany it, disclaim any liability, loss, or risk resulting directly or indirectly from the suggested procedures and theory, from any undetected errors, or from the reader's misunderstanding of the text. It is the reader's responsibility to stay informed of any new changes or recommendations made by any federal, state, and local agency as well as by his or her employing health care institution or agency.

Library of Congress Cataloging-in-Publication Data

Cox-Stevens, Kay, 1939–
  Being a health unit coordinator / Kay Cox.—5th ed.
    p. ; cm.
  At head of title: Hospital Research and Educational Trust.
  Includes bibliographical references and index.
  ISBN 0-13-091612-9
  1. Hospital ward clerks. I. Hospital Research and Educational Trust. II. Title.
  [DNLM: 1. Personnel, Hospital. 2. Hospital Records. 3. Hospital Units—organization &
  administration. 4. Medical Records. WX 159 C877b 2001]
  RA972.55.C69 2001
  362.1′1′068—dc21

                                        2001025872

Publisher: Julie Alexander
Executive Editor: Maura Connor
Senior Acquisitions Editor: Barbara Krawiec
Assistant Editor: Michael Sirinides
Managing Editor: Patrick Walsh
Production Management: Bookworks
Production Editor: Karen Fortgang
Interior Design: Rosemarie Votta
Director of Manufacturing and Production: Bruce Johnson
Manufacturing Buyer: Patrick Brown

Creative Director: Cheryl Asherman
Design Coordinator: Maria Guglielmo
Composition: BookMasters, Inc.
Marketing Manager: David Hough
Production Information Manager: Rachele Triano
Printer/Binder: Banta Company, Harrisonburg, VA
Copy Editor: Barbara Liguori
Proofreader: Pat Wilson
Cover Design: Kevin Kall

To my wonderful family, and to health unit coordinators everywhere.

Pearson Education LTD.
Pearson Education Australia PTY, Limited
Pearson Education Singapore, Pte. Ltd
Pearson Education North Asia Ltd
Pearson Education Canada, Ltd.
Pearson Educación de Mexico, S.A. de C.V.
Pearson Education—Japan
Pearson Education Malaysia, Pte. Ltd

10 9 8 7 6 5
ISBN 0-13-091612-9

Contents

Preface

As we begin the new millennium the health care industry will be faced with many challenges and opportunities. Today's sophisticated world of medicine places many demands on health care workers. Advanced technology, government regulations, and the increasingly complex nature of medical care have resulted in a critical need for competent, well-trained, and responsible personnel.

The fifth edition of *Being a Health Unit Coordinator* continues to provide the basic, easy-to-understand, current information necessary to perform the duties of a health unit coordinator. It is designed for students enrolled in unit coordinating programs and as a reference for employed unit coordinators.

ORGANIZATION

The text is organized into nineteen chapters and is logically arranged, moving from the simple to the complex. The first nine chapters provide a core of information considered necessary for all medical–clerical workers. The next eight chapters focus on subject matter more specific to the performance of health unit coordinating procedures. Chapter 18 discusses reviewing for the national certification examination, and Chapter 19 contains numerous sets of physicians' orders for order transcription practice.

The objectives are clearly stated and vocabulary words are listed at the beginning of each chapter; key ideas are highlighted; lists of medical terminology and abbreviations are included; and review questions and activities appear at the end of each chapter.

NEW FEATURES OF THE FIFTH EDITION

New abbreviations have been added, and new medications have been included and old ones deleted. Chapter 5, Introduction to Body Structure and Function, has been considerably revised and reorganized, and new information has been included. Sets of review questions have been added throughout the chapter to supplement the Learning Activities at the end of the chapter. Chapter 3, The Hospital Departments, also has been reorganized. New information on hepatitis and AIDS has been included in Chapter 6. Chapter 16, Diagnostic and Therapeutic Department Orders, has been extensively revised, with many new tests and treatments added.

This edition contains a list of vocabulary words and their definitions at the beginning of each chapter. Many new learning activities and critical thinking questions as well as new computer assignments using the Internet have been added at the end of the chapters. New artwork has been added to give the book a fresh appearance.

This fifth edition retains the many sets of physicians' orders (many in actual handwritten form) and instructions for scenarios that give students classroom opportunities for real-life practice performing health unit coordinator procedures.

The field of health care is one of rapid change. A textbook cannot be updated as often as new procedures or equipment are adopted by modern health care institutions, nor is it possible for this text to describe every procedure, form, or exact method your hospital will use. However, your instructor keeps informed of these changes and knows the specific ways of doing things in your hospital and in your community.

Now you are ready to study, to think, and to practice. The work you will learn to do is important work. Mastering it will be an accomplishment of which you can be proud.

ACKNOWLEDGMENTS

I would like to express my utmost gratitude to the wonderful people at South Coast Medical Center in South Laguna, California, for their generosity in helping me with this revision. I would also especially like to thank NAHUC president Sandy Ayres for her gracious assistance. Thanks also to the people at Brady, Barbara Krawiec, Executive Editor, Health Professions; and Michael Sirinides, Editorial Assistant.

KAY COX-STEVENS, R.N., M.A.

ABOUT THE AUTHOR

This edition of *Being a Health Unit Coordinator* is once again prepared by Kay Cox-Stevens, R.N., M.A. She is a Professor of Health Sciences at Saddleback College in Mission Viejo, California, and owns a consulting business, Achiever's Development Enterprises. She is a former instructor of health unit coordinators. She is a founding member of NAHUC (The National Association of Health Unit Coordinators) and a former regional representative and Director of Education of that organization. She is the series editor for the Medical Clerical Series and for the Clinical Allied Health textbook series for Career Publishing.

CHAPTER 1

Introduction to Being a Health Unit Coordinator

VOCABULARY

Accuracy	The quality of exactness or correctness
Career ladder	A route for advancement, often through education
Certification	That which vouches for or affirms that certain standards have been met
Certified Health Unit Coordinator (CHUC)	A unit coordinator who has passed the NAHUC-sponsored certification examination
Clinical tasks	Patient care tasks performed at the bedside
Coordination	The act of bringing into order parts of a whole
Cross training	The training of employees in more than one job
Dependability	Trustworthiness; the capability to be counted on
Empathy	The ability to put oneself in another person's position and to understand that person's feelings or experience
Evolution	The process of unfolding, growing, or developing, which usually happens by slow stages
Health care team	All the people who provide care for the patient
Health unit coordinator (HUC)	An unlicensed health care worker who performs the nonclinical (clerical, reception, communication, and coordination) tasks for the nursing unit
Hygiene	Principles of health and sanitation
Job description	A written description of the work requirements for a particular position
Legible	Easily read
National Association of Health Unit Coordinators (NAHUC)	A national organization that promotes professionalism, competence, and education for health unit coordinators
Personnel policies	Rules and regulations that relate to employment
Recertification	The completion of the requirements prescribed by the certifying board in order to remain certified

When you have completed this chapter, you will be able to:

- Define the terms listed in the vocabulary.
- List desirable characteristics for health unit coordinators.
- Name and state the purpose of the National Association of Health Unit Coordinators.
- Use the NAHUC web site to answer questions about NAHUC membership and certification.
- State the importance of good hygiene and of a dress code.
- Discuss the importance of accuracy and dependability in your daily work.
- State the three main categories of a health unit coordinator's duties and list the basic tasks you will perform.
- Describe methods for growth and advancement in your job.

A **health unit coordinator** is a very important member of the **health care team.** The health unit coordinator performs the clerical, reception/communication, and co-ordination tasks for the nursing unit, leaving more time for the nursing staff to perform the clinical or patient care duties. Through your performance as a health unit coordinator, you will make a valuable contribution to the care of the patient.

As a health unit coordinator you will be working with the medical and nursing teams doing the work of one of the most respected professions in the world: caring for the sick and promoting wellness. This is rewarding work that deserves careful attention and the determination to do a good job. During your training and while you are at work remember that the *most important person* in the hospital is the PATIENT.

*H*ISTORY OF HEALTH UNIT COORDINATING

Before the **evolution** of the health unit coordinator position, the registered nurse performed not only the clinical but also the clerical and reception tasks necessary to render care to the hospitalized patient. During World War II, nurses were in short supply, and it became necessary to train others on the job to assist the registered nurse. The clerical and reception tasks were designated to persons called ward clerks (the job title in the 1950s) and the patient care or **clinical tasks** to persons now called nursing assistants. The first reference to the use of unit coordinators is in an article published in 1940 in a journal called *The Modern Hospital.* Abraham Oseroff, a hospital administrator described the use of a "new helper" called a floor secretary. Rapid advances in medicine have resulted in an expanded role for ward clerks, and has grown into the responsible and challenging position it is today.

In the past, the only training for health unit coordinators occurred on the job. Today there are educational programs in vocational schools and colleges throughout the nation.

*N*AHUC

In recognition of the importance of the health unit coordinator's role, a professional association was formed on August 23, 1980, in Phoenix, Arizona. At the invitation of Myrna Lafleur Brooks, who became the founding president, a small group of educators and practitioners from throughout the nation attended that first meeting. The founding members in addition to Myrna Lafleur Brooks were Kay Cox, Helga Hegge, Carolyn Hinken, Estelle Johnson, Connie Johnston, Kathy Jordan, Velma Kerschner, Jane Pedersen, and Winifred Starr. At that meeting the National Association of Health Unit Clerks-Coordinators (NAHUC) was born. At a second meeting, hosted by Kay Cox in San Juan Capistrano, California, the constitution was ratified and the new association's officers were elected. In 1990 the NAHUC membership voted to change its name and drop the word *Clerk*. Figure 1.1 shows the NAHUC logo.

August 23 has been named Health Unit Coordinator Day, and it has been listed in the American Hospital Association Calendar of Health Observance Days.

The first national convention was held in June 1982 in San Antonio, Texas, hosted by Velma Kerschner, where the Code of Ethics and Standards of Practice for Health Unit Coordinators were adopted.

The **National Association of Health Unit Coordinators,** as it is now known, provides opportunities for local, state, regional, and national participation. It is a professional organization that promotes the professionalism and competence of health unit coordinators. Membership includes both individual and institutional members.

Another contribution of NAHUC is the development of a national **certification** examination. When certified, a health unit coordinator is called a **certified health unit coordinator (CHUC).** There are over 15,000 CHUCs in the United States. The examination is offered throughout the nation to anyone who is a health unit coordinator, has completed health unit coordinating training, or is involved in activities related to health unit coordinating. Membership in NAHUC is not required, but applicants must have a high school diploma or a GED.

For more information on NAHUC write to NAHUC, 1947 Madron Road, Rockford, IL 61107, or call 888-22-NAHUC or locally, 215-545-1985. Fax: 215-545-8107; http://www.nahuc.org

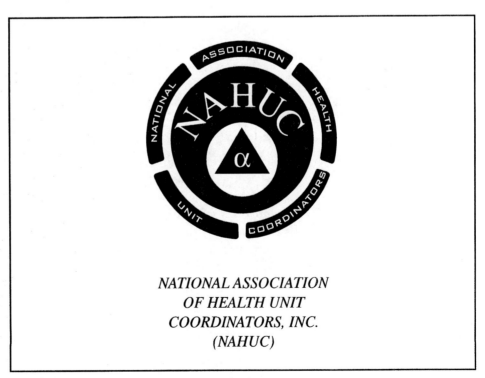

*NATIONAL ASSOCIATION
OF HEALTH UNIT
COORDINATORS, INC.
(NAHUC)*

FIGURE 1.1 The NAHUC logo (Courtesy of NAHUC.)

PERSONAL QUALIFICATIONS

You have chosen to become a health unit coordinator and you want to do the best possible job. What kind of a person makes a good health unit coordinator? Certain traits, attitudes, and habits are regularly seen in people who are successful in their work in the health care institution. Some of these traits are already part of one's personality. Other traits can be learned through practice and *become* part of one's *improved* personality.

Go through this list and see where you stand. Review those qualities you already have. Check those you think you could learn and incorporate. You have the qualifications if:

- You are trustworthy and dependable.
- You enjoy working with people.
- You get along well with others.
- You are considerate and tactful.
- You want to help people.
- You try to be gracious and polite at all times.
- You show **empathy** and patience with others.
- You like to communicate with others.
- You are a good listener.
- You like clerical work and attention to detail.
- You like to be organized.
- You strive for accuracy.
- You have reasonably good reading **comprehension.**
- You have good spelling ability.
- You have neat and **legible** handwriting.
- You can work under pressure.
- You always try to control your temper.
- You believe that you are doing important work.
- You can follow rules and instructions.
- You want to improve your performance.
- You like to learn new things.
- You don't let your private life interfere with your work.
- You are interested in the medical field.

Dependability

Your hospital is organized to function efficiently when a certain number of people are on the job. Your absence could deprive a patient of needed care.

Your absence may also cause your fellow workers to have an overload of work. It is essential that you arrive promptly every day unless you are ill. If you *are* sick, you must always notify the nursing office or appropriate supervisor as soon as possible so arrangements can be made for a replacement for you.

Dependability, however, means more than coming to work on time and coming to work every day. It also means that when you are asked to do something, you can be relied on to do it at the proper time and in the proper way.

Accuracy

Accuracy and dependability are closely related (Fig. 1.2). In a hospital you are concerned with human lives. What might appear to you as a tiny mistake or oversight

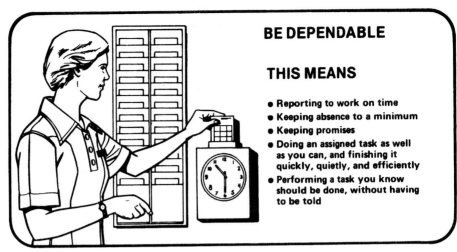

BE DEPENDABLE

THIS MEANS

- Reporting to work on time
- Keeping absence to a minimum
- Keeping promises
- Doing an assigned task as well as you can, and finishing it quickly, quietly, and efficiently
- Performing a task you know should be done, without having to be told

FIGURE 1.2

could delay the recovery of the patient. Whether you are recording a temperature, taking off doctor's orders and inputting them into the computer, or answering the telephone, it is vitally important that you stay alert, follow instructions, and be accurate. Try never to make mistakes; however, *should you make a mistake,* correct it at once and, when appropriate, report the error to your supervisor. If you do not understand, ask again. There is a reason for every step in the routine of the hospital. Remember, accuracy in this job is not just important—it is essential!

Following Rules and Instructions

Every business has its own rules and regulations. Rules and regulations governing a hospital are even more significant to know and follow than those of most other businesses because life-and-death situations are often involved. There are *specific* policies that will guide your work or conduct in the hospital. Most of these rules are in writing. Learn the rules, and if you do not understand something, ask your instructor or the nurse in charge.

A hospital staff is concerned with human lives. Instructions may be given to you very quickly and in tense situations. You must be able to follow instructions carefully and accurately and be ready to adjust quickly to any new situation.

Rules and regulations that relate to employment are called **personnel policies.** Following is a list of personnel practices and employment matters about which your hospital is likely to have precise instructions and regulations. As you consider employment in a hospital you will want to become informed about these regulations.

1. Miscellaneous regulations:
   - Locker assignment and use
   - Permission to leave during working hours
   - Policy for lost and found items

2. Time assignments:
   - Tours of duty (shift rotation or working on different units) and hours
   - Off-duty days
   - Use of the time clock

3. Salary administration:
   - Wage scales
   - Payday: time and place
   - Cashing personal checks

- Payroll deductions
- Salary differentials for various tours of duty
- Overtime pay
- Increases in salary, with advancement for certified health unit coordinators (CHUC)

4. Appearance:
   - Regulations on uniforms
   - Identification badges
   - Laundering of uniforms
   - General cleanliness and good grooming

5. Meals:
   - Assigned areas for eating or snacking
   - Meal hours and breaks
   - Cafeteria and coffee shop hours, prices, and employee discounts
   - Assigned coffee breaks and rest periods

6. Personal health:
   - Physical examinations including tuberculosis, hepatitis B, rubella, and other infectious disease screening and immunizations
   - Employee health service
   - Use of outpatient or clinic facilities
   - Sick leave
   - Absence from work because of illness, including going off duty because of illness and reporting ill from home

7. Employee benefits:
   - Vacations
   - Holidays
   - Hospitalization and medical insurance
   - Pension and retirement plans
   - Social Security and unemployment compensation insurance
   - Pharmacy prescriptions
   - Leaves of absence, with pay and without pay
   - Education stipends

8. Job status improvement:
   - Transfers
   - Promotions
   - Inservice education

9. Termination of employment:
   - Dismissals, including causes for dismissal and regulations concerning salary and benefits
   - Resignations, including length of notice required and whether notice must be in written form

10. Personnel records:
    - Applications
    - Incident reports
    - Performance evaluations
    - Letters of resignation
    - Changes of address, marital status, and dependents
    - Health record

11. Personnel–management relations:
    - Causes for disciplinary action
    - Grievance procedures

- Personnel committee
- Union affiliation

12. Personal conduct:
    - Smoking regulations
    - Confidential information
    - Hazards of noise
    - Other unprofessional behavior, such as noisiness, rowdiness, and gum chewing

There are certain general standards and regulations to be aware of. They are:

- Use of alcohol and other drugs: Consumption of alcohol or drugs or being under the influence of these substances while on duty is strictly forbidden.
- Solicitation and canvassing: Solicitation for unauthorized charitable contributions is forbidden. Authorized collections for charitable purposes, such as that for United Way, will be conducted by the hospital administration. In such instances, employees will be so notified. No employee is permitted to solicit other employees, patients, or visitors on hospital property to sell articles or services of any kind.
- Statements to the press: No statement or report of any kind concerning the hospital, its policies, or its patients is to be made by hospital staff to the press. All inquiries from the press are to be referred directly to the appropriate administrator. No staff member will pose for photographs at any time without first obtaining permission.
- Telephone calls: Adequate telephone service must be available for hospital purposes at all times. Employees must keep incoming calls at a minimum, both in number and in duration. Personal long-distance calls are forbidden. The use of hospital telephones for local calls of a personal nature is prohibited except in an emergency, and then only with the permission of the employee's supervisor.
- Use of hospital address: Employees, other than those living on the premises, are prohibited from using hospital mail facilities for receipt of personal mail. The messenger and mail facilities are reserved for hospital use only.
- Gifts and gratuities: Personnel are discouraged from accepting gifts from patients and visitors. Staff members are prohibited from accepting gifts in the form of money.

PERSONAL HYGIENE AND APPEARANCE

The health unit coordinator, as the receptionist of the nursing unit, regularly meets the public and so must apply the rules of **hygiene** and maintain a pleasant, neat, and businesslike appearance at all times. Most hospitals have a dress code for health unit coordinators. Follow the dress code of the health care institution where you work. Wear neat, clean clothes every day, repair rips and hems, and replace missing buttons on your clothing. Wear comfortable, businesslike low-heeled shoes with nonskid soles and heels. Keep jewelry at a minimum. Women should use makeup conservatively, and men should keep facial hair trimmed. Wear your name pin and assigned hospital identification (such as your picture). Don't chew gum.

Cleanliness is the most essential ingredient of any dress code. Bathe daily and use a deodorant. Keep your hair clean and neatly combed. Keep your mouth clean and your teeth in good condition. Keep your nails short, clean, and in good repair. Because you will be working closely with others, you must avoid fragrances such as cologne, perfume, or aftershave lotion.

JOB DESCRIPTION

Health care institutions use various titles for the position of health unit coordinator. These include ward clerk, unit clerk, ward secretary, unit secretary, and service coordinator. Whatever the title, the fundamental tasks and procedures you, as a health unit coordinator, will be accountable for will be found in the **job description** given to you by your hospital.

Working primarily at the desk on a nursing unit, you will be within easy reach of the unit telephones, computer, intercom system, and files. The health unit coordinator deals with both licensed and unlicensed nursing personnel, members of the medical staff, personnel from the other hospital departments, patients, and with visitors to the nursing unit. The health unit coordinator's duties fall under three main categories:

- Clerical
- Reception/communication
- **Coordination**

Everything the health unit coordinator does will be under the supervision of a registered nurse (Fig. 1.3).

FIGURE 1.3

Clerical Duties

- Transcribes doctors' orders and uses the computer to process these orders
- Maintains an orderly office environment
- Completes admission, transfer, discharge, preoperative, postoperative, and other patient records
- Keeps daily and interval records and reports
- Maintains patients' charts including filing of patient data in the chart holder
- Orders the daily diets
- Maintains an up-to-date bulletin board
- Requisitions supplies and services from various hospital departments as required
- Operates certain equipment at the nurses' station such as the computer and imprinter (to stamp the patient's name on different forms)

Reception/Communication Duties

- Answers, places, and transfers telephone calls
- Answers the intercom
- Records and relays messages
- Receives and directs visitors
- Receives and assists patients within prescribed limits
- Maintains communications (by telephone, intercom, computer, mail, fax, or messenger) within the nursing unit and between the nursing unit and other hospital departments
- Assists doctors and other health personnel as needed at the nurses' station

Coordination Duties Through communication, requisitioning, and management of supplies and equipment, the health unit coordinator coordinates the activities of the nursing staff, the patient, the doctor, other hospital departments, and visitors to the nursing unit (Fig. 1.4).

The Health Unit Coordinator and the Patient. The health unit coordinator does not perform direct patient care but aids in the care of the patient by performing such procedures as requisitioning tests, treatments, medications, and supplies that the doctor has ordered.

The health unit coordinator greets new patients and relays patient requests to nursing personnel, to doctors, and to other hospital departments.

The Health Unit Coordinator and Nursing. The health unit coordinator is usually a member of the nursing department and works under the supervision of a registered nurse and with other registered nurses, licensed practical or vocational nurses, nursing assistants, and other health unit coordinators.

The Health Unit Coordinator and the Doctor. The health unit coordinator has a great deal of contact with doctors both in person and by telephone. When doctors arrive on the nursing unit, the health unit coordinator greets them, handles their clerical requests, places and receives their calls, and relays messages for them to nursing personnel and other departments.

The health unit coordinator transcribes the doctor's orders. This means that after the doctor has written an order on the patient's chart, the health unit coordinator completes the necessary forms, orders the necessary equipment or services by computer, telephone, fax, and/or in writing, and communicates the orders to nursing personnel.

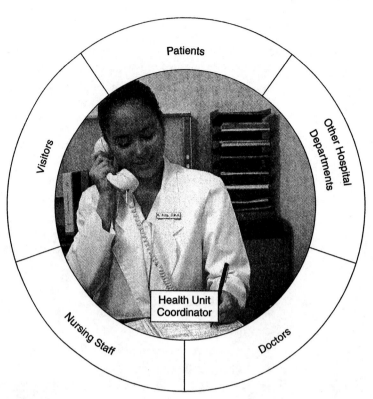

FIGURE 1.4

The Health Unit Coordinator and Other Departments. The health unit coordinator is in frequent communication with the many other hospital departments ordering tests, supplies, equipment, and other services. Messages by telephone, by computer, and in writing are sent, received, and relayed by the health unit coordinator.

The Health Unit Coordinator and the Patient's Visitors. The health unit coordinator greets and directs visitors, informs them of hospital rules as necessary, relays messages, and locates other hospital staff as requested.

OPPORTUNITIES FOR ADVANCEMENT

To keep up with new advances in the medical field, all health care workers are expected to take refresher courses and study new medical developments that affect their employment all their working lives. As you continue to learn, your job will become more interesting and rewarding personally and professionally.

You can continue to learn while you are on the job and expand your knowledge of the health care field. You can find better ways to do your work. All this can make you a more effective health unit coordinator. This means you will become more secure in your job.

Within the hospital, you will find classes offered for nursing and other health care personnel through the Department of Inservice Education. You may use this department as a resource to seek out classes best suited to enhance and enrich your learning on the job.

Classes offered through vocational schools, adult education, and community colleges in medical terminology, typing, computer skills, business skills, and management can help you make the lateral and vertical moves you desire; however, if you do not have a high school diploma, that should be your first goal. Adult education programs

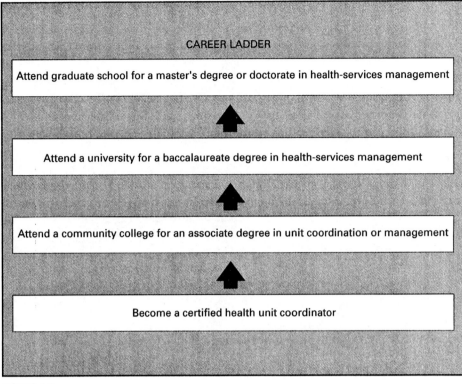

CAREER LADDER

Attend graduate school for a master's degree or doctorate in health-services management

Attend a university for a baccalaureate degree in health-services management

Attend a community college for an associate degree in unit coordination or management

Become a certified health unit coordinator

FIGURE 1.5

at local high schools offer basic education programs that lead to a high school equivalency diploma, which can help you start up the **career ladder** (Fig. 1.5).

Because NAHUC, like other professional organizations, requires contact hours for **recertification,** a variety of continuing education opportunities are available through NAHUC.

*O*THER CAREER OPPORTUNITIES

The education and experience gained through health unit coordinating provides a sound foundation for exploring other career opportunities. Many departments within a hospital and in other health care settings utilize the skills of an HUC.

Cross training is a popular trend in today's hospitals. By learning to perform other jobs or parts of other jobs the employee is able to function in more than one position. For the health unit coordinator this might include performing some admitting or transcription tasks.

*L*EARNING ACTIVITIES

Complete the following.

1. The most important person in the hospital is the _____.

2. The name of the national professional association for health unit coordinators is the _____.

3. List 10 qualifications of an excellent health unit coordinator.
   (a) _____
   (b) _____
   (c) _____
   (d) _____
   (e) _____
   (f) _____
   (g) _____
   (h) _____
   (i) _____
   (j) _____

4. Rules and regulations that relate to employment are called _____.

5. The most essential ingredient of any dress code is _____.

6. List four other titles for the position of health unit coordinator.
   (a) _____   (c) _____
   (b) _____   (d) _____

7. The fundamental tasks and procedures for which you will be accountable in your work will be found in the _____ _____ given to you by your employing hospital.

8. The health unit coordinator's duties fall under three main categories, which are
   (a) _____
   (b) _____
   (c) _____

9. As a health unit coordinator you will be under the supervision of a
   _____.

10. The quality of exactness or correctness is _____.

11. Coming to work every day on time and doing what is asked at the proper time and in the proper way is called _____.

12. A method of advancement through experience and education is called a
    _____.

13. CHUC stands for _____.

14. Go to the NAHUC web site and answer the following.
    (a) Today health unit coordinating is considered a profession. According to Wilson and Neuhauser in their book *Health Services in the U.S.,* for a group to become a profession they must meet certain criteria. According to the NAHUC web page, what are the criteria?
        (1) _____
        (2) _____
        (3) _____
        (4) _____
        (5) _____

        (6) _____
            _____
            _____

    (b) What benefits does NAHUC membership offer?
        (1) _____

(2) _____
(3) _____
(4) _____

(c) The NAHUC FAQ page says that one should become certified because of _____.

(d) In what should you take pride?

(1) _____
(2) _____
(3) _____

15. Use the following form to list those things about you that you feel will make you good at your job. Also list any traits you feel need improvement. Finally, list what you can do to improve in those areas.

My TRAIT INVENTORY

Strong	Need Improvement	What I Can Do to Improve

16. Why have you chosen this class? What do you think you will like about being a health unit coordinator? Is there anything you think you won't like? What are the pros and cons of working in a hospital?

_____
_____
_____

17. Why is it important to know and follow a hospital's rules? What is it about a hospital that makes it the same as another business/industry? What is different?

_____
_____
_____

18. How do you think you will feel if someone, perhaps a nurse or doctor, gives you instructions very quickly and doesn't say please or thank you?

_____
_____
_____

CHAPTER 2

The Working Environment

Acuity A measure of how sick a patient is and/or how much nursing care is required

Accreditation A voluntary process by which an institution is granted approved status by having met established standards

Case management The process of monitoring a patient's hospital stay and services to ensure that they are appropriate

Diagnosis related groups (DRGs) A complex classification system that provides the basis for payment to hospitals for Medicare, Medicaid, and some commercially insured patients; it categorizes patients who are medically related in terms of diagnosis and treatment into one of over 500 categories and pays the hospital a flat rate based on the DRG assigned

Health maintenance organization (HMO) A prepaid system of managed care that provides comprehensive medical care to enrolled groups at a fixed rate

Joint Commission on Accreditation of Healthcare Organizations (JCAHO) An agency that accredits hospitals

Managed care A system of health care designed to control costs

Medicaid A federal and state program that provides medical care for certain low-income patients

Medicare National insurance for persons 65 or older, the blind, and the disabled; Part A provides benefits for hospitalization, and Part B for medical care

Nursing unit Patient care areas within a hospital that are staffed with nurses and other personnel and the supplies and equipment needed to care for the patients admitted to that unit

Patient care assignment sheet A form that shows which nurse or other health care worker is caring for which patient

Prospective payment system (PPS) A system of payment to hospitals that treat Medicare patients that reimburses the hospital based on predetermined rates for each patient's illness determined by diagnosis

Provider An individual or organization such as a physician or hospital that delivers health care

Team leader A licensed nurse who directs the activities of the nursing team

Team nursing A method of organizing patient care that divides the nursing staff on a nursing unit into teams who then, under the direction of a team leader, care for a certain number of patients assigned to each team member

*T*HE HEALTH CARE INSTITUTION

When you have completed this chapter, you will be able to:

- Define the terms listed in the vocabulary.
- Explain the purposes, organization, and classifications of hospitals.
- Define Medicare Part A and Part B and the benefit period.
- Discuss how the business side of health care affects the health unit coordinator.
- Discuss the responsibilities of the medical staff.
- Define common medical specialties.
- Discuss the responsibilities of various levels of nursing personnel.
- Identify abbreviations and definitions of the various nursing units.
- Describe two ways of organizing the nursing health care team.
- Discuss the purpose and some contributions of the volunteer services.

*H*OSPITAL HISTORY

The history of medicine and surgery dates to the earliest ages, since there has been some form of hospital for centuries. The word *hospital* stems from the Latin *hospitalis* (relating to a quest)—one of the most ancient expressions of people's concern for a stranger. In ancient Greece, temples were used to house the sick, and the first church hospital was built in A.D. 369 at Ceesarea (now a part of Turkey). As Christianity spread, the sick became the concern of the church. Monasteries established hospitals for lepers, cripples, the blind, and the poor.

The first established hospitals were founded in the United States in the early eighteenth century. As medical knowledge grew, hospitals developed from the early crude establishments to our modern sophisticated institutions.

Today's hospital is a health team, a source of hope, a center for community health, an educational institution, and a laboratory; it is a provider of many different types of service—all of them important.

*F*UNCTIONS AND PURPOSES OF HOSPITALS

There are several basic functions and purposes of health care institutions, all of them having to do either with the immediate care of patients or with the health of the community—present and future (Fig. 2.1). These purposes include:

- Giving expert care to the sick and injured
- Preventing disease
- Promoting individual and community health
- Providing facilities for the education of health workers
- Promoting research in the sciences of medicine and nursing

FIGURE 2.1

*A*CCREDITATION

Hospitals that are accredited have met a standard by complying with a variety of rules and regulations set forth by the accrediting agency.

The **Joint Commission on Accreditation of Healthcare Organizations (JCAHO)** is a highly coveted **accreditation.** A JCAHO health care institution has been visited by a team of surveyors, evaluated, and approved as a hospital that is meeting high standards of operation.

There are several other accreditation agencies also that survey and evaluate health care institutions. Licensing of hospitals is usually a function of the State Department of Health.

Preparation for accreditation can be a stressful time for a hospital, and the health unit coordinator must appreciate the seriousness of the event and assist in any way possible. JCAHO accredits over 16,000 hospitals and other health care facilities.

*C*LASSIFICATIONS

Hospitals are classified most commonly by ownership or type of service offered.

Ownership Hospitals may be privately owned (groups of doctors, corporations) and operated for profit, community operated, owned by churches and fraternal organizations, or owned and operated by the government.

Type of Service There are many different kinds of hospitals. The most common is the general hospital that offers a variety of patient care services to persons of all ages. Specialized hospitals restrict their services to certain age groups (e.g., children or the elderly) or to those requiring a specialized type of care (e.g., orthopedic, maternal, psychiatric).

$\mathcal{T}$HE BUSINESS SIDE OF HEALTH CARE

Hospitals must be very business minded in their delivery of health care. In response to skyrocketing health costs, the government, insurance companies, and employers have placed intense pressure on hospitals and doctors to provide health care in a cost-effective manner. There have been and will continue to be significant changes in the way health care is provided and financed in this nation.

Many of the patients in the hospital will be insured under Medicare. **Medicare** is a federal insurance program administered by the Health Care Financing Administration (HCFA) that was created by the 1965 amendments to the Social Security Act. Medicare covers eligible people over 65, the blind, the disabled, children and adults with end-stage renal disease (ESRD) requiring dialysis or kidney transplant, and certain organ donors.

Medicare Part A is hospital insurance, and Part B is medical insurance. Medicare Part A patients must follow certain guidelines that relate to benefit periods. A benefit period begins with the day a patient enters the hospital and ends when the patient has not been an inpatient in a hospital or skilled nursing facility (SNF) for 60 consecutive days. Medicare insurance payments are renewed each time a new benefit period begins, and a patient may have unlimited benefit periods as long as the criterion for a benefit period is met. There is also a one-time 60-day reserve benefit.

For the first 60 days of hospitalization Medicare pays all but a little under $800. From the 61st to the 90th day of hospitalization the patient's portion of the bill is almost $200 a day, and the longer the patient is hospitalized, the more the patient must pay. If a patient was to be hospitalized for 5 months and had not managed to remain out of the hospital for the 60-day period so that a new benefit period could start, Medicare would pay nothing. Very close attention is paid to the medical necessity of hospitalization, and patients are moved out of an acute-care hospital as quickly as possible. Without supplemental or Medigap insurance, few patients can afford the out-of-pocket expenses that are a part of Medicare.

Medicare beneficiaries may receive health care through managed care plans that contract with Medicare. Usually, patients must receive services from hospitals that are contracted by the plan. Medicare + choice is a term used to describe the various health plan options available to Medicare beneficiaries.

Because cost containment is such a major concern, the government in 1983 implemented a payment system requiring that Medicare payments for hospital inpatient services be paid under a **prospective payment system (PPS)** based on **diagnosis related groups (DRGs).** With DRGs, patients' diseases and disorders are clustered into over 500 groups with a payment level specified for each group. Hospitals are reimbursed a flat rate that allows both payers and the hospital to predict reimbursement before the care is provided (prospectively). DRGs provide a basis for payment to hospitals for care of Medicare, **Medicaid,** and an increasing number of patients with commercial insurance. It serves as an important tool in cost containment and in hospital utilization (how long patients stay in the hospital).

Managed care is a system of health care designed to control costs. There are many types of managed care organizations (MCOs) and arrangements. Some common examples include:

- *Health Maintenance Organizations (HMOs)*—systems of health care in which a fixed sum is prepaid and after which health services are made available to the patient at a reduced rate. The kinds of services available and the reimbursement levels are outlined in the contract with the HMO. HMOs emphasize preventive medicine.

- *Preferred Provider Organizations (PPOs)*—a non-HMO type of managed care that contracts to provide care at a reduced rate that is usually more than for an HMO patient but less than regular commercial insurance would pay.
- *Independent Practice Association (IPA)*—A type of HMO in which an organization of providers who contract with payers at a discounted or capitated rate. (Money is paid based on number of enrolled patients rather than on number of services rendered.)
- *Point-of-Service Plan (POS)*—a plan that allows the patients considerable leeway in their choice of providers but provides greater reimbursement if they use a network **provider.**

Many people in the United States are without insurance. Consequently, there is tremendous financial stress on hospitals that continue to provide care to the uninsured.

All health care workers must realize that cost-containment practices are an essential part of their job. The health unit coordinator should understand that because of DRGs and managed care, hospitals must do everything possible to legally obtain the reimbursement they are due. From admission to discharge great care must be taken by the hospital personnel to properly record charges and follow policies and procedures set forth by the hospital so that it can be reimbursed for the care that is given. A hospital simply cannot survive without this cooperation from its staff.

$\mathcal{T}$HE HOSPITAL BILLING PROCESS

Because the business side of health care is so important, it is useful for the health unit coordinator to have a basic understanding of the admission review and hospital billing processes.

The Admitting Office is responsible for obtaining admitting information from the patient. This information includes personal information such as name, address, and telephone number as well as all insurance information. An admitting diagnosis is also recorded, which may change or be modified during hospitalization. Various legal forms are signed by the patient including a consent for treatment, a permission for release of information, an arbitration agreement, and a statement of financial responsibility.

The patient is then taken to his or her room and begins to receive medical care from the hospital and in the process, to accumulate many charges. Increasing numbers of patients' hospitalizations are paid for by some type of managed care program that functions under a variety of contracts and federal and state regulations. Hospitals negotiate managed care contracts and agree to give discounts to obtain increased numbers of patients.

In the case of Medicare patients, admissions must be carefully monitored, and the documentation in the medical record must show that the patient's diagnosis meets Medicare's criteria to be certified for reimbursement. The hospital's Utilization Review Department (UR) will review the admission, and if it is found to be necessary, it will be certified. The physician gives a tentative diagnosis so that a DRG can be assigned. As the patient's condition changes a new DRG may be assigned. DRGs are assigned using an automated system called a *DRG grouper.* There is ongoing review of the admission as the physician continues to document in the patient's chart the necessity for the admission and all care that is given.

Under the law, for a hospital to be eligible for Medicare reimbursement it must contract with a peer review organization. These organizations are made up of physicians who evaluate the quality of the care given by other physicians. They are responsible for the review of various aspects of the admission.

ADMITTING DEPARTMENT

↓

Patient Admitted

↓

Patient Receives Hospital Services

↓

Charges from Hospital Departments

↓

HOSPITAL BILLING DEPARTMENT

↓

Insurance Claims Sent

↓

Payments Received and Posted

FIGURE 2.2 The Hospital Billing Process

Case management is a process of monitoring a patient's hospital stay and services to ensure that they are appropriate. The case manager reviews the records of currently admitted patients to be sure that the severity of the illness and the level of services that are being given meet the criteria for acute care. If they do not, the case manager will talk with the attending physician to find options to acute hospital care. The case manager works with all the patient's caregivers to ensure that appropriate discharge planning occurs. Most insurance companies require that the case manager notify them of the results of the review before they will authorize continued hospitalization or payment of the bill.

Charges are recorded by computer from the various hospital departments that provided services for the patient. This information is organized by the billing department and transmitted electronically to the payers such as Medicare, Medicaid, commercial payers, health maintenance organizations, the Blue Plans (Blue Cross and Blue Shield), and some workers' compensation carriers. If a form is used to bill for services it is the Uniform Bill Claim Form, or UB-92. When payment is received by the hospital it is posted to patients' accounts. When appropriate, patients are billed for the portion not paid by insurance (Fig. 2.2).

𝒯RENDS AFFECTING HEALTH CARE

There are other trends that affect the way health care is provided. The American population as a whole is getting older. According to the American Association of Retired People (AARP), since the turn of the century the percentage of people in the United States over 65 has tripled. People over the age of 65 are expected to represent 20 percent of the population by the year 2030. The fastest-growing group of people are those over age 85 (29 times larger than in 1900). The implications of these statistics are fairly clear. The longer people live, the more health care services will be needed. This will result in more demand for community-based programs and increased public pressure for protection against the costs of long-term care. More and more emphasis will be placed on preventive health care. We have already seen the shift from inpatient to ambulatory care settings, which has resulted in a high acuity level for hospitalized patients. **Acuity** refers to how sick a patient is and/or how much nursing care is required.

There is competition for patients today, and health care workers must realize that marketing of the hospitals' services has become increasingly important. Hospitals strive constantly to identify, understand, and meet the needs of their patients and expand their visibility in the community.

The business side of health care affects health care workers who strive to provide quality care in a rapidly changing environment. The health unit coordinator must recognize that cost-containment practices are an essential part of the job and understand the importance of such procedures as coding (the assignment of numbers and letters to diagnose and procedures for billing purposes) and utilization review (the determination of the appropriateness of care and length of service for a hospitalized patient) that are performed by other members of the hospital staff.

Changes in health care delivery systems may create new duties for the health unit coordinator, with greater emphasis on business and management practices and increasing use of information systems.

ORGANIZATION

Health care institutions are comparable to business organizations in their division of functions. Most are governed by a board of directors (i.e., persons from the business and professional community who establish general policies, approve the budget, and hire the hospital administrator).

The hospital administrator, or chief executive officer (CEO), is in charge of the hospital and functions much as the president of a business does. With the aid of one or more assistant administrators, often called vice presidents, the hospital administrator handles the day-to-day operation of the hospital and carries out the policies of the board.

Each hospital will have its own organizational chart that will vary somewhat depending upon the type and ownership of the facility (Fig. 2.3).

THE MEDICAL STAFF
RESPONSIBILITIES

The medical staff is responsible for the diagnosis and treatment of the hospitalized patient. It is the doctor who orders the laboratory tests, the radiographs, and other diagnostic examinations; the doctor also prescribes the patient's medications and other therapy.

In many hospitals you will be working with licensed physicians, residents, interns, and medical students who serve a clinical clerkship, and are allowed to perform certain limited procedures and activities to gain hospital experience. However, the care of all private patients is assumed by attending physicians—that is, by licensed physicians who are either family practitioners or specialists.

EDUCATION

To practice medicine, a doctor must meet rigid educational standards. Although there are some variations, commonly a doctor must have graduated from college, completed a four-year course in medical school, and served for one year as a resident gaining hospital experience. After this, the doctor may be licensed as a physician by passing a state board examination.

Many physicians decide to specialize in some particular field of medicine. To do so the doctor must devote several years gaining further experience in the specialty he or she has chosen. The doctor then becomes recognized to practice medicine in that specialty by passing a national board examination (Fig. 2.4).

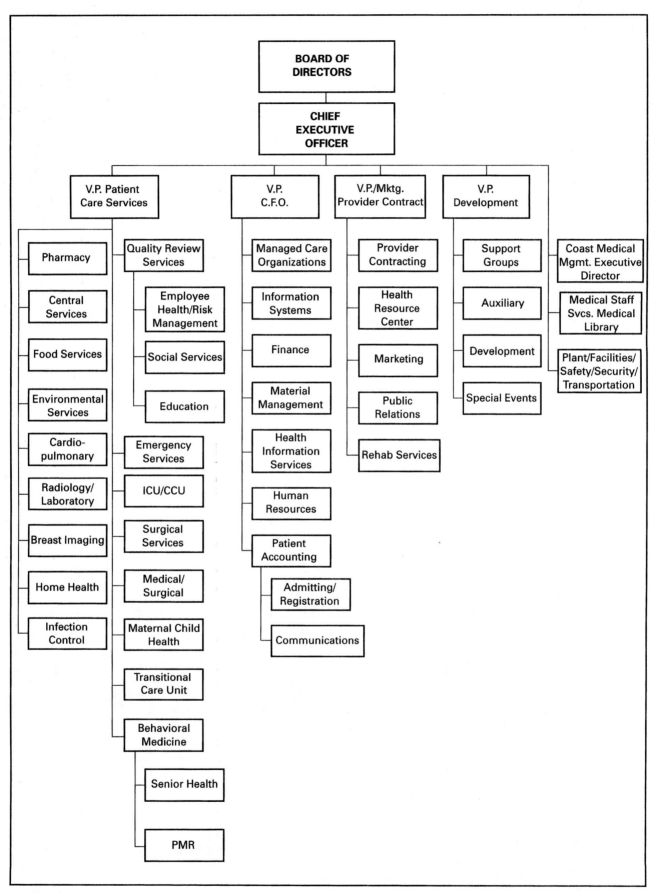

FIGURE 2.3 Hospital organizational chart.

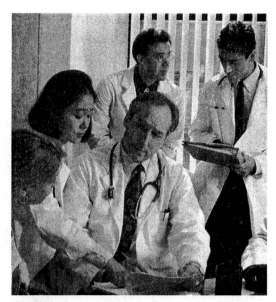

FIGURE 2.4

$\mathcal{M}$EDICAL SPECIALTIES

A medical specialty is a branch of knowledge concerning a certain part of the body or body system—its diseases, conditions, and treatments. A medical specialist is a physician who is devoted to a single branch of medical knowledge. You will hear medical specialties referred to in conversation by doctors, nurses, and other hospital personnel. Since the health unit coordinator has a great deal of interaction with the medical staff, it will be helpful for you to know the definitions of the terms you will hear.

Table 2.1 lists definitions of most of the present-day medical specialties and the standard title of the physician practicing in those specialties.

$\mathcal{O}$THER HEALTH PROFESSIONALS

Not all doctors with whom the health unit coordinator will come in contact are M.D.'s (medical doctors). Table 2.2 lists other specialties. State law and your hospital will have strict policies regarding the scope of practice for these individuals.

TABLE 2.1 $\mathcal{M}$EDICAL SPECIALTIES

Specialty	Physician's Title	Description
Allergies	Allergist	A subspecialty of internal medicine dealing with diagnosis and treatment of body reactions resulting from unusual sensitivity to foods, pollens, dust, medicines, or other substances
Anesthesiology	Anesthesiologist	Administration of various forms of anesthesia in operations or procedures to cause loss of feeling or sensation
Cardiovascular diseases; Cardiology	Cardiologist	A subspecialty of internal medicine involving the diagnosis and treatment of diseases of the heart and blood vessels
Dermatology	Dermatologist	Diagnosis and treatment of diseases of the skin
Emergencies	Emergency physician	Deals with immediate, urgent care of patient in emergency rooms and emergency clinics

Continued

TABLE 2-1 CONTINUED		
Specialty	**Physician's Title**	**Description**
Endocrinology	Endocrinologist	Diagnosis and treatment of diseases of the hormone-secreting ductless glands
Family practice	Family practitioner	Diagnosis and treatment of disease by medical and surgical methods for all members of the family regardless of age
Gastroenterology	Gastroenterologist	A subspecialty of internal medicine concerned with diagnosis and treatment of disorders of the digestive tract
Gerontology	Geriatrician	Diagnosis and treatment of diseases and disorders of the elderly
Gynecology	Gynecologist	Diagnosis and treatment of diseases of the female reproductive organs
Hematology	Hematologist	Diagnosis and treatment of diseases of the blood and blood-forming tissues
Internal medicine	Internist	The diagnosis and nonsurgical treatment of adults
Neonatology	Neonatologist	The care and treatment of newborns
Nephrology	Nephrologist	The diagnosis and treatment of diseases of the kidney
Neurological surgery	Neurosurgeon	Diagnosis and surgical treatment of brain, spinal cord, and nerve disorders
Neurology	Neurologist	Diagnosis and treatment of diseases of brain, spinal cord, and nerves
Obstetrics	Obstetrician	The care of women during pregnancy, childbirth, and the interval immediately following
Oncology	Oncologist	Diagnosis and treatment of cancer
Ophthalmology	Ophthalmologist	Diagnosis and treatment of diseases of the eye, including prescribing glasses
Orthopedics	Orthopedist	Diagnosis and treatment of disorders and diseases of the muscular and skeletal systems
Otolaryngology	Otolaryngologist	Diagnosis and treatment of diseases of the ear, nose, and throat
Pathology	Pathologist	Study and interpretation of changes in organs, tissues, cells, and alterations in body chemistry to aid in diagnosing disease and determining treatment
Pediatrics	Pediatrician	Prevention, diagnosis, and treatment of children's diseases
Physical medicine and rehabilitation	Physiatrist	Diagnosis of disease or injury in the various systems and areas of the body and treatment by means of physical procedures as well as treatment and restoration of the convalescent and physically handicapped patient
Plastic surgery	Plastic surgeon	Corrective or reparative surgery to restore deformed or mutilated parts of the body or to improve the appearance of a part of the body (cosmetic surgery)
Proctology	Proctologist	Diagnosis and treatment of diseases of the rectum
Psychiatry	Psychiatrist	Diagnosis and treatment of mental disorders
Radiology	Radiologist	Use of radiant energy including x-rays, radium, cobalt, and other radioactive materials, in the diagnosis of disease
Rheumatology	Rheumatologist	Diagnosis and treatment of rheumatic disorders such as arthritis, gout, bursitis, and other conditions
Surgery	Surgeon	Operative treatment of disease and injury
Therapeutic radiology	Radiologist	The use of radiant energy, including x-rays, radium, and other radioactive substances in the treatment of diseases
Thoracic surgery	Thoracic surgeon	Operative treatment of the lungs, heart, or the large blood vessels within the chest cavity
Urology	Urologist	Diagnosis and treatment of diseases or disorders of the kidneys, bladder, ureters, urethra, and of the male reproductive organs

TABLE 2.2 *O*THER HEALTH PROFESSIONALS

Doctor of Osteopathy (DO)	A health professional who has earned a degree by satisfactorily completing a course of education in an approved college of osteopathy. Osteopathic physicians follow almost identical courses of training and practice as medical physicians but emphasize treatment that involves manipulation of structures and the study of mechanical derangement of tissues as a cause of disease.
Doctor of Chiropractic (DC)	Provides treatment through the mechanical manipulation of the spinal column, physiotherapy, and diet. May diagnose through the use of radiology but does not employ surgery or drugs. Completes at least two years of premedical school followed by four years of education in an approved chiropractic school.
Podiatrist (DPM)	A health professional licensed to diagnose and treat diseases of the feet. Performs surgery, prescribes drugs and physical therapy. Completes at least two years of premedical courses and four years of study in an accredited college of podiatry and is awarded a DPM (Doctor of Podiatric Medicine).
Psychologist	A professional who specializes in the study of behavior and the processes of the mind, especially in regard to the environment, both social and physical. A clinical psychologist has earned a graduate degree in psychology and training in clinical psychology and is qualified to provide testing and counseling services.
Optometrist	Holds a degree of Doctor of Optometry (OD) and is licensed after at least two years of college and four years in an approved college of optometry to test the eyes for visual acuity and prescribe corrective lenses.
Dentist	Practices the prevention and treatment of diseases and disorders of the teeth and oral cavity. Can prescribe pain medications, antibiotics, and some other medications that require prescriptions. Completes at least two years of undergraduate study and three to four years at an approved dental college and then may be awarded a DDS (Doctor of Dental Surgery). There are eight recognized specialties that require advanced training.

*T*HE NURSING STAFF

*N*URSING STAFF RESPONSIBILITIES

Nursing personnel are responsible for carrying out the doctors' orders and giving nursing care to the patient. The nursing service plans and implements nursing care, observes the patient and records these observations, coordinates care and activities performed by other departments, conducts family and patient teaching, and works closely with the doctor in the care and rehabilitation of the hospitalized patient. Nursing Service is the largest department within a hospital.

Recent revisions to nurse practice acts have expanded the role of the registered nurse, and broader definitions of nursing interpret the nurse as a colleague of the physician rather than as an assistant.

As a health unit coordinator you are usually part of the nursing department. It is important that you understand the structure and function of nursing service and the roles of nursing service personnel (Figs. 2.5 and 2.6).

*N*URSING SERVICE ADMINISTRATIVE PERSONNEL

Administrative nursing personnel are registered nurses who usually have obtained advanced degrees such as BSN (Bachelor of Science in Nursing), MSN (Master of Science in Nursing), or doctorate degrees.

It is not uncommon for there to be changes in terminology to denote certain responsibilities within a hospital. For example, some hospitals refer to the head of the

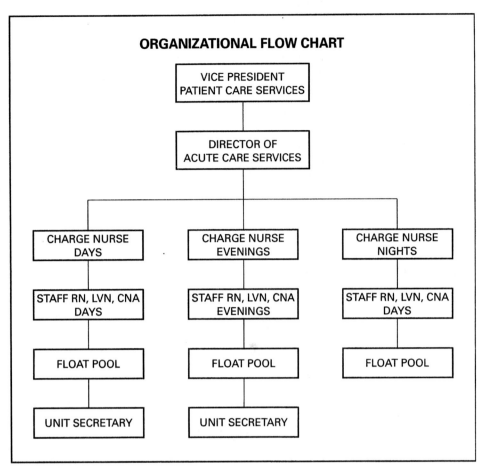

FIGURE 2.5

nursing department as the **Director of Nursing (DON),** whereas others call that position the **Vice President of Patient Care Services.** Figures 2.5 and 2.6 show two examples of organizational charts for nursing.

The Vice President of Patient Services (or Director of Nursing) is responsible for the administration of Nursing Service and is accountable to the hospital's president or chief executive officer. An Assistant Vice President of Patient Services (or Assisted Director of Nursing) assists the Director of Nursing and assumes those duties when the director is absent.

A **nursing supervisor** assists the Director of Nursing in carrying out administrative responsibilities and is responsible to the Director of Nursing. A hospital, depending on its size, will employ several nursing supervisors to work on each shift so that nursing administration is represented at all times.

The **Director of Education** is responsible for the continuing education and staff development of nursing service personnel and the orientation of new nursing service personnel, and may be responsible for all hospital staff inservice. The Director of Education is responsible to the Director of Nursing.

*N*URSING UNIT PERSONNEL

A **registered nurse (RN)** is a graduate of a two- to four-year school of nursing, has passed a state board examination, and is licensed by the state in which he or she is practicing nursing. Many registered nurses are college graduates who have obtained the

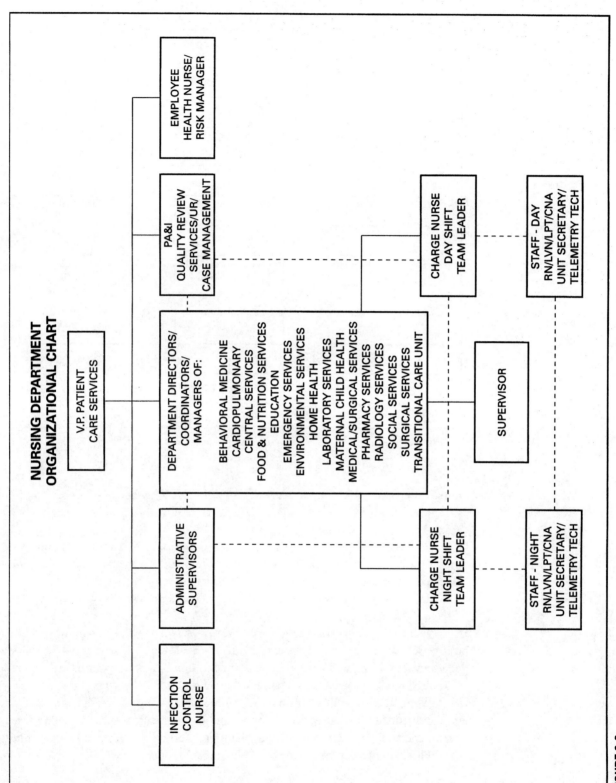

NURSING DEPARTMENT ORGANIZATIONAL CHART

V.P. PATIENT CARE SERVICES

INFECTION CONTROL NURSE

ADMINISTRATIVE SUPERVISORS

PA&I QUALITY REVIEW SERVICES/UR/ CASE MANAGEMENT

EMPLOYEE HEALTH NURSE/ RISK MANAGER

DEPARTMENT DIRECTORS/ COORDINATORS/ MANAGERS OF:

BEHAVIORAL MEDICINE
CARDIOPULMONARY
CENTRAL SERVICES
FOOD & NUTRITION SERVICES
EDUCATION
EMERGENCY SERVICES
ENVIRONMENTAL SERVICES
HOME HEALTH
LABORATORY SERVICES
MATERNAL CHILD HEALTH
MEDICAL/SURGICAL SERVICES
PHARMACY SERVICES
RADIOLOGY SERVICES
SOCIAL SERVICES
SURGICAL SERVICES
TRANSITIONAL CARE UNIT

CHARGE NURSE DAY SHIFT TEAM LEADER

STAFF - DAY RN/LVN/LPT/CNA UNIT SECRETARY/ TELEMETRY TECH

SUPERVISOR

CHARGE NURSE NIGHT SHIFT TEAM LEADER

STAFF - NIGHT RN/LVN/LPT/CNA UNIT SECRETARY/ TELEMETRY TECH

FIGURE 2.6

BSN, MSN, or other advanced degrees. Many nursing specialties require certification. An ACLS means that the nurse is qualified in Advanced Cardiac Life Support. A CCRN is a registered nurse who is certified by the American Association of Critical Care Nurses Certification Corporation.

Licensed Nurses

A **head nurse** (nurse manager or coordinator) is a registered nurse who has managerial responsibilities for a particular **nursing unit** throughout the 24-hour day. The head nurse usually works the day shift and is responsible to nursing administration.

A **charge nurse** assumes managerial responsibility for a particular unit on the evening or night shift or on the day shift in the absence of the head nurse. The charge nurse is directly responsible to the head nurse.

A **staff nurse** is a registered nurse who is able to do complete patient care and all nursing diagnosis, treatments, and other procedures, and often functions as a team leader.

A **graduate nurse (GN)** is one who is working while waiting for the results of the state board examination to become a registered nurse.

A **licensed vocational nurse (LVN)** or **licensed practical nurse (LPN)** is a graduate of a one-year nursing program, has passed a state board examination for vocational nurses, and is licensed in the state in which he or she practices. This level of nurse works under the supervision of a registered nurse and provides patient care including treatment and administration of medications prescribed by the physician. Many states have career ladder programs that offer the LVN or LPN the opportunity, with further education, to take the RN state board examination and advance to the status of registered nurse.

Nonlicensed Nursing Personnel

Nursing assistants perform basic patient care and bedside tasks for the patient under the supervision of a registered nurse.

An **orderly** is a male nursing assistant who usually performs the same tasks as a nursing assistant but may have expanded duties such as responsibility for orthopedic equipment and certain male surgical preps (shaves) and catheterizations.

PROFESSIONAL NURSING SPECIALTIES

Certified Registered Nurse Anesthetist (CRNA)	A registered nurse who has been specially trained through postgraduate training and can administer various types of anesthetics.
Nurse Practitioner	Has acquired advanced skills through education and training. If specialization is in family health, may be called Family Nurse Practitioner (FNP); if in pediatrics, Pediatric Nurse Practitioner (PNP).
Nurse-Midwife	Specializes in care of the pregnant woman from conception through the postpartum period. A registered nurse who has completed an approved nurse-midwifery program may be called a Certified Nurse Midwife (CNM). Certification denotes the passing of an examination.
Community Health Nurse	A public health nurse who works in the community to promote and provide health care.
Clinical Nurse Specialist	A registered nurse with advanced training and knowledge with a master's degree in nursing and a high degree of competence in a specialized area of nursing.
Clinician	A registered nurse with demonstrated expertise in nursing practice and a baccalaureate degree in nursing.
Nurse Epidemiologist or Infection Control Nurse	A registered nurse trained in the tracking and prevention of nosocomial (hospital-acquired) infections.

Nursing assistants and orderlies are trained on the job, through a vocational school, or at the beginning level of a career ladder program at a community college.

Certified Nursing Assistants (CNAs) have graduated from a training program with prescribed hours and have met certain other standards and passed a certification examination (Fig. 2.7).

Patient Care Technician (PCT) may be referred to as an advanced nursing assistant. The PCT provides basic care to the patient as well as being able to perform other procedures such as electrocardiograms, drawing blood (phlebotomy), and performing simple testing of specimens at the bedside. Additional tasks of the PCT may include certain procedures requiring the use of sterile technique such as simple dressing changes. The PCT may obtain skills that allow him or her to perform certain HUC functions in the absence of the health unit coordinator.

*N*URSING UNITS

Hospitals are divided into various **nursing units** according to the type of service provided to the patient (Tables 2.3 and 2.4). As a health unit coordinator, you will be assigned to a nursing unit, and during the course of your employment, you may work on several different ones. Some health unit coordinators are not assigned to a single unit but move throughout the hospital as the need arises. The term for this is *floating,*

THE NURSING HEALTH CARE TEAM

PROFESSIONAL REGISTERED NURSE

Four-year university education with a bachelor's degree
or
Two-year junior or community college education with an associate degree
or
Three-year diploma from a hospital nursing school
and
Passed state board examinations

LICENSED PRACTICAL NURSE (LPN)
or
LICENSED VOCATIONAL NURSE (LVN)

One-year training program

Passed state board examinations

PLPN–Pharmaceutical Licensed Practical Nurse is one who administers drugs or medications after taking a special course and passing a special examination

CERTIFIED NURSING ASSISTANT

NURSING ASSISTANT

NURSE'S AIDE

HOME HEALTH AIDE

GERIATRIC AIDE

ORDERLY

PATIENT CARE TECHNICIAN

All are names used for the nonprofessional worker who, under the direction and supervision of the registered nurses, carries out basic bedside nursing functions

HEALTH UNIT COORDINATOR

Works at the desk of the nurses' station
–Does clerical work
–Answers the telephone at the nurses' station
–Helps to direct traffic on the floor
–Processes doctor's orders

FIGURE 2.7

TABLE 2.3 𝒩URSING UNITS	
Unit	**Function**
Behavioral Medicine	Care of patients receiving care for behavioral and mental disorders. May include: ■ *Alcohol and Drug Rehabilitation*—Care of patients receiving treatment for alcohol and/or drug abuse ■ *Psychiatry (Psych)*—Care of patients with mental and emotional disorders
Eyes, Ears, Nose, and Throat (EENT)	Care of patients with medical and surgical conditions in these parts of the body
Gynecology (GYN)	Care of women with diseases of the female reproductive system
Intensive Care Unit (ICU)	Care of patients who are critically ill and in need of constant supervision and specialized nursing care. May be further divided into: ■ *Coronary Care Unit (CCU)*—Care of critically ill patients with heart and related diseases ■ *Medical Intensive Care Unit (MICU)*—Care of critically ill medical patients ■ *Pediatric Intensive Care Unit (PICU)*—Care of critically ill children ■ *Surgical Intensive Care Unit (SICU)*—Care of critically ill surgical patients ■ *Neonatal ICU*—Intensive care of newborn
Medical (Med)	Care of patients with medical (nonsurgical) conditions
Neurology (Neuro)	Care of patients with diseases of the nervous system
Nursery	Care of newborn infants
Obstetrics (OB)	Care of women who are having, or have had, babies
Orthopedics (Ortho)	Care of patients with injury or disease of the musculoskeletal system
Pediatrics (Peds)	Care of children
Rehabilitation (Rehab)	Care of patients receiving treatment for physical handicaps
Surgical (Surg)	Care of patients who will undergo or have undergone surgery
Telemetry	Care of patients on cardiac monitors whose ECG is being observed at the nurses' station
Transitional Care Unit (TCU)	Care of patients requiring a reduced level of care. May be called Stepdown Unit.
Urology	Care of patients with diseases of the urinary system and males with diseases of the reproductive tract

TABLE 2.4 𝒮PECIALIZED UNITS	
Unit	**Function**
Emergency Department (ED)	Care of patients needing emergency treatment for diseases or injuries that have occurred outside the hospital.
Labor and Delivery (L&D)	Care of women who are in labor or are delivering babies.
Medical Short Stay Unit (MSSU)	Care of medical patients requiring care and stabilization for less than 24 hours.
Operating Room (OR)	Care of patients undergoing surgery.
Outpatient Department (OPD)	Care of patients seen in a clinic setting for disorders not requiring hospitalization.
Outpatient Surgery	Care of patients having minor surgery that does not require overnight hospitalization. Also called Same Day Surgery (SDS) or Ambulatory Surgery.
Postanesthetic Care Unit (PACU)	Also called the Recovery Room. Provides care of patients immediately after surgery until condition stabilizes and they can return to nursing unit.
Renal Dialysis	Care of patients with kidney disorders who require artificial devices to maintain kidney function and sustain life.
Trauma Unit	Immediate surgical care of injured patients by special team of physicans and nurses.

and the unit coordinator who is given the opportunity to float will learn many new and interesting things about the medical field.

A large hospital may include even more divisions than those that have been listed. In all the units thus described, the hospitalized patient is an inpatient and will receive 24-hour nursing care. There are other specialized units within a hospital in which a health unit coordinator may be employed where a patient will receive care before being either transferred to one of the units listed or in some cases discharged.

PATIENT CARE ASSIGNMENTS

Since health unit coordinators frequently need to communicate information to the nurse caring for a patient, they need to be aware of the type of patient care assignment used by the nursing unit. The nursing health care team in your hospital may be organized in one of the following ways:

Primary Nursing or Total Patient Care Primary nursing is a method of patient care delivery in which the professional nurse is responsible and accountable for the entire nursing care of the patient. This is a patient-oriented system, and the purpose is to ensure that the professional nurse works directly with the patient—planning, implementing, and evaluating the patient's nursing care. Primary nursing is usually the type of patient care assignment employed in the critical care units.

Team Nursing In **team nursing** the head nurse or charge nurse divides the staff into teams. Each team has a **team leader.** The head nurse or charge nurse assigns a group of patients to each team. The team leader (usually an RN) then assigns patients for each team member to care for during the shift. Team members may be RNs, LPNs or LVNs, NAs, orderlies, or students. The team leader is teacher, adviser, and helper to all team members.

Whatever the method of patient care assignment, as a health unit coordinator you must know *which nurse is caring for which patient.* To determine this, you will refer to a **patient care assignment sheet,** which is made out each day for each shift indicating the member of the nursing team that is assigned to each patient. These assignment sheets are posted at the nurse's station for your easy reference (Fig. 2.8).

Unless your hospital utilizes primary nursing or total patient care assignments and employs only RNs, you must take this process one step further. You must be able to determine which information and requests to communicate to the RN, which to the LVN or LPN, and which to the NA.

To help you in these decisions you must know what these individuals with various levels of education in nursing may do. Remember:

- **Registered nurses** perform all nursing care procedures and treatments, give medications, start and monitor IVs (intravenous administration), and take and implement doctors' orders verbally, in writing, and by telephone. Registered nurses supervise other nursing personnel.
- **LVNs and LPNs** perform most of the procedures that RNs perform. In acute care hospitals, LVNs and LPNs are usually not in supervisory positions; however, in extended care facilities in some states, LPNs/LVNs may function in that capacity. You must learn the policies of your hospital and determine the policy of your unit so that you will know which information to communicate to the LVN/LPN and which to the RN.

```
┌─────────────────────────────────────────────────────────┐
│              PATIENT CARE ASSIGNMENT SHEET                │
│                                                           │
│  Head Nurse                          Date                 │
│                                                           │
│  Health Unit Coordinator             Shift                │
├───────────────────────────┬───────────────────────────────┤
│          TEAM 1           │           TEAM 2              │
```

Team Leader - J. Jones, R.N.

Rm. 130
131
132 } T. Smith N.A.
133

134A
B
C } L. Grace N.A
135

136
137 } T. Johnson L.P.N.
138

Team Leader - P. Pearl, R.N.

Rm. 139A
B
C } D. Stevens N.A.
140
141

142
143 } G. Bullock N.A.
144
145

146
147 } S. Tall N.A.
148

(NOTE: Patient names are often included on the assignment sheet as well as room numbers.)

FIGURE 2.8

- **Nursing assistants** perform basic patient care. They *do not* give medication, *do not* take doctors' orders, *do not* perform sterile techniques, and *do not* start IVs. Also, they do not function in supervisory roles.
- **Volunteers** give their services without pay. Although they do not actually care for the patients, they contribute to the patients' comfort and well-being in many ways such as arranging flowers, reading to patients, and writing letters. Candy stripers and other high school students give their time after school and on weekends. Adult volunteers may escort patients, deliver messages, or run library and gift carts. They also raise money for the hospital through gift shops and hospital benefits.

LEARNING ACTIVITIES

Complete the following.

1. List the five functions and purposes of a hospital.
   (a) _____
   (b) _____
   (c) _____
   (d) _____
   (e) _____

2. List the two ways in which hospitals are most commonly classified.

(a) _____

(b) _____

3. The meeting of an official standard by a hospital is called _____.

Match the medical specialists in Column A with the description of the specialty in Column B.

Column A

(a) Allergist

(b) Anesthesiologist

(c) Cardiologist

(d) Oncologist

(e) Dermatologist

(f) Internist

(g) Orthopedist

(h) Neurologist

(i) Obstetrician

(j) Gynecologist

(k) Ophthalmologist

(l) Pathologist

(m) Pediatrician

(n) Psychiatrist

(o) Plastic surgeon

(p) Radiologist

(q) Urologist

(r) Geriatrician

(s) Neonatologist

Column B

_____ The care of women during pregnancy, childbirth, and the interval immediately following

_____ Diagnosis and treatment of mental disorders

_____ A subspecialty of internal medicine dealing with diagnosis and treatment of body reactions resulting from unusual sensitivity to foods, pollens, dust, medicines, or other substances

_____ Diagnosis and treatment of diseases of the elderly

_____ The care and treatment of newborns

_____ Diagnosis and treatment of diseases of the kidneys, bladder, ureters, urethra, and of the male reproductive organs

_____ Diagnosis and treatment of diseases of the eye, including prescribing glasses

_____ A subspecialty of internal medicine involving the diagnosis and treatment of disease of the heart and blood vessels

_____ Use of radiant energy including x-rays, radium, cobalt, and the like in the diagnosis of disease

_____ Administration of various forms of anesthesia in operations or diagnosis to cause loss of feeling or sensation

_____ The diagnosis and nonsurgical treatment of illnesses of adults

_____ Diagnosis and treatment of cancer

_____ Diagnosis and treatment of disorders and diseases of the muscular and skeletal systems

_____ Prevention, diagnosis, and treatment of children's diseases

_____ Diagnosis and treatment of diseases of brain, spinal cord, and nerve disorders

_____ Diagnosis and treatment of diseases of the female reproductive organs

_____ Corrective or reparative surgery to restore deformed or mutilated parts of the body

_____ Study and interpretation of changes in organs, tissues, cells, and alterations in body chemistry to aid in diagnosing disease and determining treatment

_____ Diagnosis and treatment of diseases of the skin

Complete the following statements regarding nursing personnel.

1. The _____ is responsible for the overall administration of nursing service.

2. The _____ is responsible for the continuing education and staff development of nursing service personnel and the orientation of new nursing service personnel.

3. The _____ has managerial responsibilities for a particular nursing unit throughout the 24-hour day.

4. The _____ has graduated from a one-year program and is licensed by the state to give direct patient care and perform less technical skills than the RN.

5. The _____ is not licensed and performs basic treatments and bedside tasks for the patient.

Write the correct abbreviation for each of the following nursing units in the space provided.

1. Medical _____
2. Surgical _____
3. Obstetrics _____
4. Gynecology _____
5. Orthopedics _____
6. Pediatrics _____
7. Neurology _____
8. Psychiatry _____
9. Intensive care _____
10. Coronary care _____
11. Operating room _____
12. Emergency department _____
13. Transitional care unit _____

Complete the following.

1. List two ways in which the nursing health care team in your institution may be organized.
    (a) _____
    (b) _____

2. To determine which nurse is caring for which patient, the health unit coordinator will refer to the _____.

3. List four things the health care worker should know about the business side of healthcare.
   (a) _____
   (b) _____
   (c) _____
   (d) _____

True or False. Circle T if the statement is true and F if it is false.

(a) T F RNs act in supervisory positions.

(b) T F Requests for pain medications should be referred to the nursing assistant.

(c) T F Calls from doctors should be referred to the RN.

(d) T F The registered nurse may start IVs.

(e) T F LVNs and LPNs perform many of the procedures performed by RNs.

(f) T F Nursing assistants do not take doctors' orders.

(g) T F Patient care technicians are usually nursing assistants with advanced training.

In the space to the left, check the health professionals who hold the degree of M.D.

_____ Rheumatologist

_____ Hematologist

_____ Osteopath

_____ Nephrologist

_____ Psychologist

_____ Podiatrist

_____ Chiropractor

_____ CRNA

Complete the following.

1. Medicare Part A is _____ insurance; Medicare Part B is _____ insurance.

2. A benefit period for a Medicare patient begins with the day a patient _____ the hospital and ends when the patient has not been an inpatient in a hospital or skilled nursing facility for _____ consecutive days.

Match the terms in Column A with their definitions in Column B

Column A

(a) HMO

(b) Medicare

(c) Medicaid

(d) Case management

(e) Managed care

(f) DRGs

Column B

_____ A system that classifies patients that are medically related and provides the basis for payment to hospitals by Medicare

_____ A process for monitoring a patient's stay and services to be sure they are appropriate

_____ National insurance for persons 65 and older, the blind, and the disabled

_____ A prepaid system of managed care that provides medical care to enrolled groups at a fixed rate

_____ A federal and state program that provides medical care for certain low-income patients

_____ A system of health care designed to control costs

1. Choose any physician specialty that interests you from the list provided in the text. Find out all that you can about it. Why does it interest you? What kinds of diseases and disorders does this kind of doctor treat? Be prepared to discuss your answer in class.

    _____
    _____
    _____
    _____
    _____
    _____
    _____
    _____
    _____
    _____
    _____
    _____

2. What do you see as the benefits of managed care? As the disadvantages?

    _____
    _____
    _____
    _____
    _____
    _____
    _____
    _____
    _____
    _____
    _____
    _____

CHAPTER 3

The Hospital Departments

VOCABULARY

Abstract	To select and remove data from a medical record for the purpose of gathering statistics
Alleviate	To relieve or to make easier
Capitation	Payment by managed care plans of a fixed amount of money to a provider (hospital, physician, pharmacy, and so on) for each patient enrolled, whether services are given or not
Diagnostic and procedural codes	Codes taken from the ICD-9-CM, CPT, and HCPCS code books that describe the patient's diagnosis and procedures and services rendered, for insurance and statistical purposes
Endoscopy	The process of visualization of the inside of the body through an instrument called an endoscope
Enteral therapy	Feeding of special formulas through a tube that leads to the digestive tract
Inservice training program	Education and training provided to hospital personnel
Interface	To form a common boundary
Intravenous	Into a vein
Medical transcription	The word processing of a physician's dictated records
Neurodiagnostic department	Department that performs certain diagnostic procedures on the nervous system such as the electroencephalogram (EEG)
"Old charts"	The medical records of a patient from previous admissions
Parenteral therapy	Treatment given by a route other than the gastrointestinal tract; the intravenous provision of all of the patient's nutritional needs
Pathology	The study of disease
Pharmacist	A health care professional licensed to prepare and dispense drugs
Phlebotomist	One who draws blood
Provider contracting	Negotiations between the hospital and managed health plans concerning the details and monitoring of managed care plan contracts
Pulmonary function tests	Various tests to determine how well the lungs are exchanging oxygen and carbon dioxide
Rehabilitation	The process of helping a disabled person obtain maximum function
Reimbursement	A payment for services rendered
Requisitions	A formal request such as for supplies or services
Termination interview	Exit interview held when an employee quits or is fired
Third-party payer	Insurer who pays the hospital bill for the patient as agreed on by contract

When you have
completed this chapter,
you will be able to:

- Define the terms listed in the vocabulary.
- Describe the primary functions of the various hospital departments.
- Discuss the health unit coordinator's responsibilities as they relate to the various departments
- Describe the purpose of discharge planning.
- Give examples of types of "special orders" that might be placed through the dietary department.

Many departments within a hospital contribute to the care of the patient. Working in these departments are many people with various levels and types of skills. Each department is important, and the health unit coordinator in his or her coordination role must understand the functions and organization of the departments and how he or she **interfaces** with them in performing the health unit coordinator's duties.

An overview of the common departments follows. More information will be given in the chapters on medications, and diagnostic and therapeutic orders.

For the purpose of study, the departments are grouped into three main categories:

- Administrative and Business Services
- Operational Services
- Patient Care Services

THE ADMINISTRATIVE AND BUSINESS SERVICES
THE BUSINESS OFFICE

Departmental Organization and Services

The business office manages the hospital's business activities. This office also keeps the administration informed of the financial condition of the institution. A partial list of the business office activities follows.

- Records all charges to be made to each patient's account, including nursing care, the use of supplies and equipment, diagnostic tests, treatments, and special services (e.g., telephone or television rental)
- Handles payroll records of and payment to all hospital employees
- Assists in preparing budgets, taking into account the estimated needs of each department
- Secures patient valuables in a safe located in the business office
- Bills **third-party payers** and patients, and collects payments including **capitation** payments
- Determines patient's ability to pay and verifies insurance eligibility

The business department is usually headed by a controller or chief financial officer. The department itself has many subdivisions and may employ accountants, cashiers, bookkeepers, insurance billing specialists, clerks, and a stock room manager to accomplish the various duties.

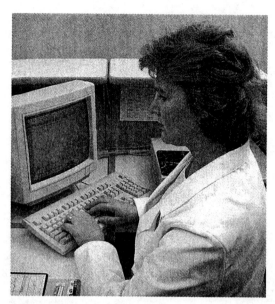

FIGURE 3.1

Provider contracting may be a function of this department, or there may be a separate department responsible for these duties.

Execution of Forms

Because the business office issues the final bill to each patient, records of any **requisitions** for supplies or other items to be charged to the patient must be directed to this office. These records are computer generated and sent from the department performing the service on completion of the test or treatment or electronically transferred via computer. Your instructor will explain whatever responsibilities you may have regarding the business office.

It is possible that you may be required to notify the business office (usually by telephone or computer) of patients about to be discharged so that their bills can be prepared.

It is obviously very important that all charges to the patient are recorded accurately and completely (Fig. 3.1).

*T*HE ADMITTING DEPARTMENT

The admitting department is responsible for admitting patients to the hospital. Admitting personnel interview patients, complete necessary forms and obtain patients' signatures, explain hospital admitting procedures to patients, and notify nursing units or departments of the patients' arrival. The patient identification bracelet, addressograph plate, and face sheet for the chart usually originate in this office. Preadmissions, inpatient and outpatient admissions, emergency department registration, insurance verification, and cashiering may all be part of the duties of this department.

*T*HE COMMUNICATIONS DEPARTMENT

Some hospitals may call the communications department the telephone switchboard. Telephone operators handle incoming and outgoing calls and operate the doctors' paging or signal light system. In some hospitals the communications department may also act as an information station for visitors to the hospital.

*T*HE HUMAN RESOURCES DEPARTMENT

The human resources or personnel department is responsible for interviewing and often hiring hospital employees. Human resources maintains employee records and conducts **termination interviews.** Information and records regarding employee benefits such as sick leave, insurance, vacations, the credit union, and retirement can be found in this department.

*T*HE PUBLIC RELATIONS DEPARTMENT

The public relations department works to market the hospital and to promote community relations with the hospital and provides the community with information about hospital activities. Many hospitals sponsor health fairs and offer many other community outreach programs such as seminars, CPR classes, and Meals on Wheels—nutritional meals prepared at the hospital and delivered each day to the homes of persons who might not otherwise enjoy a hot meal. The public relations department publicizes these activities and may also publish a newsletter for hospital employees.

*T*HE TRANSPORTATION DEPARTMENT

The transportation department may deliver mail, specimens, and reports throughout the hospital as well as pick up and deliver patients to the various departments. This service may include the transportation of patients being admitted or discharged.

*T*HE HEALTH INFORMATION SERVICES DEPARTMENT

Health information services or medical records is responsible for all the charts or records of persons who have been patients in the hospital. After discharge, the patient's records are sent to this department, where they are carefully reviewed by specialists to make sure that each chart is complete, accurate, and signed by all appropriate personnel. If the records are not complete, the health information services department will contact staff members and require that additional charting or signatures be added. After a certain period of time, the patient's chart is put on film called microfiche and may be viewed by the physician on a special machine in the medical records department.

One of the most important functions of health information services is the assigning of **diagnostic and procedural codes.** This is done to gather statistics and especially to obtain **reimbursement** for the hospital. Since 1983 the HCFA has required the use of DRGs for Medicare patients. If a coder does not select the correct code, reimbursement to the hospital may be reduced. Another function performed by health information services is **abstracting.** This is the process of collecting information from the medical record for the purpose of gathering statistics. The hospital then uses this information to determine how different physicians utilize the hospital, to analyze staffing needs, and to report required data to government agencies.

When a patient is admitted and the doctor requests the "**old charts,**" those charts will be obtained from this department (Fig. 3.2).

Medical transcription (the word processing of dictated records by the physician) is done in medical records. The health unit coordinator then files these typewritten reports (such as histories, physical examinations, consultations, surgical and pathology reports) on the patient's chart.

FIGURE 3.2

$\mathcal{T}$HE INFORMATION SYSTEMS DEPARTMENT

The information systems department is responsible for the computers within a hospital. The information systems department provides and works to improve computer hardware and software, provides support for systems operations, and assists hospital personnel with computer education. Working within this department are clinical data systems (CDS) analysts.

$\mathcal{T}$HE CENTRAL SUPPLY DEPARTMENT

Most medical and nursing equipment and supplies—probably the most frequently used items in the hospital—are stored in the central supply section. This department is also responsible for preparing and issuing the equipment and supplies. The central supply department stocks commonly used items such as cotton, bandages, dressings, and a variety of trays needed for different procedures. It may also supply more specialized appliances such as air mattresses, bed cradles, orthopedic frames, and soak machines. Central supply is also the center of sterilization; such items as surgical instruments and a variety of trays and equipment are wrapped and sterilized there (Fig. 3.3).

Requisitions

There are generally two types of requests on orders to central supply, which is often done by computers.

1. Requisitions for equipment and supplies to be charged to the unit include standard equipment used in routine nursing care (e.g., tongue blades, bandages, sterile pads, and cotton). In some hospitals, stock is replenished routinely by the central supply department, through scheduled checking and delivery.

2. Requisitions for equipment or supplies to be charged to the patient include special items needed by the individual patient, who must be charged for their use. Suction apparatus and special trays for nonroutine patient care are examples of nursing supplies that would be charged to the patient.

SUPPLIES CHARGED TO
THE NURSING UNIT
FIGURE 3.3

Most nursing supplies and equipment are charged to the patient, and the health unit coordinator must be sure that all charges are made accurately.

Many central supply departments stock disposable, chargeable patient supplies on the nursing unit and attach a CS requisition to each article stating the type of supply. When nursing uses a supply, they will bring the requisition to you. You should stamp the patient's addressograph plate and then route it to CS.

Another system central supply may use is to keep a CS Kardex in the supply or clean utility room on the nursing unit with a CS card for each patient. Each CS item has a sticker. Nursing affixes the sticker to the patient's individual central supply Kardex when the supply is used. Central supply tabulates the charges from each CS Kardex daily for each unit. Other hospitals are using computers to accomplish this purpose. You will learn the procedure utilized in your health care institution.

Figure 3.4 illustrates a partial list used for stocking the supply cart on a medical/surgical floor.

Nondisposable equipment and supplies are also requisitioned from central supply (Fig. 3.5).

All equipment used for patient treatment must be charged for as well. After the initial order has been placed, central supply staff may be responsible for daily tracking of use so that accurate charges may be made.

It is exceedingly important to a hospital's financial health that it be reimbursed for care that is rendered. Every hospital employee must assist in this process.

Nursing procedure orders are discussed in Chapter 15.

*T*HE PURCHASING DEPARTMENT

As you can imagine, buying and storing huge quantities of equipment and supplies needed by the hospital is a big job, that requires planning and organization. The hospital must always have a sufficient quantity of all the things it needs, and it must obtain new and better equipment as it is developed. The hospital must never run out of essential items; nor can such items be so overstocked that space and funds are not available for new purchases.

Medical Surgical Floor

		Upper Cabinet
	2	Bx small latex gloves
	2	Bx medium latex gloves
	2	Bx large latex gloves
	2	Bx limb holders
	2	Arterial hand aids
	6	Posey soft belts
	10	Urinals

Drawer

	2	Bx IVAC covers
	6	Oral thermometers
	6	Rectal thermometers

Lower Cabinet

	10	Bedpans
	10	Sanpans
	20	Emesis basins
	5	Urine strainers
	5	Wash basins
	8	Fracture pans
	8	Graduates

Cart

	15	Admit kits
	10	Suction canisters
	4	Kangaroo bags
	15	Suction kits
	10	Suction tubing
	10	Wall tubing
	10	Yankauer suction tips

Medicine Room

	4	1/2" steri-strips
	2	Bx alcohol preps
	1	Bx Betadine preps
	4	Suture removal kits
	2	Staple removal kits
	4	Disposable scissors
	4	Sterile Kellys
	2	Needle holders
	1	Bx 19ga × 1" needles
	1	Bx 19ga × 1 1/2" needles
	1	Bx 20ga needles
	1	Bx 23ga needles
	1	Bx 25ga needles
	1	Bx 20ga syringes
	1	Bx 22ga syringes
	1	Bx 23ga syringes
	1	Bx 25ga syringes
	1	Bx 10cc syringes
	1	Bx 5cc syringes
	1	Bx insulin syringes
	1	Bx TB syringes
	20	IV start kits

In Kitchen

	10	Water pitchers

* * 5 IV pumps standby * *

Fourth Floor Circle Cart

Top Shelf

	2	Eggcrate mattress
	4	Sterile water
	4	Sterile saline
	1	Suction canister
	1	Bx isolation masks

Second Shelf

	4	Baby powder
	4	Lotion
	4	Shampoo
	4	Mouthwash
	4	Dental kits
	4	Tissues
	4	Ivory soap w/ dish
	4	Razors
	4	Shave cream
	4	Odor eliminators
	6	Oral swabs
	4	Specimen cups
	2	U-bags
	2	Urine strainers

Third Shelf

	1	Sitz bath
	1	Ring cushion
	5	Chux
	5	Bedpads
	10	Adult pampers

Bottom Shelf

	1	Urinemeter w/foley
	1	Urinemeter
	1	16fr foley cath tray

FIGURE 3.4 Nursing care items are restocked by central supply as they are used.

Fourth Floor Circle Cart

	1	18fr Foley cath tray
	1	Irrigation tray
	1	Drainage tray
	1	Urethral cath tray
	1	Trach care kit
	1	Bx latex gloves small
	1	Bx latex gloves medium
	1	Bx latex gloves large
	1	Bx limb holders

Drawer #1

	2	Large slippers
	2	Medium slippers
	5	Combs
	1	Enema fleet
	1	Enema oil
	1	Enema bucket
	4	Lemon swabs

Drawer #2

	2	1/8" steri-strips
	2	1/4" steri-strips
	2	1/2" steri-strips
	2	1" steri-strips
	2	Kerlix rolls
	2	2" kling
	2	3" kling
	2	4" kling
	2	6" kling
	2	Small opsite
	2	Medium opsite

	2	Large opsite
	2	Vaseline gauze
	1	Bx spot Band-Aids
	1	Bx 1" Band-Aids
	1	Bx 2" Band-Aids

Drawer #3

	1	Bx IVAC covers
	1	Shroud
	2	Denture cups
	2	Lab cups
	5	Skin wipes
	2	1" micropore tape
	2	2" micropore tape
	2	1" transpore tape
	2	2" transpore tape

Drawer #4

	1	Bx sterile 2 × 2 dressing
	1	Bx sterile 4 × 4 dressing
	2	4 × 4 tubs

Drawer #5

	2	Suction tubing
	2	Wall tubing
	2	Yankauer suction tips
	2	60cc cath tip syringes
	2	ABG kits
	2	Culturettes
	1	Small condom cath
	1	Medium condom cath
	1	Large condom cath
	2	Cath adapters

Drawer #6

	2	Ea. Sterile gloves			
	6.0		6.5		7.0
	7.5		8.0		8.5
	10	White towels			
	1	Shave prep			
	1	Sterile basin			
	1	Peri-bottle			
	5	Sterile Q-tips			
	5	Sterile tongue blades			
	5	Safety pins			
	5	K-Y			
	5	Belongings bags			

In Cabinet

	4	Urinals
	4	Washbasins
	4	San pans
	4	Graduates
	4	Bedpans
	4	Fracture pans
	4	Water pitchers
	4	Admit kits

FIGURE 3.4 (Continued)

FIGURE 3.5

In most hospitals, all supplies, equipment, and materials used in the hospital, from pencils to the most complicated heart–lung machine, are bought by the purchasing department (or material management department) in cooperation with the business department. Each hospital department regularly submits a list of the supplies it needs. These supplies are then delivered on scheduled dates. Emergency requests, of course, are handled in a different manner and are delivered as soon as possible.

Forms and Requisitions

The purchasing department usually has a variety of forms to be used in requisitioning supplies. A sample form used in requesting stationery supplies is shown in Fig. 3.6.

THE OPERATIONAL SERVICES

THE ENVIRONMENTAL SERVICES DEPARTMENT

Functions

The environmental services or housekeeping department is responsible for maintaining the clean, sanitary, and pleasant environment that is so important to the medical and nursing care of the patient and to the entire hospital staff as well. An environment housing ill and infected people must be kept as clean as possible to aid in restoring them to good health and to prevent the spread of disease.

- Members of the environmental services staff perform the daily routine tasks that keep the various areas of the hospital (e.g., the wards, halls, restrooms, and dayrooms) clean and orderly at all times.
- They also do special cleaning chores such as window washing, floor waxing, and cleaning light fixtures, on a regular basis.

OFFICE SUPPLY REQUISITION
•STOREROOM STATIONERY ONLY

DATE	COST CENTER NO.	DEPT. NAME	DIRECTOR'S SIGNATURE X

QTY. ORDERED	UNIT	STOCK NO. NAME	QTY. ORDERED	UNIT	STOCK NO. NAME
	EA	0448 BATTERY, AA		EA	5150 OUTLET 6 PLUG
	EA	0465 BATTERY, AAA		PD	5640 PAD, POST-IT NOTE 1 1/2 × 2
	EA	0455 BATTERY, C		PD	5642 PAD, POST-IT NOTE 3 × 3
	EA	0460 BATTERY, D		PD	5585 PAD, SCRATCH 3 × 5
	EA	0472 BATTERY, 6v, J		PD	5595 PAD, SCRATCH 5 × 8
	EA	0471 BATTERY, 8.4v		PD	5600 PAD, STENO 6 × 9 GREGG 60
	EA	0474 BATTERY, 9v		PD	5580 PAD, YEL. RULED 8 1/2 × 11
	EA	6055 BINDER DATA 14 7/8 × 11 #LbC1411NJ		PD	5565 PAD, WIRE BOUND 8 1/2 × 11
	EA	5555 BINDER, 3/RG, BE, 8 1/2 × 11, 1"		RM	5662 PAPER, COPY MACHINE 8 1/2 × 11
	EA	5560 BINDER, 3/RG, BE, 8 1/2 × 11, 2"		RL	5646 PAPER, FAX F/SHARP
	BX	5745 CARD, PATIENT, BLU., PLASTIC		DZ	5675 PEN, BALL BK, F
	BX	5120 CLIP, PAPER, JUMBO		DZ	5680 PEN, BALL BK, M BIC ROUND
	BX	5115 CLIP, PAPER, REGULAR		DZ	5690 PEN, BALL RD, M
	EA	5110 CLIPBOARD. LTR, BN, 9 × 12 1/2		DZ	5700 PENCIL, BK #2 #600
	EA	5370 CORRECT FLUID, WE 1/2 OZ.		EA	5765 PROTECTOR, SHEET 8 1/2 × 11
	EA	5374 CORRECT FLUID, COPIER		EA	5845 RIBBON, COR., SEL III
	BX	5125 DISKETTE, 3.5, DS, DD, 10/BX		EA	5846 RIBBON, COR., SEL II
	BX	5126 DISKETTE, 3.5, DS, HD, 10/BX		EA	5775 RIBBON, DIGITAL #LA75
	BX	5185 ENVELOPE, CLASP, 6 1/2 × 9 1/2		EA	5770 RIBBON, DIGITAL #LA424
	BX	5190 ENVELOPE, CLASP, 9 × 12		EA	5786 RIBBON, F/OKIDATA ML390/931 BK
	BX	5195 ENVELOPE, CLASP, 10 × 13		EA	5785 RIBBON, F/OKIDATA ML84
	EA	5177 ENVELOPE, INTER-DEPT., 5 × 11 1/2		BX	5890 RUBBER BANDS, 1/4#, REVERE 18, SMALL
	EA	5178 ENVELOPE, INTER-DEPT., 10 × 13		BX	5895 RUBBER BANDS, 1/4#, REVERE 64, LARGE
	BX	5200 ENVELOPE, NO CLASP, 9 × 12		EA	5915 RULER, OFFICE 12"
	EA	5215 ENVELOPE, PADDED, 9 1/2 × 12		EA	5926 SHEARS, BLACK, HANDLE 7"
	EA	5220 ENVELOPE, PATIENT VALUABLES		EA	6010 STAPLE REMOVER
	EA	5245 ERASER, PENCIL TIP		EA	6015 STAPLER, FULL BK
	BX	5252 FASTENER, BASE #22		BX	6025 STAPLES, STD FULL 5M/BX
	BX	5268 FILM, Sx70		RL	6038 TAPE, ADDING MACHINE 2 1/4
	BX	5261 FILM, 779BC		EA	6057 TAPE, CASSETTE 60 MIN.
	PK	5270 FILM, SPECTRA		RL	6125 TAPE, DBL STICK .75 × 1296
	BX	5295 FOLDER, FILE 1/3 ASSORT.		EA	5847 TAPE, LIFTOFF, SEL II
	BX	5294 FOLDER, FILE 1/3 1st POS		RL	4374 TAPE, MASK 1"
	BX	5296 FOLDER, FILE, PENDAFLEX, LTR		RL	4375 TAPE, MASK 2"
	BX	5297 FOLDER, TABS, PENDAFLEX		RL	6105 TAPE, MENDING 1/2
	ST	5320 INDEX, RG/BK 8CR 8 1/2 × 11		RL	6110 TAPE, MENDING 3/4
	PK	5050 INDEX CARD, WE 3 × 5, RULED		EA	6135 TAPE, VIDEO 120
	RL	5445 LABEL, ALLERGIC, RED		BTL	5649 TONER CARTRIDGE, COPIER #SF830NTI
	BX	5375 LABEL, CONT. COMPUTER 3 1/2 × 1, 5M/BX		EA	5651 TONER CARTRIDGE, FAX #F033NTI
	BX	5380 LABEL, FILE FOLDER		EA	5020 TONER CARTRIDGE F/ LASERJET IIP, IIIP, IIP PLUS
	RL	5475 LABEL, MEDICATION, RED		EA	5030 TONER CARTRIDGE F/ LASERJET IIISi
	RL	5400 LABEL, PRECUT, PLN, 2 1/2 × 1 1/2		EA	5035 TONER CARTRIDGE #92295A
	RL	5500 LABEL, RM, PT, DR, WHITE		EA	5650 TONER SF 7350
	EA	5535 MARKER, FELT, BLK		BTL	5648 TONER, SHARP SF80TI
	EA	5550 MARKER, FELT, RED		BTL	5645 TONER, TOSHIBA T50P
	EA	5695 MARKER, HIGHLIGHTER, PINK			
	EA	5696 MARKER, HIGHLIGHTER, YELLOW			
	EA	5532 MARKER, SHARPIE, BLK			
	EA	5533 MARKER, SHARPIE, RED			

DO NOT WRITE IN THIS SPACE
This request for storeroom stationery must be presented to Purchasing by 9:00 A.M. on your order day.
See reverse side for numerical listing for cross reference.

FIGURE 3.6

- In many hospitals, environmental services aides dispense clean linen and make necessary mending repairs.
- Environmental services cleans rooms of discharged patients, makes up the bed, and prepares the unit for the next patient.

You have undoubtedly seen environmental services aides at work performing these and a variety of other tasks. In all the work they do, they must show the same consideration for the patient as is shown by the entire hospital staff. Housekeeping personnel do their jobs quietly and efficiently, disturbing the patients as little as possible. The result of their work is a clean, neat, and safe hospital (Figs. 3.7 and 3.8).

Departmental Organization

The director of environmental services directs all the activities of this department and its staff. The director of environmental services supervises the daily routine cleaning and also has an overall plan so that the larger chores are performed on a regular schedule. Other related responsibilities:

- Selecting new furnishings and recommending redecorating as the need arises
- Planning and directing an **inservice training program** for environmental services personnel

In large hospitals, the director of environmental services usually has an assistant. The rest of the housekeeping staff work under their direction to maintain high standards of cleanliness.

The Environmental Services Department and the Health Unit Coordinator

Although you will see environmental services aides at work on your unit every day, it is quite possible that you will have very little to do with the department as a whole. It is important, however, that you know and understand the extent of its responsibilities

FIGURE 3.7

POTENTIAL HAZARD

NOTIFY HOUSEKEEPING OF...

TRASH

SPILLED MEDICINE

WET FLOORS

NOTIFY LAUNDRY OF...

LAUNDRY CHUTE

EXCESSIVE LAUNDRY

FIGURE 3.8

in your hospital so that when special situations arise, you will know the appropriate section or person to call.

Some conditions require prompt attention from environmental services personnel. You may be responsible for telephoning environmental services in the following situations:

- When there is a large spill of some sort that can't be easily cleaned up by nursing
- When dripping umbrellas have made the halls wet and slippery

- When accumulations of trash have created a messy and potentially danger-ous situation
- When patients have inadvertently hemorrhaged, vomited, urinated, or defe-cated (had a bowel movement) on the floor

*T*HE LAUNDRY DEPARTMENT

Functions

The laundry department collects and launders all hospital linens and maintains an adequate supply of clean, sanitary linen for all departments. Linen includes not only sheets and pillowcases but may also include patient gowns, employee uniforms, tow-els, and many other items.

Departmental Organization

In some hospitals, the position of laundry manager may be combined with that of ex-ecutive housekeeper. In others, it is a separate department. The laundry manager su-pervises the laundry workers, schedules the work loads so that the entire laundering process moves efficiently, and inspects equipment frequently, making any necessary minor repairs. The rest of the staff is made up of washers, marker-sorters, ironers, and tumbler (dryer) operators. The laundered items are inspected to be sure that they are clean and well ironed before they are distributed to the various hospital departments. In many hospitals, the laundry is sent out to a commercial laundry, and the laundry department coordinates this activity.

Health Unit Coordinator Responsibilities

It is unlikely that you will have frequent association with this department. Should an un-usual amount of laundry accumulate on your unit between scheduled pickups, however, you might be asked to request that a member of the laundry staff come to collect it.

*T*HE ENGINEERING AND MAINTENANCE DEPARTMENT

Function

The maintenance department provides continuous upkeep of the hospital's buildings and grounds and the safe, efficient operation of all its utilities. Among the many re-sponsibilities of this department are:

- To service and maintain all the lighting and heating equipment in the hospital
- To make any necessary carpentry, plastering, painting, and plumbing repairs
- To repair all type of equipment, from boilers to furniture
- To keep electrically operated equipment, (e.g., elevators) in good running order
- To landscape and care for the hospital grounds
- To transport medical supplies and equipment, building materials, furniture and fixtures, and trash, and to service the trucks used for this purpose
- To train new employees in these tasks

Departmental Organization

The maintenance department is usually under the direction of a superintendent of buildings and grounds. In large hospitals, he or she may delegate some of his or her duties to a chief engineer and a maintenance supervisor.

```
┌─────────────────────────────────────────────────────────┐
│           REPAIR REQUISITION FOR MAINTENANCE              │
│                   STAFF REPAIRS ONLY                      │
│                 NOT FOR NEW ARTICLES                      │
│                                                           │
│  The following repairs are required in _____   │
│        Location _____  │
│  Description _____  │
│  _____ │
│  _____ │
│  _____ │
│  _____ │
│  Date _____                        │
│  Supervisor _____  │
│  Mark "URGENT" in red ink if repair is so indicated.      │
│  Job completed _____  │
│        Name _____  │
│        Date _____                  │
│    SEND BOTH COPIES TO FRONT OFFICE WHEN REPAIRS ARE NEEDED.│
└─────────────────────────────────────────────────────────┘
```

FIGURE 3.9

The number of personnel in this department depends on the size and needs of the hospital but will generally include carpenters, painters, masons, plumbers, electricians, mechanics, repair persons, gardeners, and truck drivers. These people work together to provide and maintain safe and efficient conditions as well as an attractive, pleasant environment for patients, staff, and visitors.

Health Unit Coordinator Responsibilities

In Chapter 9 you will learn about some of the hazards that may occur in the hospital. Some examples include nonfunctioning lights, faulty electrical equipment, and jammed windows. All these and many other situations are ordinarily corrected by the maintenance department staff. A typical form used to request repairs that may be needed in your unit is shown in Fig. 3.9. In many hospitals all ordering for maintenance is computerized.

PATIENT CARE SERVICES

DISCHARGE PLANNING AND HOME HEALTH SERVICES

For some patients, illness causes problems that cannot be solved by medical and nursing care alone. Many hospitals employ nurses who have the responsibility of discharge planning with the doctor's consent. These nurses interview certain patients in need of auxiliary services following discharge and help arrange for these services. Auxiliary services are offered to **alleviate** the anxieties and difficulties that frequently accompany a hospitalization. Referral forms and other forms that may be issued for auxiliary

SPIRITUAL NEEDS

FIGURE 3.10

services contain information regarding the patient's illness, medications provided or prescribed, and instructions for follow-up care. These forms must be completed by a nurse or physician. Your hospital's routine for filling out and validating the forms will be explained by your instructor.

Home health services include assisting the patient in obtaining needed supplies and equipment as well as providing nursing care and assisted care through the use of home health nurses and home health aides (HHA).

Home health care has grown, and today a great deal of care is provided to patients in their homes by nurses and home health aides (Fig. 3.10).

$\mathcal{T}$HE SOCIAL SERVICES DEPARTMENT

The financial problems that often accompany a hospitalization can cause more suffering than the pain of illness. Worrying about money, a disrupted family life, or unemployment can easily delay a patient's recovery. The social service agency gives assistance to patients beset by these and other difficulties.

Some health care institutions have their own medical social services department that perform patient services. These services include those for outpatients with financial problems. The social services department assists them in finding new jobs if illness has rendered them no longer suitable for their previous employment, secures the aid of specialized resources such as home health agencies, and generally makes available the many community resources (such as vocational rehabilitation counseling) that may be helpful in recovery from illness and adjustment to life's circumstances.

$\mathcal{P}$ASTORAL CARE

This department provides spiritual support to the patient and family members during their time of need. Some hospitals maintain a program for members of the clergy who wish to become hospital chaplains (Fig. 3.11).

SPIRITUAL NEEDS

FIGURE 3.11

*T*HE HOSPITAL PHARMACY

The hospital pharmacy is operated under the direction of the chief **pharmacist,** a person who has graduated from a school of pharmacy and is fully trained and licensed in compounding and dispensing medicines and preparations according to prescriptions written by physicians. The pharmacist must be licensed by the state in which he or she works. Figure 3.12 shows a pharmacy organizational chart.

Working with the pharmacist are pharmacy technicians who, under the direct supervision and control of a registered pharmacist, perform a variety of tasks related to the processing of a prescription in a licensed pharmacy but do not perform duties restricted to a registered pharmacist.

The pharmacy provides a variety of services to the hospital and its patients, such as the following:

- Compounds prescriptions and dispenses medications needed for individual patient care
- Maintains supply of stock medications that are administered to the patients as needed

FIGURE 3.12

- Dispenses controlled drugs and keeps records for inspection
- Dispenses **intravenous (IV)** solutions and often the various IV tubings
- Adds medications to IV solutions
- Distributes information about new drugs and often provides other educational materials
- Usually stocks emergency supply cabinets or carts in specified areas of the hospital.

Medication orders are discussed in Chapter 14.

$\mathcal{T}$HE LABORATORY

The director of laboratories, in most hospitals, is a physician with special training in pathology. **Pathology** is a branch of medical science dealing with the nature of disease. The director is responsible for the total operation of the laboratory service, which includes testing of body specimens such as blood, urine, wound drainage, sputum, stool, and samples of tissues taken from the body. **Autopsies** are also a function of this department. The director may also direct teaching and research activities in which the department is engaged. Figure 3.13 shows a typical organizational chart for the laboratory.

The laboratory staff may include:

- Other pathologists or residents in pathology who assist the director
- Laboratory technicians
- Medical technologists trained and licensed to perform the more complicated laboratory tests
- **Phlebotomists** who draw blood from patients and commonly perform routine tests and duties
- Histology technician who sections, stains, and mounts tissue for microscopic study
- Clerical personnel who maintain records and reports
- Auxiliary personnel who perform such tasks as transporting patients, delivering laboratory results, and collecting requisitions (Fig. 3.14).

FIGURE 3.13

FIGURE 3.14 Hospital laboratory.

RADIOLOGY

The radiology department provides diagnostic and therapeutic services to in-hospital patients and to patients on an outpatient basis. The department is under the direction of a **radiologist,** a doctor who specializes in the diagnosis and treatment of diseases by the use of x-rays, radioactive isotopes, and ionizing radiation. The radiologist is responsible for all radiological examinations and treatments and also interprets radiographs.

Radiologic technologists and technicians work with the doctor and operate equipment, perform many of the x-ray procedures, develop the film, and assist in other related duties. Frequently the staff also includes a group of personnel who transport the patients to and from the radiology department.

There are several major divisions of the radiology department:

- X-rays—with or without the use of contrast media and with or without special preparation
- Nuclear medicine
- Radiation therapy
- Ultrasonography
- Computerized tomography—CT scan (Fig. 3.15)
- MRI—magnetic resonance imaging

CARDIOLOGY

This department is responsible for both noninvasive and invasive diagnostic studies of the heart. Noninvasive tests of the heart include the electrocardiogram (ECG), the treadmill stress test, echocardiograms, and testing using the Holter monitor. Cardiac catheterization is an invasive examination done through this department in some hospitals. ECG technicians and cardiovascular technologists work under the supervision of a cardiologist, a physician specializing in the diagnosis and treatment of diseases of the heart.

Cardiac rehabilitation, consisting of prescribed exercises and other therapy for patients who have had heart attacks or have other heart disorders, is often a division of cardiology (Fig. 3.16).

FIGURE 3.15 CT brain scanning.

Respiratory or Inhalation Therapy

Oxygen and other gases are used in inhalation therapy as a treatment for pulmonary (lung) difficulties. These gases may be administered by face mask, cannula, or tent. Respiratory therapists manage respirators, draw and analyze arterial blood gases, perform **pulmonary function tests,** and supervise pulmonary treatment.

Physical Therapy

Physical therapy includes the use of exercises and massage, as well as light, heat, cold, water, and electricity in the treatment of disease and injury. The physical therapy department will ordinarily have equipment such as whirlpools, parallel bars, ramps,

FIGURE 3.16

crutches, wheelchairs, braces, and prostheses (artificial limbs, etc.). Trained physical therapists help patients overcome or adjust to their disabilities through instruction and supervised practice.

*O*CCUPATIONAL THERAPY

Occupational therapy consists of directed activities, such as games and work projects. These activities aid in the treatment and **rehabilitation** of patients confined to the hospital. The program is adapted to suit the particular needs of each patient to provide him or her with the sort of diversion and skills that will best contribute to his or her physical and emotional progress. In this department, partially disabled patients learn to develop and explore new vocational possibilities. In many instances, the activities of the occupational therapy department are coordinated with those of the physical therapy department so that patients may develop skills both at work and in recreation.

*E*LECTROENCEPHALOGRAPHY SECTION

An electroencephalogram (EEG) is a mechanical tracing of brain waves, used to help determine the presence and location of tumors or other brain disorders.

If the hospital is not large enough to have a **neurodiagnostic department** and to require the services of a full-time neurologist—a doctor specializing in diseases of the nervous system—and an electroencephalograph technician, a technician may bring the equipment in from outside the hospital to take the tracing and perform the test.

*E*NDOSCOPY DEPARTMENT

An **endoscopy** is an examination of the body with the use of an instrument. *Endo* means "inside"; *scopy* means "to examine or visualize." This is a diagnostic procedure done by a doctor. In large hospitals endoscopies may be done in the endoscopy department. In smaller hospitals (depending on the type of endoscopy) it may be done in an examination room on the nursing unit.

*T*HE DIETARY DEPARTMENT

Department Organization

Registered dietitians are professionals who are accredited by the Commission of Dietetic Registration, the credentialing agency of the American Dietetic Association. Their training and education is at the bachelor's and often master's degree level. Dietitians are an integral part of the health care team. They perform nutrition assessments, educate patients on therapeutic diet needs, and consult on **enteral** (by mouth or tube) and **parenteral** (by other than the digestive tract) **therapies.**

The chief dietitian supervises all personnel concerned with the preparation and serving of food and those concerned with training in the department (Fig. 3.17).

Some hospitals have a large central kitchen where all the food is prepared. In other hospitals, there are smaller kitchens on each floor where the meals for the patients on that floor are prepared. There may be cooking facilities on each floor even if complete meals are not prepared; this permits nursing personnel to serve supplemental nourishments to the patients.

FIGURE 3.17

Functions of the Dietary Department

The responsibilities of the dietary department include:

- Planning general diets for patients and employees
- Planning menus for patients on special diets
- Preparing and serving food to patients and employees
- Training students and employees
- Preparing a diet manual
- Preparing and distributing infant formulas

The dietary department also ordinarily provides the following services for the patients:

- Members of the dietary staff often visit patients in their rooms to determine their food preferences. In this way, the patient whose diet has been restricted to certain types of foods has the opportunity to select those most appealing to him or to her.
- Dietary personnel also give advice and instruction to patients with special dietary problems at the time the patients are ready to be discharged from the hospital. With this help, the patients can continue the proper diet after they return home.
- The dietary staff also cooperates with the medical staff in planning, preparing, and serving experimental diets in a continuing effort to improve the entire dietary program.

STOCK NOURISHMENT

FIGURE 3.18

Special Orders

In addition to the regular meals served to patients, the dietary department handles certain special orders. These generally include:

■ Extra meals for visitors, so that a friend or family member may eat with the patient on occasion

■ Supplemental nourishments for the patients, such as crackers, milk, and juices, served midmorning, midafternoon, and evening

■ Stock nourishments, such as tea, coffee, milk, and crackers, served as required or desired by the patient (Fig. 3.18)

■ Hold diets, for patients who must have tests or treatments that either conflict with mealtime hour or that must be completed before the patient is allowed to eat

Diagnostic and therapeutic orders are discussed in Chapter 16.

*L*EARNING ACTIVITIES

Match the department in Column A with the brief description of its services in Column B.

Column A

(a) Health information services

(b) Environmental services

(c) Radiology

(d) Pharmacy

(e) Purchasing

Column B

____ Handles patients' accounts

____ Dispenses drugs and IV solutions

____ Community outreach

____ Incoming and outgoing calls

____ X-rays, radiation therapy, nuclear medicine

(f)   Human resources   _____ Prepares, stocks, and issues nursing supplies

(g)   Business office

(h)   Engineering and maintenance   _____ Performs tests on blood and other body specimens

(i)   Laboratory

(j)   Cardiology   _____ Reviews and maintains patients' charts after discharge

(k)   Central supply   _____ Buys hospital supplies and equipment

(l)   Physical therapy

(m)   Communications   _____ Provides clean, neat, safe hospital environment

(n)   Public relations

_____ Maintains buildings and grounds

_____ Interviews, facilitates hiring, employee benefits

_____ Rehabilitation

_____ Electrocardiograms

Complete the following.

1. List two examples of home health services that may be available to help the patient after discharge.
   (a) _____
   (b) _____

2. Pastoral care provides _____
   _____
   _____

3. List three responsibilities of the clinical dietitian.
   (a) _____
   (b) _____
   (c) _____

4. For the purpose of study, the hospital departments may be grouped into what three categories?
   (a) _____
   (b) _____
   (c) _____

5. Write the correct department in the following spaces. You may use each answer more than once.

admitting	business office	human resources
health information services	information systems	central supply
purchasing	environmental services	engineering and maintenance

   (a) The elevator has stopped running. _____
   (b) A patient is discharged and the room must be cleaned. _____
   (c) You need to order office supplies. _____

(d) You are having trouble with the computer. _____
(e) Nursing needs a Foley catheter tray. _____
(f) The doctor requests the patient's "old charts." _____
(g) You need the face sheet and addressograph plate for the new patient. _____
(h) You need information on your employee benefits. _____
(i) The doctor has not received his dictated history and physical for the patient's chart. _____
(j) You have a question about your paycheck. _____
(k) You have an order for an air mattress for a patient's bed. _____
(l) A patient has just vomited a very large amount in the hall. _____
(m) The sink in the women's restroom is plugged. _____

6. Define the following terms.
(a) Phlebotomist _____
(b) Third-party payer _____
(c) Requisition _____
(d) Pharmacist _____
(e) Pathology _____
(f) Capitation _____
(g) Enteral therapy _____
(h) Termination interview _____
(i) Neurodiagnostic department _____
(j) Inservice training program _____

7. List three examples of special orders that may be requested through the dietary department.
(a) _____
(b) _____
(c) _____

8. List three responsibilities of the pharmacist.
(a) _____
(b) _____
(c) _____

9. What is the purpose of discharge planning? _____

10. How important do you think it is for the health unit coordinator to communicate effectively with the various departments? _____

11. List some ways you feel you could establish and maintain good relationships with the personnel in the hospital departments.
    (a) _____
    (b) _____
    (c) _____

12. Do you think it would be interesting to work in any of the departments discussed in this chapter? If so, which department or departments would you find most interesting and why? _____

_____

_____

_____

Medical Terminology

VOCABULARY

Abbreviation	A shortened form of a word or phrase used to represent the complete word or phrase
Acronym	A word or abbreviation formed by combining the first letter of several words, such as AIDS for acquired immune deficiency syndrome or CBC for complete blood count
Adjective	A word used to modify a noun
Combining form	A root plus a combining vowel
Combining vowel	A vowel (usually an o) that is frequently added to link a root to another root or a root to a suffix
Eponym	A person or place or thing after whom or which something is named, such as a disease, surgical procedure or instrument, or body organ
Noun	A word used as a person, place, or thing
Prefix	A word element added to the beginning of a word that changes or adds to its meaning
Root	The simple element from which a word is derived the meaning of the word
Suffix	An element added to the end of a word to change or to add to its meaning
Word element	A word part or component

OBJECTIVES

When you have completed this chapter, you will be able to:

- Define the terms listed in the vocabulary.
- Correctly spell, pronounce, and define the medical terms in this chapter.
- Recognize word elements, abbreviations, and their meanings.
- Recognize singular and plural forms of terms.
- State the rules for formulating medical terms.

Correct spelling, pronunciation, and definition of words are vitally important in a hospital. The medical staff will depend on you to transcribe doctors' orders and fill out charts, records, and reports with accuracy. It is essential for you to have a good working knowledge of terms describing diseases and medical and surgical treatments. Understanding medical terminology will also make your work more meaningful and the performance of your duties more efficient.

In this chapter, you will learn the important rules for forming various medical terms and you will be introduced to many of the terms in common usage in modern hospitals. The formation of new words is not an exact science; there are exceptions to every rule. Learning medical terminology is comparable to learning another language. The rules of everyday English do not always apply.

The following material is designed to help you recognize **word elements** and their meanings. Time, thought, and practice are required before you can become proficient in the language of medicine. Your efforts will help you attain the goal of all hospital workers: better patient care.

𝒢UIDE TO PRONUNCIATION

New medical terms included in this chapter are followed by simple guides to their pronunciation. Only long vowels are marked in the pronunciation guides. Pronunciation of other vowel sounds is indicated only on words that are especially difficult to pronounce correctly. As an exercise and using the following rules, pronounce each new word aloud.

Accents: The principal accent is written in capital letters. *Example:* DOC tor.

Syllables: Division between syllables is indicated by a slash (/). *Example:* gas/TRI/tis.

Vowels: (see following table)

Symbol	Example	Name
ā	-āle	long a
ă	ādd	short a
ē	ēve	long e
ĕ	ĕnd	short e
ī	īce	long i
ĭ	ĭll	short i
ō	ōld	long o
ŏ	ŏdd	short o
ū	cūbe	long u
ŭ	ŭp	short u

𝒲ORD ELEMENTS

Many medical terms are composed of several smaller, simpler words or word elements. The three main word elements that are frequently combined to form medical terms are the **prefix,** the **suffix,** and the **root** (Fig. 4.1).

The *root* is the body or main part of the word and denotes the meaning of the word as a whole.

The *prefix* is a word element combined with the root that changes or adds to its meaning. A prefix is always added to the beginning of a root.

The *suffix* is also a word element used to change or add to the meaning of the root. It is always added to the end of the root.

Examples of prefixes are followed by a hyphen (e.g., pre-).

Examples of suffixes are preceded by a hyphen (e.g., -ectomy).

In addition, a **combining vowel** (usually an *o*) is frequently added to link a root to another root or a root to a suffix for ease in pronunciation. The combining vowel is not used if a suffix begins with a vowel (enteritis, not enteroitis), but, as previously stated, it is used between two roots.

The **combining form** is the root plus the combining vowel (*arthr + o = arthro*), the combining form meaning joint.

Prefix	Combining Vowel	Root	Suffix	Word
dis-		agree	-able	disagreeable
		war	-like	warlike
un-		pardon	-able	unpardonable
inter-		nation	-al	international
speed-	o	meter		speedometer
		beauty	-ful	beautiful

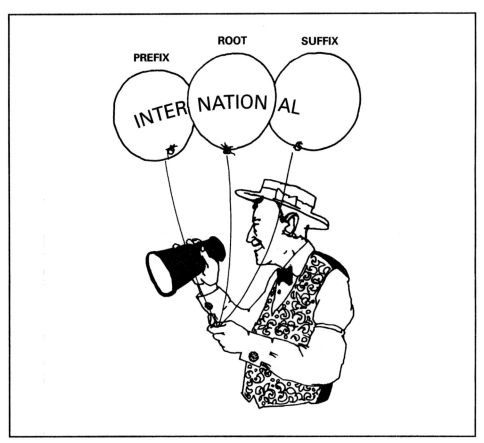

FIGURE 4.1

The word elements of medical terms work very much like the preceding examples. The main difference is that most medical word elements are derived from foreign languages, chiefly Latin and Greek. Thus, before you will be able to recognize easily the definitions of medical terms, you will need to learn the English meanings of the word elements in those terms. An alphabetical list of common word elements in medical terminology with their meanings and guides to pronunciation is given in this chapter.

COMBINING WORD ELEMENTS

Medical terms (like many English words) do not necessarily contain all word elements (Figs. 4.2 and 4.3).

■ The medical term may be a combination of a prefix and a root:

Medical Term		Prefix	Root
ectoderm	EC/to/derm	ecto-	derm
retropubic	RE/trō/pū/bic	retro-	pubic*
endoskeleton	EN/dō/skel/e/ton	endo-	skeleton
hemiplegic	he/mi/PLĒ/jic	hemi-	plegic*
hypertension	hȳ/per/TEN/sion	hyper-	tension

*-ic is a suffix that means "pertaining to"

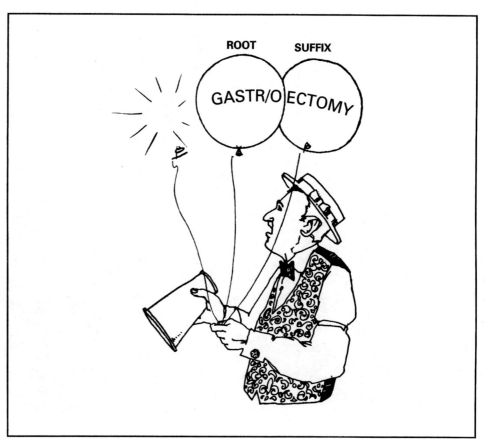

FIGURE 4.2

■ In other medical terms, the root may be combined with only a suffix:

Medical Term		Root	Suffix
colostomy	co/LOS/to/mē	col (o)	-stomy
gastrectomy	gas/TREC/to/mē	gastr	-ectomy
myasthenia	mȳ/as/THĒ/nē/a	my	-asthenia
osteoma	os/tē/Ō/ma	oste	-oma

■ Some medical terms may be formed by using prefixes and suffixes alone:

Medical Term		Prefix	Suffix
diarrhea	dī/a/RRHĒ/a	dia-	-rrhea
endoscopy	en/DOS/co/pē	endo-	-scopy
excise	ex/CĪSE	ex-	-cise
epilepsy	EP/i/lep/sē	epi-	-lepsy
polyuria	pol/ē/Ū/rē/a	poly-	-uria

■ Some medical terms are formed by combining two roots. The resulting word describes the disease or treatment more accurately:

Medical Term		1st Root	Comb. Vowel	2nd Root
bronchopneumonia	bron/chō/pneu/MŌ/nia	bronch	(o)	pneum (o)
gastroenteritis	gas/trō/en/ter/Ī/tis	gastr	(o)	enter
osteoarthritis	os/tē/ō/ar/THRĪ/tis	oste	(o)	arthr
pyelonephritis	pȳ/e/lŏ/ne/PHRĪ/tis	pyel	(o)	nephr

FIGURE 4.3

$\mathcal{W}$ORD VARIATIONS

There are a few special problems you may encounter as you begin your study of medical terminology.

- First, a word that has been formed from several different word elements may *omit, change,* or *add* certain letters so that it conforms to rules of spelling and pronunciation:

Prefix	Root	Comb. Vowel	Suffix		Word
em-	py		-ema	empyema	em/pȳ/Ē/ma
endo-	arteri		-itis	endarteritis	end/ar/ter/Ī/tis
	neur	(o)	-logy	neurology	neu/ROL/o/jē
supra-	renal			suprarenal	sū/pra/RĒ/nal
	stomat		-itis	stomatitis	stō/ma/TĪ/tis

- Second, some suffixes are used to create **nouns;** others are used to create **adjectives.**

Noun Suffixes	Adjective Suffixes
-ax	-al
-ium, um	-ic
-on, ion	-ac
-y, -ity	-ar
-us	-ous

WORD ELEMENTS SIMILAR IN SPELLING
BUT HAVE DIFFERENT MEANING.

CYT/O   CYST/O

FIGURE 4.4

All the adjective suffixes listed on page 65 mean "pertaining to."

■ Third, many of the word elements with which you must be familiar are similar in spelling but quite different in meaning (Fig. 4.4). The following is a list of word elements that often present difficulties. Examine this list carefully.

Prefix or Combining Form	Example	Meaning
ante-	*ante*febrile	*before* onset of fever
anti-	*anti*febrile	used *against* fever
a-	*a*dipsia	*absence* of thirst
ad-	*ad*renal	*near* the kidney
a-, an-	*an*uria	*absence* of urine
ano	*ano*rectal	pertaining to *anus* and rectum

Prefix or Combining Form	Example	Meaning
ad-	*ad*oral	*near* the mouth
aden	*aden*itis	*gland*ular inflammation
cyt/o	*cyto*genesis	production (origin) of the *cell*
cyst/o	*cysto*gram	x-ray record of the *bladder*
di-	*di*atomic	containing *two* atoms
dia-	*dia*gnosis	state of complete knowledge
dis-	*dis*sect	to cut *apart*
dys-	*dys*menorrhea	*difficult* or painful menstruation
en-	*en*cephalitis	inflammation *of* the brain
enter/o	*entero*plasty	operative revision of *intestines*

Prefix or Combining Form	Example	Meaning
hem-	*hem*angioma	tumor consisting of *blood* vessels
hemi-	*hemi*analgesia	pain relief in *half* of body
hem/o	*hemo*toxin	a *blood* poison
hyper-	*hyper*tension	*high* blood pressure
hypo-	*hypo*tension	*low* blood pressure
ile/o	*ileo*cecum	parts of *small* and *large intestine*
ili/o	*ilio*sacrum	part of hip bone and vertebral column
inter-	*inter*stitial	lying *between* spaces
intra-	*intra*cranial	*within* the skull
macro-	*macro*scopy	seen *large,* as with the naked eye
micro-	*micro*scopy	seen *small,* as by microscope
my/o	*myo*logy	study of *muscle*
myel-	*myel*oma	tumor of the *bone marrow*
necr-	*necr*osis	state of tissue *death*

Prefix or Combining Form	Example	Meaning
nephr-	*nephr*osis	condition of the *kidneys*
neur-	*neur*osis	*nervous* condition
oste-	*osteo*logy	study of *bone*
ot/o	*oto*logy	study of the *ear*
per-	*per*cussion	a striking *through* the body
peri-	*peri*cardial	*around* the heart
pre-	*pre*clinical	*before* the onset of disease
py/o	*pyo*genic	*pus* producing
pyr/o	*pyro*genic	*fever* producing

■ Finally, two groups of suffixes contain quite similar word elements, each of which has a specific meaning.

Suffix	Word	Definition
-gram	electrocardio*gram*	*record* of heart action
-graph	electrocardio*graph*	*machine* that makes record
-graphy	electrocardio*graphy*	*process* of making record

Electrocardiography is performed by a technician who connects parts of the patient's body to an **electrocardiograph,** which produces a record of the patient's heart action called an **electrocardiogram.**

Suffix	Word	Definition
-ectomy	gast*rectomy*	surgical *removal* of the stomach
-stomy	gastro*stomy*	surgical *opening* into the stomach
-tomy	gastro*tomy*	surgical *incision* into the stomach

An infant who swallowed a pin requires a **gastrotomy** to remove the pin from the stomach; a patient unable to take food by mouth has a **gastrostomy** and is fed by tube directly into the stomach; the doctor performs a **gastrectomy** on a patient with bleeding ulcers (Fig. 4.5).

FIGURE 4.5

LIST OF WORD ELEMENTS

The following list of word elements is arranged alphabetically. Word elements that are most often used as prefixes are followed by a hyphen (ambi-); suffixes are preceded by a hyphen (-algia). Remember that sometimes a term changes its function (a prefix is used as a root, for example) when it is used in a different word.

- Repeat aloud each of the word elements and its meaning.
- Pronounce the words given as examples.
- Try to figure out the meaning of the sample word with the help of information given in the list. For example, the third word on the list is *adrenal; ad* means "near," "toward." Now look up *renal.* You will find that it means "kidney." Therefore, adrenal means "near the kidney."

Prefix, Suffix, or Combining Form	Refers to or Means	Example	
A-, AN-,	without, lack of, absent, deficient	asepsis anemia	ā/SEP/sis an/Ē/mē/a
AB-, ABS-	from, away	abnormal abscess	ab/NORM/al ABS/cess
AD-	near, toward	adrenal	ad/RĔN/al
ADEN/O	gland	adenopathy	ad/en/OP/a/thē
AER/O	air	anaerobe	an/ĂER/ōbe
ALB	white	albuminuria	al/BŪ/mi/nur/ē/a
-ALGESIA, -ALGIA	pain	analgesia	an/al/JĔ/sia
AMBI	both	ambidextrous	am/bi/DEX/trous

Prefix, Suffix, or Combining Form	Refers to or Means	Example	
ANGI/O	vessel (blood or lymph)	angioma	an/jē/Ō/ma
ANTE-	before	antenatal	an/tē/NĂ/tal
ANTI-	against	antiseptic	an/ti/SEP/tic
ARTERI/O	artery	arteriosclerosis	ar/ter/ē/ō/scle/RO/sis
ARTHR/O	joint	arthroplasty	AR/thro/plas/tē
-ASTHENIA	weakness	myasthenia	mī/as/THĒ/nē/a
AUTO-	self	autopathy	au/to/PATH/ē
BI-	two, twice	bicellular	bi/CELL/ū/lar
BLEPHAR/O	eyelid	blepharoplasty	ble/pha/RŌ/plas/tē
BRADY-	slow	bradycardia	bră/di/CAR/dē/a
BRONCH/O	bronchus	bronchitis	bron/KĪ/tis
CARCIN/O	cancer of epithelial tissue	carcinogen	car/CI/no/jen
CARDI/O	heart	myocardium	mī/o/CAR/dē/um
-CELE	tumor, swelling, hernia, sac	enterocele	EN/ter/ō/cēle
-CENTESIS	puncture	thoracentesis	thor/a/cen/TĒ/sis
CEPHAL/O	head	hydrocephaly	hy/drō/CE/pha/lē
CHOL/E	gall	cholelithiasis	chō/le/lith/Ĭ/a/sis
CHOLECYST/O	gallbladder	cholecystectomy	chō/le/cys/TEC/to/mē
CHOLEDOCH/O	common bile duct	choledochostomy	chō/le/do/KOS/to/mē
CHONDR/O	cartilage	chondroma	chon/DRŌ/ma
-CIDE	kill	germicide	GERM/i/cīde
CIRCUM-	around	circumcision	cir/cum/CI/sion
-CISE	cut	excise	ex/CĪSE
COL/O	colon	colitis	co/LĬ/tis
COLP/O	vagina	colporrhaphy	col/POR/rha/phē
CONTRA-	against	contraception	con/tra/CEP/tion
COST/O	rib	intercostal	in/ter/COS/tal
CRANI/O	skull	craniotomy	crā/nē/OT/o/mē
CYAN/O	blue	cyanotic	cȳ/a/NO/tic
CYST/O	urinary bladder	cystogram	CYS/to/gram
CYT/O	cell	monocyte	MON/o/cȳte
DE-	down, from	decubitus	de/CŬ/bi/tus
DENT/I	tooth	dentistry	DEN/tis/trē
DERM/O, DERMAT/O	skin	dermatology	derm/a/TOL/o/jē
DEXTR/O	right	dextrocardia	dex/tro/CAR/dē/a
DI-	two	diplopia	dip/LŌ/pē/a
DIA-	through, between, across, apart	diarrhea	dī/a/RRHĒ/a
DIS-	apart	dissect	dis/SECT
DYS-	painful, difficult, disordered	dysmenorrhea	dys/meno/RRHĒ/a
ECTO-	outer, on the outside	ectocytic	ec/to/SȲ/tic
-ECTOMY	surgical removal	prostatectomy	pros/ta/TEC/to/mē
-EMESIS	vomiting	hematemesis	hem/at/EM/ē/sis
-EMIA	blood	leukemia	leu/KĒ/mē/a
EN-	in, inside	encapsulated	en/CAP/su/lā/ted
ENCEPHAL/O	brain	encephalitis	en/ceph/a/LĬ/tis
ENDO-	within, inner, on the inside	endometrium	en/do/MĒ/trē/um
ENTER/O	intestine	enteritis	en/ter/Ĭ/tis
EPI-	above, over	epigastric	ep/i/GAS/tric
ERYTHR/O	red	erythrocyte	e/ryth/RO/cȳte
-ESTHESIA	sensation	anesthesia	an/es/THĒ/sia
EX-	out	extrahepatic	ex/tra/hep/A/tic
EXTRA-			
FEBR/I	fever	afebrile	ā/FE/brĭle
FIBR/O	connective tissue	fibroma	fī/BRŌ/ma

(continued)

Prefix, Suffix, or Combining Form	Refers to or Means	Example	
GASTR/O	stomach	gastrocele	GAS/trō/cēle
-GENE, -GENIC	production, origin	neurogenic	neu/ro/JEN/ic
GLOSS/O	tongue	glossalgia	glos/SAL/jē/a
GLUC/O, GLYC/O	sugar, sweet	glycosuria	glȳ/cō/SUR/ē/a
-GRAM	record	myelogram	MȲ/e/lō/gram
-GRAPH	machine	electroencephalograph	e/lec/trō/en/CE/pha/lo/graph
-GRAPHY	practice, process	ventriculography	ven/tri/cū/LOG/ra/phē
GYNE	woman	gynecology	gy/ne/COL/o/jē
HEMAT/O, HEM/O	blood	hematology	hē/ma/TO/lo/jē
HEMI-	half	hemiplegia	he/mi/PLĒ/jēa
HEPA, HEPAT/O	liver	hepatitis	he/pa/TĪ/tis
HERNI/O	rupture	hernioplasty	HER/nē/o/plas/tē
HIST/O	tissue	histology	his/TOL/o/jē
HYDR/O	water	hydronephrosis	hy/dro/ne/PHRŌ/sis
HYPER-	over, above, increased, excessive	hypertension	hȳ/per/TEN/sion
HYPO-	under, beneath, decreased	hypotension	hȳ/pō/TEN/sion
HYSTER/O	uterus	hysterectomy	hys/te/REC/to/mē
-IASIS	abnormal condition of	urolithiasis	ūr/o/li/THI/a/sis
IATR/O	treatment	iatrogenic	ī/a/tro/JE/nic
ICTER/O	jaundice	icterogenic	IC/ter/o/je/nic
ILE/O	ileum (part of small intestine)	ileitis	il/ē/Ī/tis
ILI/O	ilium (part of hip)	iliosacrum	il/i/ō/SĀ/crum
INTER-	between	intercellular	inter/CEL/lū/lar
INTRA-	within	intramuscular	in/tra/MUS/cū/lar
-ITIS	inflammation of	appendicitis	ap/pen/di/CĪ/tis
LAPAR/O	abdomen	laparotomy	la/pa/RO/to/mē
-LEPSY	seizure, convulse	narcolepsy	NAR/co/lep/sē
LEUK/O	white	leukorrhea	leu/ko/RRHĒ/a
LIP/O	fat	lipoma	lī/PŌ/ma
LITH/O	stone, calculus	lithocystotomy	li/thō/cys/TO/to/mē
-LOGY	study of	neurology	neu/RO/lo/jē
-LYSIS	loosen, dissolve	hemolysis	he/mo/LY/sis
MACRO-	large, long	macrocyte	MA/cro/cȳte
MAL-	bad, poor, disordered	malabsorption	mal/ab/SORP/tion
-MANIA	insanity	kleptomania	klep/to/MĀ/nēa
MAST/O	breast	mastectomy	mas/TEC/to/mē
MEG/A	large	splenomegaly	sple/nō/ME/ga/lē
MEN/O	month	menstruation	men/strū/Ā/tion
MESO-	middle	mesocardia	me/so/CAR/dē/a
-METER	measure	thermometer	ther/MO/me/ter
METR/O	uterus	metrorrhagia	mē/tro/RRHĀ/jea
MICRO-	small	microscope	MĪ/cro/scōpe
MONO-	single one	monocyte	MO/no/cȳte
MUC/O	mucous membrane	mucocutaneous	mū/cō/cū/TĀ/nē/ous
MYC/O	fungus	mycosis	my/CŌ/sis
MYEL/O	spinal cord, bone marrow	myelomeningocele	mȳ/el/ō/me/NIN/go/cēle
MY/O	muscle	myopathy	mȳ/O/pa/thē
NARC/O	stupor	narcotic	nar/CO/tic
NAS/O	nose	nasopharynx	nā/sō/PHAR/ynx
NAT/I	birth	prenatal	pre/NĀ/tal
NECR/O	death	necropsy	NE/crop/sē
NEO-	new	neoplasm	NĒ/o/plasm
NEPHR/O	kidney	nephritis	ne/PHRĪ/tis
NEUR/O	nerve	neuralgia	neu/RAL/jē/a
NON-	no, not	nontoxic	non/TOX/ic
OCUL/O	eye	oculomycosis	O/cū/lo/mȳ/cō/sis
-OMA	tumor	carcinoma	car/ci/NŌ/ma

Prefix, Suffix, or Combining Form	Refers to or Means		Example
OOPHOR/O	ovary	oophorectomy	ō/o/pho/REC/to/mē
OPHTHALM/O	eye	ophthalmoscope	oph/THAL/mo/scōpe
-OPIA	vision	photopic	phot/Ō/pic
ORCHI/O	testicle	orchipexy	OR/chi/pe/xē
ORTH/O	straight	orthopedics	or/tho/PĒ/dics
-OSIS	abnormal condition	neurosis	neu/RŌ/sis
OSTE/O	bone	osteoma	os/tē/Ō/ma
OT/O	ear	otolith	Ō/tol/ith
-PARA	to bring forth or to bear	multipara	MUL/ti/pa/ra
PARA-	alongside of, abnormal	paraplegia	para/a/PLĒ/jē/a
PATH/O	disease	pathology	pa/THO/lo/jē
PED/O (Latin)	foot	pedograph	PE/do/graph
PED/O (Greek)	child	pediatrics	pe/dē/A/trics
-PENIA	too few	leukopenia	leu/ko/PĒ/nē/a
PERI-	around, covering	pericarditis	pe/ri/car/DĪ/tis
-PEXY	to sew up in position	nephropexy	NE/phro/pe/xē
PHARYNG/O	throat	pharyngoplasty	phar/YN/go/plas/tē
PHLEB/O	vein	phlebitis	phle/BĪ/tis
-PHOBIA	fear, dread	photophobia	pho/to/PHŌ/bē/a
PHOT/O	light	photolysis	phō/TO/ly/sis
-PLASTY	operative repair	rhinoplasty	RHĪ/no/plas/tē
-PLEGIA	paralysis	quadriplegia	qua/dri/PLĒ/jē/a
-PNEA	breathing	orthopnea	or/thop/NĒ/a
PNEUM/O	air, lungs	pneumonia	pneu/MŌ/nia
POLY-	much, many	polyuria	po/lē/UR/ē/a
POST-	after	postpartum	post/PAR/tum
PROCT/O	rectum	proctoscopy	proc/TOS/co/pē
PRE-	before	preoperative	prē/OP/er/a/tive
-PTOSIS	falling	nephroptosis	ne/phrop/TŌ/sis
PYEL/O	pelvis of kidney	pyelonephritis	pȳ/e/lō/ne/PHRĪ/tis
PY/O	pus	pyogenic	pȳ/o/JE/nic
PYR/O	heat, temperature	pyrexia	pȳ/REX/ē/a
REN/O	kidney	suprarenal	sū/pra/RĒ/nal
RETRO-	behind, backward	retrosternal	re/tro/STER/nal
RHIN/O	nose	rhinopathy	rhī/NO/pa/thē
-RRHAGE	profuse bleeding, flow	hemorrhage	HE/mo/rrhij
-RRHAPHY	to suture/to repair a defect	herniorrhaphy	her/nē/OR/raph/ē
-RRHEA	flow	diarrhea	dī/a/RRHĒ/a
SALPING/O	oviduct	salpingectomy	sal/pin/JEC/to/me
SCLER/O	hardening	scleroderma	scler/o/DER/ma
-SCOPE	instrument to view	cystoscope	CYS/to/scōpe
-SCOPY	look into, see	esophagoscopy	e/so/pha/GOS/co/pē
SECT/O	to cut	transect	tran/SECT
SEMI-	half	semicircular	se/mē/CIR/cū/lar
SEPT/I	poison, infection	septicemia	sep/ti/CĒ/mē/a
SPLEN/O	spleen	splenocele	SPLE/nō/cēle
STOMAT/O	mouth	stomatitis	stō/ma/TĪ/tis
-STOMY	surgical opening	colostomy	co/LOS/to/mē
SUB-	under	subacute	sub/a/CŪTE
SUPRA-, SUPER-	above	suprapubic	sū/pra/PŪ/bic
-THERAPY	treatment	hydrotherapy	hȳ/dro/THER/a/pē
-THERMY	heat	diathermy	DĪ/a/ther/mē
THORAC/O	chest	thoracotomy	thor/a/CO/to/mē
THROMB/O	clot	thrombosis	throm/BŌ/sis
THYR/O	thyroid gland	thyroxin	thȳ/ROX/in

(continued)

Prefix, Suffix, or Combining Form	Refers to or Means		Example
-TOME	instrument to cut	dermatome	DER/ma/tōme
-TOMY	incision, surgical cutting	gastrotomy	gas/TRO/to/mē
TRANS-	across	transfusion	trans/FŪ/sion
UNI	one	unicellular	ū/ni/CELL/ū/lar
UR/O	urine	uremia	ū/RĒ/mē/a
-URIA, -URIC	condition of, presence in urine	glycosuria	glȳ/cō/SŪR/ē/a
VAS/O	blood vessel	vasoconstriction	vā/sō/con/STRIC/tion

*F*ORMING MEDICAL TERMS

Careful study will increase your familiarity with Latin and Greek roots and the English words that come from them (Table 4.1; Figs. 4.6, 4.7, and 4.8).

TABLE 4.1   *D*EFINITIONS OF LATIN AND GREEK ROOT WORDS BY BODY SYSTEM

Word Element or Combining Form	Refers to
Integumentary system (skin)	
derm/o, dermat/o	skin
muc/o	mucous membrane
hist/o	tissue
Musculoskeletal system	
my/o	muscle
myocardi/o	heart muscle
myocolp/o	vaginal muscle
myometr/o	uterine muscle
oste/o	bone
chondr/o	cartilage
fibr/o	connective tissue
arthr/o	joint
cost/o	rib
crani/o	skull
ili/o	hipbone, ilium
sacr/o	sacrum
myel/o	bone marrow
rachi/o	spinal column; vertebrae
inguin/o	groin
Respiratory system	
aer/o	air
nas/o, rhin/o	nose
pharyng/o	throat
trache/o	windpipe
thorac/o	chest
bronch/o	bronchus
pneum/o	lung
Circulatory system	
cardi/o	heart
hemat/o, hem/o	blood
vas/o	blood vessel
arteri/o	artery
phleb/o	vein
lymph/o	lymphatic system
angi/o	blood and lymphatic vessels
erythr/o	red
leuk/o	white
cyan/o	blue

TABLE 4.1 CONTINUED	
Word Element or Combining Form	**Refers to**
Digestive system	
stomat/o	mouth
dent/i	teeth
gloss/o	tongue
pharyng/o	pharynx, throat
esophag/o	esophagus, food pipe
gastr/o	stomach
enter/o	small intestine
hepat/o	liver
cholecyst/o	gallbladder
chol/e	bile, gall
lip/o	fat
choledoch/o	common bile duct
ile/o	ileum
col/o	large intestine
append/o	appendix
proct/o	rectum
an/o	anus
lapar/o	abdomen
Nervous system	
encephal/o	brain
myel/o	spinal cord
neur/o	nerve
ocul/o, ophthalm/o	eye
ot/o	ear
radicu/o	nerve root
Endocrine system	
aden/o	gland
adren/o	adrenal gland
thyr/o	thyroid
glyc/o, gluc/o	sugar
hypophys/o	pituitary gland
Urinary system	
nephr/o, ren/o	kidney
pyel/o	kidney pelvis
hydr/o	water
ur/o	urine
ureter/o	ureter
cyst/o	urinary bladder
Reproductive system	
andr/o	man
gynec/o	woman
orchi/o, orchid/o	testicles
oophor/o	ovary
hyster/o, metr/o	uterus, womb
salping/o	oviduct
colp/o	vagina
mast/o, mamm/o	breast
prostat/o	prostate
gravid/o	pregnancy

Word Element: path

When the word element *path* is found in a medical term, it always means "disease." Examine the word *pathology*. The suffix *-logy* means the "study of"; *pathology* therefore means the "study of disease." Now, use the word element *path* as a suffix to formulate a whole category of medical terms.

arterio*pathy*   any disease of the arteries
pneumono*pathy*   any disease of the lungs
uro*pathy*   any disease affecting the urinary tract

FIGURE 4.6

Word Element: itis

The study of medical terminology can aid you in understanding the name of the specific disease for which the patient has been hospitalized. The suffix *-itis* means "inflammation." Almost every organ in the body is subject to infection by disease organisms that will cause an inflammatory reaction. The word to describe a diagnosis of this nature is formed simply by adding the suffix *-itis* to the word for the body organ so affected.

appendic*itis*	inflammation of the appendix
dermat*itis*	inflammation of the skin
hepat*itis*	inflammation of liver tissue
rhin*itis*	inflammation of nasal mucosa
stomat*itis*	inflammation of the mouth

Other Word Elements

Many terms concerned with a disease, its many symptoms, the tools and procedures used to diagnose it, and the diagnoses themselves are formed in the manner just described. Study and learn the following terms in common usage.

Word Element or Combining Form	Example	Definition
-algia	neur*algia*	*pain* along the nerves
-centesis	thora*centesis*	*puncture* of chest wall to remove fluids
-emia	ur*emia*	urinary wastes in the *blood*
febr/o	a*febr*ile	absence of *fever*
-genic	pyo*genic*	*producing* pus
-iasis	cholelith*iasis*	gallstone *condition*
lith/o	nephro*lith*	*stone* in the kidney
-oma	lip*oma*	fatty *tumor*
-scopy	ano*scopy*	*visualization* of the anus
-osis	nephr*osis*	abnormal *condition* of the kidney
-plegia	hemi*plegia*	*paralysis* of half of the body
-pnea	a*pnea*	absence of *breathing*
py/o	*pyo*derma	skin disease caused by *pus*-forming bacteria
-therapy	hydro*therapy*	water used in *treatment* of disease
-uria	poly*uria*	excessive *urine* production and urination

FIGURE 4.7

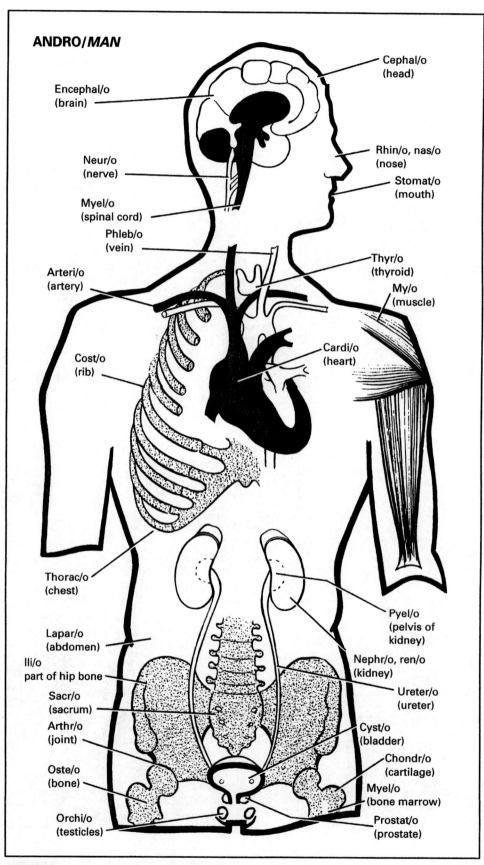

ANDRO/MAN

Cephal/o
(head)

Encephal/o
(brain)

Rhin/o, nas/o
(nose)

Stomat/o
(mouth)

Neur/o
(nerve)

Myel/o
(spinal cord)

Phleb/o
(vein)

Thyr/o
(thyroid)

My/o
(muscle)

Arteri/o
(artery)

Cardi/o
(heart)

Cost/o
(rib)

Thorac/o
(chest)

Pyel/o
(pelvis of
kidney)

Lapar/o
(abdomen)

Nephr/o, ren/o
(kidney)

Ili/o
part of hip bone

Ureter/o
(ureter)

Sacr/o
(sacrum)

Cyst/o
(bladder)

Arthr/o
(joint)

Chondr/o
(cartilage)

Oste/o
(bone)

Myel/o
(bone marrow)

Orchi/o
(testicles)

Prostat/o
(prostate)

FIGURE 4.8

SURGICAL PROCEDURES

When you are working on a surgical floor, you will encounter another large group of medical terms. These describe surgical procedures. You will need to have some idea of the type of surgery done on a patient. For this you must learn the word elements used in the names for surgical procedures.

Word Element: ectomy

The suffix *-ectomy* means *surgical removal*. When used in combination with any word element denoting an organ or other body part, the term formed means that the organ or body part has been removed. The terms *excision* and *resection* also mean to remove.

gastr*ectomy*	surgical removal of the stomach
thyroid*ectomy*	surgical removal of the thyroid gland
col*ectomy*	surgical removal of the large intestine

In many cases, an organ may be removed only partially. To indicate this procedure, other words are used to modify the medical term. For example:

subtotal thyroidectomy   *partial* cystectomy

Other modifying words may precede the medical term to identify the surgery performed even more accurately.

left salpingo-oophor*ectomy*	removal of the left ovary and oviduct
vaginal hyster*ectomy*	removal of the uterus through the vagina
transurethral prostat*ectomy*	removal of the prostate through the urethra
total abdominal hyster*ectomy*	removal of the entire uterus through the abdomen

OTHER WORD ELEMENTS USED IN SURGICAL PROCEDURES

Word Element	Example	Definition
-rrhaphy	herniorrhaphy	*suturing* of a hernia
-stomy	ureterostomy	*formation of an opening* for ureteral drainage
-tomy	colpotomy	*surgical incision* into the vagina
-pexy	cystopexy	*fixation of bladder* to the abdominal wall
-plasty	rhinoplasty	*surgical repair* of the nose
-tripsy	lithotripsy	*crushing* of a stone in the kidney, bladder, or urethra

EPONYMS

Many medical terms are based on **eponyms.** Eponyms are persons, whether real or legendary; places; or things after whom or which things are named. Diseases such as Rocky Mountain spotted fever and Lyme disease are named after geographical areas. The Epstein–Barr virus is named after two physicians who discovered it in 1964. Many parts of the body are named after the scientist who discovered or described them. The fallopian tubes are named after Gabrielle Fallopio, an Italian anatomist. Bowman's capsule, a part of the kidney, is named after Sir William Bowman, a British physician. Surgical procedures, diagnostic tests, instruments, and equipment may also be named after or derived from eponyms.

FORMING PLURALS

Certain rules apply for forming plurals from the singular form of a word.

- If the word ends in *a,* keep the *a* and add *e.*

Singular	Plural
vertebr*a*	vertebr*ae*

- If the word ends in *ex* or *ix,* drop the *ex* or *ix* and add *ices.*

Singular	Plural
ap*ex*	ap*ices*

- If the word ends in *is,* drop the *is* and add *es.*

Singular	Plural
cris*is*	cris*es*

- If the word ends in *um,* drop the *um* and add *a.*

Singular	Plural
ov*um*	ov*a*

- If the word ends in *us,* drop the *us* and add *i.*

Singular	Plural
nucle*us*	nucle*i*

ABBREVIATIONS

Many facilities have approved lists of **abbreviations** that they use, and lists can be found in many medical texts. Although abbreviations are used constantly, there is a lack of consistency among these sources. Some use periods or capitalization; others may not (cc, c.c. = cubic centimeter; CC, C.C. = chief complaint). One abbreviation may have several meanings (e.g., CD = carbonate dehydratase, cardiac disease, cystic duct, and communicable disease). Some abbreviations are **acronyms** (words formed from the first letters of other words or parts of words), such as A/AIDS105 and CBC. Some are symbols and some are abbreviations of a word or words. Some are from Greek and Latin, and others are from English, but all are shorter terms for longer words.

The health unit coordinator must be familiar with many abbreviations. Study the approved list from your hospital and the lists that follow. When in doubt about the meaning of any abbreviation, always remember to ask.

Add to the following list any new abbreviations commonly used in your health care institution.

Abbreviation	Meaning	Abbreviation	Meaning
		A	
ā	before	AMA	against medical advice, American Medical Association
a̅a̅	of each, equal parts		
AA	Alcoholics Anonymous		
AAA	abdominal aortic aneurysm	Amb	ambulatory
@	at	Amp	ampule
AB	abortion	Amt	amount
Abd	abdomen	ANA	antinuclear antibodies
ABG	arterial blood gas	A&P repair	anterior and posterior repair
ABR	absolute bed rest	Anes	anesthesia
ac	before meals	Ant	anterior
Acid phos	acid phosphatase	AP&L	anterior, posterior, and lateral
ACL	anterior cruciate ligament	Approx	approximately
ACTH	adrenocorticotropic hormone	Appy	appendectomy
		aPTT	activated partial thromboplastin time
AD	admitting diagnosis, right ear		
A&D	admission and discharge	Aq	aqueous
ADL	activities of daily living	aqua	water, H_2O
Ad lib	as desired	ARC	AIDS-related complex
Adm	admission	ARDS	acute respiratory distress syndrome
adm spec	admission specimen		
AED	automatic external defibrillator	ARF	acute renal failure
		AS	left ear
AFB	acid fast bacillus	ASAP	as soon as possible
AFP	alpha-fetoprotein	ASCVD	arteriosclerotic cardiovascular disease
$AgNO_3$	silver nitrate		
A/G	albumin/globulin ratio	ASHD	arteriosclerotic heart disease
AIDS	acquired immune deficiency syndrome	ATH	acute toxic hepatitis
		ATN	acute tubular necrosis
AKA	also known as, above-the-knee amputation	AU	both ears
		AV	atrioventricular
A-Line	arterial line	A&W	alive and well
alk phos	alkaline phosphatase	AWOL	away without leave
ALS	amyotrophic lateral sclerosis	AZ test	Aschheim–Zondek test for pregnancy
AM	morning		
		B	
B/A	backache	BOW	bag of water
B&B	bowel and bladder (training)	BP	blood pressure
BBB	bundle branch block	BPH	benign prostatic hyperplasia
Baso	basophil	BR	bedrest
BE	barium enema	BRP	bathroom privileges
BID	twice a day	BS	blood sugar
bkfst	breakfast	BSC	bedside commode
Bld	blood	BUN	blood urea nitrogen
BM	bowel movement	BVD	bag-valve device
BMT	bilateral myringotomy with tubes, bone marrow transplant	BW	birth weight
		Bx	biopsy
		C	
C	Celsius	C EX	cataract extraction
c̄	with	CHF	congestive heart failure
Ca	cancer, calcium	CHO	carbohydrate
CABG	coronary artery bypass graft	chol	cholesterol
CAD	coronary artery disease	chr	chronic
Cal	calorie	Cl	chloride
Cap	capsule	Cmpd	compound
CAT	computerized axial tomography	CMV	cytomegalovirus
		CNS	central nervous system
Cath	catheter or catheterize	C/O	complains of
CBC	complete blood count	CO_2	carbon dioxide
CBF	cerebral blood flow	Coag	coagulation
CC	chief complaint	Comf	comfortable
cc	cubic centimeter	Cont	continuous
CCU	Coronary Care Unit, Critical Care Unit	COPD	chronic obstructive pulmonary disease
CDC	Centers for Disease Control and Prevention	CP	cocktail privileges, chest pain

(*continued*)

Abbreviation	Meaning	Abbreviation	Meaning
CPA	carotid phonoangiography	C-section	cesarean section
CPAP	continuous positive airway pressure	CSF	cerebral spinal fluid
CPK	creatinine phosphokinase	CSS	closed system suction
CPR	cardiopulmonary resuscitation	CT	computed tomography
CPT	chest physiotherapy	CVA	cerebral vascular accident
CRRT	continuous renal replacement therapy	CVD	cerebral vascular disease
CS	Central Supply or Central Service	CVI	cerebral vascular insufficiency
		CVP	central venous pressure
C-S, C/S	cervical spine	C/W	consistent with
C&S	culture and sensitivity	CXR	chest x-ray
		Cysto	cystoscopy

D

Abbreviation	Meaning	Abbreviation	Meaning
D 5½ NS	5% dextrose in 0.45% normal saline	DKA	diabetic ketoacidosis
D 5¼ NS	5% dextrose in 0.25% normal saline	DM	diabetes mellitus
		DNA	desoxyribonucleic acid, do not awaken
D5LR	5% dextrose in lactate Ringer's	DNR	do not resuscitate
D5NS	5% dextrose in normal saline	DOA	dead on arrival
D5W	5% dextrose in water	DOB	date of birth
DAT	diet as tolerated	DOE	dyspnea on exertion
DC	discontinue	DPT	diphtheria, pertussis, tetanus
D/C	discharge	Dr.	doctor
D&C	dilation and curettage	dr or ℨ	dram
DDD	degenerative disk disease	DRG	diagnosis related group
Del. Rm. or DR	Delivery Room	DSD	dry sterile dressing
Dept.	department	Dsg	dressing
Diff	differential white blood cell count	D.T.'s	delirium tremens
		DU	duodenal ulcer
Dig	digoxin	Dx	diagnosis
Dil	dilute or dissolve		

E

Abbreviation	Meaning	Abbreviation	Meaning
E	enema	ELOS	estimated length of stay
Ea	each	EMG	electromyogram
EBL	estimated blood loss	ENT	ears, nose, throat
ECF	extended care facility	EOB	edge of bed
ECG	electrocardiogram	EOM	extraocular movement
ECHO	echogram	ER	emergency room
ECHO virus	enterocytopathogenic human orphan virus	ERCP	endoscopic retrograde cholangiopancreatography
ECT	electroconvulsive therapy	Esp	especially
ED	emergency department	ESR	erythrocyte sedimentation rate
EDC	estimated date of confinement	ESS	endoscopic sinus surgery
EDD	estimated date of delivery	Etc	et cetera
EEG	electroencephalogram	Etiol	etiology
EENT	eyes, ears, nose, throat	ETOH	alcohol
EFM	electronic fetal monitor	ETT	endotracheal tube
EGD	esophagogastroduodenoscopy	EUA	examination under anesthesia
EKG	electrocardiogram	Eval	evaluation
Elix	elixir	Exam	examination

F

Abbreviation	Meaning	Abbreviation	Meaning
F	Fahrenheit	FHR	fetal heart rate
F or Fe	female	Fib	fibrillation
FB	foreign body	FIO_2	fractional inspired oxygen
FBS	fasting blood sugar	Fld	fluid
Fdg	feeding	Fluro	fluoroscopy
Fe	iron	FM	fetal movement
$FeSO_4$	ferrous sulfate	Frac	fracture
FEF	forced expiratory flow	FS	frozen section
FEV1	forced expiratory volume 1 second	Ft	foot or feet
		F/U	follow-up
FEV3	forced expiratory volume 3 seconds	FUO	fever of undetermined origin
		FWB	full weight-bearing
FF	fundus firm, force fluids	FWW	front wheel walker
FH	family history	Fx	fracture

Abbreviation	Meaning	Abbreviation	Meaning
G		**G**	
G	gravida	GER	gastroesophageal reflux
GA	general anesthesia	Gl	gastrointestinal
Gal	gallon	Gm or g	gram
GB	gallbladder	GP	general practitioner
GBS	gallbladder series	gr	grain
GC	gonorrhea	gtt	drop
GCS	Glasgow coma scale	GTT	glucose tolerance test
GE	gastroenterology	G tube	gastric tube
GEA	general endotracheal anesthesia	GU	genitourinary
Gen	general	GYN	gynecology
H		**H**	
H/A	heated aerosol	H₂O	water
HA	headache	H₂O₂	hydrogen peroxide
HAL	hyperalimentation	H/O	history of
HAV	hepatitis A virus	HOB	head of bed
Hg	hemoglobin	H & P	history and physical
HBD	has been drinking	HP	hot packs
HBP	high blood pressure	HPI	history of present illness
HBV	hepatitis B virus	hr	hour
HCO₃	bicarbonate	hs	at bedtime
HCG	human chorionic gonadotropin	HSV	herpes simplex virus
		HT	Hubbard tank
HCl	hydrochloric acid	Ht	height
Hct	hematocrit	HVD	hypertensive vascular disease
H & H	hemoglobin and hematocrit	Hx	history
HIV	human immunodeficiency virus	Hyper	above or high
		Hypo	below or low
I		**I**	
IBD	inflammatory bowel disease	Info	information
ICD	implantable cardioverter-defibrillator	Int	internal
		I & O	intake and output
ICF	intermediate care facility	IOL	intraocular lens
ICP	intracranial pressure	IOP	intraocular pressure
ICU	intensive care unit	IPA	independent physicians association
I & D	incision and drainage		
IDDM	insulin-dependent diabetes mellitus	IPPB	intermittent positive pressure breathing
i.e.	that is	IQ	intelligence quotient
IH	infectious hepatitis	Irreg	irregular
IHD	ischemic heart disease	Irrig	irrigation
IM	intramuscular	IS	incentive spirometer
Immuno	immunology	Isol	isolation
imp	impression	IUD	intrauterine device
in.	inch	IV	intravenous
Inc	incomplete	IVC	intravenous cholangiogram
Inc Spiro	incentive spirometry	IVP	intravenous pyelogram
IND	induction of labor	IVPB	intravenous piggyback
Infx	infection		
J		**J**	
JP	Jackson–Pratt drain	Junct	junctional
Jt	joint	JVD	jugular vein distension
K		**K**	
K	potassium	KPE	Kelman phacoemulsification
KCl	potassium chloride	KS	Kaposi's sarcoma
Kg	kilogram	KUB	kidneys, ureters, bladder
KI	potassium iodide	K wire	Kirchner wire
L		**L**	
L	liter, lumbar	Lb	pound
L&A	light and accommodation	LBBB	left bundle branch block
Lab	laboratory	L&D	labor and delivery
Lac	laceration	LDH	lactic dehydrogenase
Lap	laparotomy	LE	lower extremity
Lat	lateral	LLQ	left lower quadrant

(*continued*)

Abbreviation	Meaning	Abbreviation	Meaning
LMP	last menstrual period	L/S	lumbar spine
LOA	leave of absence	L-S	lumbosacral
LOB	loss of balance	LSD	lysergic acid diethylamide
LOC	loss of consciousness	Lt or L	left
LOS	length of stay	LUQ	left upper quadrant
LP	lumbar puncture	LVN	licensed vocational nurse
LPGD	low-profile gastrostomy device	L & W	living and well
LPN	licensed practical nurse	Lymph	lymphocyte

M

Abbreviation	Meaning	Abbreviation	Meaning
m	murmur, meter	med	medication, medium
M	male	mEq	milliequivalent
MAA	macroaggregated albumin	mg	milligram
MAB	management of assaultive behavior	MG	myasthenia gravis
MAC	monitored anesthesia care	MHP	moist hot pack
MAE	moves all extremities	MI	myocardial infarction, mitral insufficiency
MAP	mean arterial pressure	Min A	minimal assist
Mat	maternity	ml	milliliter
Max	maximum	mm	millimeter
Max A	maximum assist	MMPI	Minnesota Multiphasic Personality Inventory
McB	McBurney's point	Mod	moderate
MCH	maternal child health	Mono	monocyte
MCHC	mean corpuscular hemoglobin count	MR	may repeat
mcg	microgram	MRI	magnetic resonance imaging
MCV	mean corpuscular volume	MRS	middle respiratory syndrome
MD	doctor of medicine	MS	multiple sclerosis
mec	meconium	MVP	mitral valve prolapse

N

Abbreviation	Meaning	Abbreviation	Meaning
N	nitrogen	NIL	not in labor
NA	Narcotics Anonymous	NKA	no known allergies
Na	sodium	N$_2$O	nitrous oxide
NaCl	sodium chloride	no.	number
NAD	no apparent distress	Noc	night
NaHCO$_3$	sodium bicarbonate	NP	neuropsychiatric, nursing procedure
NAS	no added salt	NPO	nothing by mouth
NB	newborn	NS	normal saline
N/C	no complaints	Nsg	nursing
NC	nasal cannula	NSR	normal sinus rhythm
Neg	negative	NSVD	normal spontaneous vaginal delivery
Neuro	neurology	NTG	nitroglycerin
N/G	nasogastric	N&V	nausea and vomiting
NHL	non-Hodgkin's lymphoma	NWB	non-weight-bearing
NICU	Neonatal Intensive Care Unit		
NIDDM	non-insulin-dependent diabetes mellitus		

O

Abbreviation	Meaning	Abbreviation	Meaning
O	none	OPG	oculoplethysmography
O$_2$	oxygen	O & P	ova and parasites
O$_2$ cap	oxygen capacity	OPR	Outpatient Recovery
O$_2$ cont	oxygen content	OPS	Outpatient Surgery
O$_2$ sat	oxygen saturation	ORIF	open reduction internal fixation
OB	obstetrics	Ortho	orthopedics
OBS	organic brain syndrome	os	mouth
Occ	occasional	OS	left eye
OCG	oral cholecystogram	OT	Occupational Therapy
OCT	oxytocin challenge test	OTC	over the counter
OD	right eye, overdose	OU	both eyes
Oint	ointment	OV	office visit
OOB	out of bed	oz or ℥	ounce
OP	operation, outpatient		
OPD	Outpatient Department		

Abbreviation	Meaning	Abbreviation	Meaning
P		**P**	
P	pulse	PM	afternoon
p̄	after	PMC	postmortem care
PA	pulmonary artery	PMH	past medical history
P & A	percussion and auscultation	PMI	point of maximal impulse
PAC	premature atrial contraction	PMS	premenstrual syndrome
PACU	Post Anesthesia Care Unit	PND	paroxysmal nocturnal dyspnea
p_2CO_2	partial pressure of CO_2 in arterial blood	PNS	peripheral nerve stimulator
p_2O_2	partial pressure of O_2 in arterial blood	P-OX	pulse oximetry
		pO_2	partial pressure of oxygen
Pap smear	Papanicolaou smear	PO	by mouth
PAT	paroxysmal atrial tachycardia	Poc	position of comfort
Path	pathology	POD	postoperative day
PAWP	pulmonary artery wedge pressure	Polys	polymorphonuclear leukocytes
PBI	protein bound iodine	Post	posterior
pc	after meals	Post-op	postoperative
PCA	patient-controlled analgesia	PP	postpartum
pCO_2	carbon dioxide pressure	PPBS	postprandial blood sugar
PCP	pneumocystis carinii pneumonia, primary care physician	PPD	purified protein derivative
		PPE	personal protective equipment
PCV	packed cell volume	Pre	before
PCXR	portable chest x-ray	Pre-op	before surgery
PD	postural drainage	Prep	preparation
PD&P	postural drainage and percussion	Prev	previous
		Prog	prognosis
PE	physical examination	PRN	when necessary
Ped	pediatric	PROM	premature rupture of membranes
PEEP	positive end expiratory pressure		
		Prot	protein
PEFR	peak expiratory flow rate	Pro time	prothrombin time
PEG	percutaneous endoscopic gastrostomy	PSA	prostatic serum antigen
		Pt	patient
Per	by, through	PT	physical therapy, prothrombin time
PERL	pupils equal and reactive to light	PTA	prior to admission
		PTCA	percutaneous transluminal coronary angioplasty
PFT	pulmonary function test		
pH	measure of acidity or alkalinity	PTL	preterm labor
PH	past history	PTT	partial thromboplastin time
Phono	phonophoresis	PTX	pneumothorax
Phos	phosphorus	PUD	peptic ulcer disease
PI	present illness	PUW	pick up walker
PICC	peripherally inserted central catheter	PVC	premature ventricular contraction
PID	pelvic inflammatory disease	PVD	peripheral vascular disease
		PVH	pulmonary venous hypertension
PIH	pregnancy induced hypertension		
		PVS	persistent vegetative state
PKU	phenylketonuria	PWB	partial weight-bearing
PLT	platelets	Px	prognosis
Q		**Q**	
q	every	qhs	every night at bedtime
qAM	every morning	q noc	every night
QC	quad care	qid	four times a day
qd	every day	qns	quantity not sufficient
qh	every hour	qod	every other day
q2h	every 2 hours	QS	quad sets
q3h	every 3 hours	qs	quantity sufficient
q4h	every 4 hours	Qt	quart
R		**R**	
R	respiration	RIA	radioimmunoassay
RA	rheumatoid arthritis	RLQ	right lower quadrant
Rad T	radiation therapy	RN	registered nurse
RBBB	right bundle branch block	R/O	rule out
RBC	red blood cell, red blood count	ROM	range of motion, rupture of membranes
RDS	respiratory distress syndrome	ROS	review of systems
Rec	recommend	RR	recovery room
Reg	regular	RSR	regular sinus rhythm
REM	rapid eye movement	Rt or R	right
Resp	respiration	RT	respiratory therapy
RF	rheumatoid factor	RUQ	right upper quadrant
Rh	rhesus factor	RVH	right ventricular hypertrophy
RHD	rheumatic heart disease	Rx	prescription

(continued)

Abbreviation	Meaning	Abbreviation	Meaning
s̄	without	**S** SOB	shortness of breath
s	sacral	Sol	solution
SA	suicide attempt	SOR	see old records
SAB	spontaneous abortion	Spec	specimen
SBE	subacute bacterial endocarditis	Sp gr	specific gravity
SBS	small bowel series	Span	spansule
Sc or Sub Q	subcutaneous	SR	sedimentation rate, system review, sustained release
SCBB	stereotactic core breast biopsy	s̄s̄	one half
SCN	Special Care Nursery	SSE	soap suds enema
SDS	Same Day Surgery	SSKI	saturated solution of potassium iodide
Sed rate	sedimentation rate	stab	stabnuclear neutrophil
SGOT	serum glutamic oxaloacetic transaminase	Staph	staphylococcus
SGPT	serum glutamic pyruvic transaminase	STAT	at once
		Stbn	stillborn
SH	social history	STD	sexually transmitted disease
SIDS	sudden infant death syndrome	STK	streptokinase
SLE	systemic lupus erythematosus	Strep	streptococcus
		STSG	split thickness skin graft
SMR	submucous resection	Subling	sublingual
SNF	skilled nursing facility	Supp	suppository
S/O	significant other	Surg	surgery
SO₂	oxygen saturation	SV	stroke volume
SOAP	subjective, objective, assessment, plan	Syr	syrup
T	temperature, thoracic	**T** TM	tympanic membrane
T & A	tonsillectomy and adenoidectomy	TMJ	temporomandibular joint
		TNM	T—primary tumor, N—nodal involvement, M—distant metastasis
Tab	tablet		
TAB	therapeutic abortion	TO	telephone order
TAH	total abdominal hysterectomy	TOB	time of birth
Talc	talcum	Tol	tolerance
TB	tuberculosis	TPA	tissue plasminogen activator
Tbsp	tablespoon	TPN	total parenteral nutrition
TCDB	turn, cough, and deep breathe	TPR	temperature, pulse, respiration
T & C	type and cross-match	Trach	tracheostomy
TCP	transcutaneous pacing	t-s, t/s	thoracic spine
TCU	Transitional Care Unit	Tsp	teaspoon
Temp	temperature	TT	tetanus toxoid
TENS	transcutaneous electrical nerve stimulation	TURP	transurethral resection of prostate
TF	to follow	TURV	transurethral vaporization of prostate
THR	total hip replacement		
TIA	transient ischemic attack	TV	tidal volume
tid	three times a day	TVH	total vaginal hysterectomy
Tinc	tincture	TWE	tap water enema
TKO	to keep open	Tx	treatment, traction
TKR	total knee replacement		
TLC	total lung capacity, tender loving care		
U	unit	**U** UPC	unit packed cells
UA	urinalysis	URI	upper respiratory infection
UCD	usual childhood diseases	US	ultrasound
UGI	upper gastrointestinal	USN	ultrasonic nebulizer
Ung	ointment	UTI	urinary tract infection
UNOS	United Network for Organ Sharing	UWB	unit whole blood
UOQ	upper outer quadrant		

Abbreviation	Meaning	Abbreviation	Meaning
		V	
V	vein	Vit	vitamin
Vag	vagina, vaginal	VO	verbal order
VC	vital capacity	Vol	volume
VD	venereal disease	V & P	vagotomy and pyloroplasty
VDRL	Venereal Disease Research Laboratory	VS	vital signs
		VSS	vital signs stable
VE	vaginal examination	VT or V tach	ventricular tachycardia
VF or V fib	ventricular fibrillation		
		W	
W/A	while awake	WNL	within normal limits
WB	whole blood	WP	whirlpool
WBAT	weight bearing as tolerated	WPW	Wolfe–Parkinson–White syndrome
WBC	white blood cell, white blood count	Wt	weight
W/C	wheelchair		
WD/WN	well developed, well nourished		
		X	
x	times	XRT	x-ray therapy
		Y	
Yd	yard	Yr	year
YO	year old		
		Symbols	
&	and	+	plus
@	at	−	minus
> or ↑	greater than	±	plus or minus
↑	increase	−	negative
< or ↓	less than	O or +	positive
↓	decrease	×	times
⇌	equal to	♀	female
O	hour	♂	male
Δ	change		

✐ EARNING ACTIVITIES

Complete the following.

1. The _____ is a word element added at the end of a word to change or add to its meaning.

2. The _____ is added to the beginning of a word.

3. The _____ is the body or main part of the word and denotes the primary meaning of the word as a whole.

4. The _____ is added sometimes for ease of pronunciation.

5. The _____ is a combination of the word elements that together make up a word.

6. An _____ is a person, place, or thing after whom or which something is named.

7. An _____ is a word or abbreviation formed by combining the first letter of several words.

8. Define the following word elements:
   (a) -gram _____
   (b) -graph _____
   (c) -graphy _____
   (d) -ectomy _____
   (e) -tomy _____
   (f) -stomy _____

9. Indicate whether each of the following words is plural (P) or singular (S) by placing the correct letter in the space provided.

   _____ appendix

   _____ metastases

   _____ metastasis

   _____ bacterium

   _____ nuclei

Study the word elements on pages 68–72 and give the meaning of the following word elements or combining forms.

1. ab- _____
2. ad- _____
3. aden/o _____
4. angi/o _____
5. arthr/o _____
6. brady _____
7. cardi/o _____
8. -centesis _____
9. cholecyst/o _____
10. chondr/o _____
11. crani/o _____
12. cyan/o _____
13. cyst/o _____
14. cyt/o _____
15. -emesis _____
16. encephal/o _____
17. enter/o _____
18. erythr/o _____
19. -esthesia _____
20. gastr/o _____

21. hem/o _____

22. hepa _____

23. hist/o _____

24. hyper _____

25. hyp/o _____

26. icter/o _____

27. lapar/o _____

28. -lepsy _____

29. leuk/o _____

30. metr/o _____

31. myel/o _____

32. -oma _____

33. ophthalm/o _____

34. -scopy _____

35. -osis _____

36. ot/o _____

37. path/o _____

38. phleb/o _____

39. -plasty _____

40. plegia _____

41. pneum/o _____

42. poly _____

43. post _____

44. proct/o _____

45. py/o _____

46. ren/o _____

47. rrhage _____

48. stomat/o _____

49. thromb/o _____

50. -uria _____

Give the meaning of the following terms. You have studied all the word elements.

1. chondroma _____

2. cardiology _____

3. arthroplasty _____

4. angioma _____

5. cholecystitis _____

    6. erythrocyte _____

    7. hematemesis _____

    8. cystogram _____

    9. craniotomy _____

    10. anesthesia _____

    11. leukorrhea _____

    12. metrorrhagia _____

    13. bronchoscopy _____

    14. orchiectomy _____

    15. myelogram _____

    16. polyuria _____

    17. apnea _____

    18. rhinopathy _____

    19. hydrotherapy _____

    20. diathermy _____

Match the abbreviation in Column A with its definition in Column B.

Column A	Column B
1. $FeSO_4$	_____ Anterior, posterior, and lateral
2. NTG	_____ Carbohydrate
3. MI	_____ Central venous pressure
4. DRG	_____ Silver nitrate
5. NKA	_____ Chest x-ray
6. Etiol	_____ Outpatient department
7. AP&L	_____ Cerebrovascular accident
8. Irrig	_____ Electromyogram
9. $NaHCO_3$	_____ No added salt
10. CHO	_____ Incision and drainage
11. CVP	_____ Central nervous system
12. CNS	_____ No known allergies
13. $AgNO_3$	_____ Transurethral resection prostate
14. OPD	_____ As soon as possible
15. EMG	_____ Shortness of breath
16. NAS	_____ Complains of
17. I&D	_____ Diagnosis
18. TURP	_____ Ferrous sulfate
19. ASAP	_____ Sodium bicarbonate

20. SOB   ＿＿ Recovery room

21. CXR   ＿＿ Magnetic resonance imaging

22. Dx   ＿＿ At once

23. CVA   ＿＿ Nitroglycerine

24. C/O   ＿＿ Etiology

25. RR   ＿＿ Tender loving care

26. ARC   ＿＿ Position of comfort

27. STAT   ＿＿ Turn, cough, deep breathe

28. TLC   ＿＿ Chronic obstructive pulmonary disease

29. POC   ＿＿ Myocardial infarction

30. TCDB   ＿＿ AIDS-related complex

31. MRI   ＿＿ Diagnosis-related group

32. COPD   ＿＿ Irrigation

Complete the following. Use a medical dictionary to learn more about these terms.

1. *Path* means ＿＿＿＿＿＿＿＿＿＿＿＿＿＿＿＿＿＿＿＿＿＿＿＿
   (a) *Pneumopathy* means any disease of the ＿＿＿＿＿＿＿＿＿＿
   (b) *Adenopathy* means any disease of the ＿＿＿＿＿＿＿＿＿＿
   (c) *Cardiomyopathy* means any disease of the ＿＿＿＿＿＿＿＿
   (d) Any disease of the arteries is called ＿＿＿＿＿＿＿＿＿＿＿
   (e) Any disease of the nerves is called ＿＿＿＿＿＿＿＿＿＿＿

2. *-itis* means ＿＿＿＿＿＿＿＿＿＿＿＿＿＿＿＿＿＿＿＿＿＿＿＿
   (a) *Stomatitis* is inflammation of the ＿＿＿＿＿＿＿＿＿＿＿＿
   (b) *Gastritis* is inflammation of the ＿＿＿＿＿＿＿＿＿＿＿＿＿
   (c) *Dermatitis* is inflammation of the ＿＿＿＿＿＿＿＿＿＿＿＿
   (d) Inflammation of the liver is called ＿＿＿＿＿＿＿＿＿＿＿＿
   (e) Inflammation of the urinary bladder is called ＿＿＿＿＿＿＿

3. *-ectomy* means ＿＿＿＿＿＿＿＿＿＿＿＿＿＿＿＿＿＿＿＿＿＿
   (a) A *cholecystectomy* is the surgical removal of the ＿＿＿＿＿
   (b) A *glossectomy* is the surgical removal of the ＿＿＿＿＿＿
   (c) The surgical removal of the uterus is a ＿＿＿＿＿＿＿＿＿＿
   (d) A subtotal thyroidectomy would be a ＿＿＿＿＿＿＿ removal of
      the ＿＿＿＿＿＿＿ gland
   (e) The surgical removal of cartilage is called ＿＿＿＿＿＿＿＿

Write the meaning of the abbreviations in the corresponding spaces.

1. Mrs. Tracy was admitted to the hospital today. Her diagnosis is (a) **CHF** and (b) **R/O** (c) **CVA.** Her admitting physician requests (d) **O₂** at 2 (e) **L** (f) **STAT,** (g) **CBC** and electrolytes, elevate (h) **HOB,** and an (i) **IV** of (j) **D5LR** (k) **TKO,** among many other orders. Mrs. Tracy has been (l) **SOB** and (m) **C/O** a severe (n) **HA** on the (o) **R** side.

  (a) ＿＿＿＿＿＿＿＿＿ (b) ＿＿＿＿＿＿＿＿＿
  (c) ＿＿＿＿＿＿＿＿＿ (d) ＿＿＿＿＿＿＿＿＿
  (e) ＿＿＿＿＿＿＿＿＿ (f) ＿＿＿＿＿＿＿＿＿
  (g) ＿＿＿＿＿＿＿＿＿ (h) ＿＿＿＿＿＿＿＿＿

(i) _____   (j) _____
(k) _____   (l) _____
(m) _____   (n) _____
(o) _____

2. Mr. Amberson was admitted with a severe (a) **UTI** and has had a (b) **cysto**
and (c) **IVP** because he has not responded to the antibiotic therapy and
continues to run a high (d) **temp.** His blood work has included a (e) **BUN,**
(f) **Na,** (g) **K,** and (h) **Cl.** He has also had a urine (i) **C&S** and a (j) **CXR.**
He has (k) **BRP** and is to (l) **FF.** He is on (m) **I&O** has an (n) **IV** of (o) **D5½
NS** (p) **@** 100 (q) **cc** an (r) **hr.**

(a) _____   (b) _____
(c) _____   (d) _____
(e) _____   (f) _____
(g) _____   (h) _____
(i) _____   (j) _____
(k) _____   (l) _____
(m) _____   (n) _____
(o) _____   (p) _____
(q) _____   (r) _____

3. The admitting (a) **Hx** for Mr. Amberson says that he is a (b) **WD/WN**
white male. He has had the (c) **UCD** and his parents are (d) **L&W.** He has
had (e) **chr.** bladder infections and noticed (f) **bld** in his urine 5 days ago.
(g) **OP** (h) **Tx** has been unsuccessful and he is now hospitalized for further
evaluation.

(a) _____   (b) _____
(c) _____   (d) _____
(e) _____   (f) _____
(g) _____   (h) _____

CHAPTER 5

Introduction to Body Structure and Function

VOCABULARY

Absorption	Passage of digested materials through the small intestine into the bloodstream
Anabolism	The building up of a body substance from simple parts to complex; the constructive phase of metabolism, as in the building of protein
Anatomy	The study of the structure of the body
Catabolism	The breaking down of complex substances into more simple parts; the destructive phase of metabolism with the resultant release of energy
Contract	To reduce in size and become smaller in diameter
Diagnosis	Determination of the nature and cause of a disease or disorder
Digestion	The change of food taken into the body by physical and chemical means so that it can be absorbed by the body
Dilate	To increase in size and become larger in diameter
Elimination	The excretion of waste products by the kidneys, skin, lungs, and intestines; in the digestive system solid waste materials or feces are expelled through the anus
Homeostasis	A state of balance or equilibrium within the body
Intake and Output	The measurement of all fluid that a patient takes into and eliminates from the body
Menopause	The cessation or stopping of menstruation
Metabolism	The total of all the physical and chemical changes that occur in the cell that involve anabolism and catabolism
Microscopic	So small as to be able to be viewed only with a microscope
Myocardial infarction	A heart attack; occurs when there is blockage of a coronary artery that leads to the heart, and there is insufficient blood and oxygen to the heart muscle
Physiology	The study of the function of the body
Prognosis	The outcome of a disease or disorder; what is going to happen to the patient in terms of recovery or lack of recovery
Pulmonary	Pertaining to the lungs
Regenerate	Repair or restoration
Tubules	Small tubes
Turgid	Swollen
Water soluble	Able to dissolve in water

OBJECTIVES

When you have completed this chapter, you will be able to:

- Define the terms listed in the vocabulary.
- Describe the structure and function of cells, tissues, organs, and systems.
- Explain how the body systems work together.
- Better understand orders and instructions which relate to particular parts of the anatomy.

HUMAN ANATOMY AND PHYSIOLOGY

In order to work intelligently as a health unit coordinator, you must acquire a basic knowledge of the human body. By understanding the structure and function of the body you can better grasp the meaning of medical terminology, physicians' orders, treatments, **diagnosis, prognosis,** surgical procedures, and instructions that you receive. Knowledge of these subjects will help you perform your duties more effectively and will make your job more interesting.

In this chapter you will be introduced to **anatomy**—the study of the body's structure, and **physiology**—the study of its function. You will learn that the living body is organized from the simple to the complex. The most basic living form is the cell. Specialized cells become tissues. Tissues group together to form organs, and these organs form systems (Fig. 5.1).

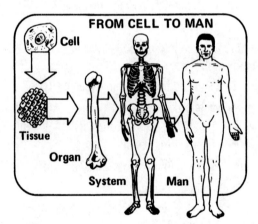

FIGURE 5.1

THE BODY'S ORGANIZATION
POSITIONAL AND DIRECTIONAL TERMS

As part of the study of the body we begin with a discussion of its organization and with the names given to body areas, positions, cavities, and planes. In any demonstration or diagram, the body or body part shown is in the anatomical position. The person is standing up straight, facing you, palms out, and feet together. When you look at a person in the anatomical position, remember that the left side is always on your right, as in a mirror. This is especially important in studying diagrams. The front of a person is referred to as the **anterior** (ventral) side. The back, containing the backbone, is called the **posterior** (dorsal) side. The areas of the body closer to the head are called **superior.** Those closer to the feet are called **inferior.** These terms may also be used to describe the position of an organ in the body. For example, the liver is inferior to the diaphragm; the shoulder is superior to the elbow.

The term **lateral** means pertaining to the side (the ears are lateral to the nose). **Medial** pertains to the middle (the nose is medial to the ears). **Distal** means farther from the point of attachment to the trunk and usually refers to the extremities (arms and legs). The wrist is distal to the elbow because the elbow is closer to where the arm attaches to the trunk of the body. **Proximal** means nearer the point of attachment to the trunk, so the knee is proximal to the ankle. When these terms are used with body organs, the portion closest to the organ above is proximal. Thus, the proximal end of the stomach attaches to the esophagus while the distal end attaches to the duodenum, the first part of the small intestine. **Deep** refers to distant from the surface, such as deep pain, and **superficial** means on or near the surface, such as a superficial wound.

BODY CAVITIES

The body has two major cavities—the **dorsal** cavity and the **ventral** cavity. The dorsal cavity is divided into the cranial and spinal cavities. The **cranial** cavity is in the head. It contains the brain, its protecting membranes, large blood vessels, and nerves. The **spinal** cavity contains the spinal cord.

The ventral cavity is divided by a large, dome-shaped muscle—called the **diaphragm**—into the thoracic and abdominal cavities. The **thoracic** cavity is in the chest. It contains the lungs, the heart, the major blood vessels, and a portion of the esophagus. The esophagus is the food tube. It penetrates the diaphragm and enters the stomach, which is in the **abdominal** cavity. The lower portion of the abdominal cavity is called the **pelvic** cavity and contains the urinary bladder and the reproductive organs.

Examples of organs in the abdominal cavity include the liver, spleen, pancreas, stomach, and small and large intestines.

The kidneys are located in the dorsal portion of the abdominal cavity. The kidneys are outside the large membrane that envelops all the other organs. This membrane is known as the **peritoneum.** When this membrane becomes infected, the disease is known as **peritonitis.** The peritoneum, like all membranes in the body, is made up of both epithelial and connective tissue. It protects organs and prevents friction when they move (Figs. 5.2 and 5.3).

BODY PLANES

Imaginary planes are used to divide the body into various sections. Operative reports often use the following terms to describe the site of the incision.

Frontal or **coronal plane**	Divides the body into front (anterior or ventral) and back (posterior or dorsal) positions.
Sagittal plane	Divides the body into right and left sides; the **midsagittal plane** divides the body exactly in half.
Transverse or **horizontal plane**	Divides the body into a top (superior) and a bottom (interior) portion.

ABDOMINAL REGIONS

The abdomen, for reference, can be divided in one of two ways, by **regions** or by **quadrants.** These reference points are used to describe the location of surgical incisions, wounds, pain, and so on.

Positional and Directional Terms

ANTERIOR
TOWARD THE FRONT

VENTRAL
ON THE BELLY SIDE

SUPERFICIAL
ON OR NEAR
THE SURFACE

DEEP
DISTANT FROM
THE SURFACE

SUPERIOR
UPPER PORTION

POSTERIOR
TOWARD THE BACK

DORSAL
ON THE BACK SIDE

INFERIOR
LOWER PORTION

FIGURE 5.2

There are nine abdominal regions:

- Right hypochondriac
- Left hypochondriac
- Epigastric
- Right lumbar
- Left lumbar
- Umbilical
- Right iliac
- Left iliac
- Hypogastric

There are four abdominal quadrants:

- Right upper quadrant (RUQ)
- Left upper quadrant (LUQ)
- Right lower quadrant (RLQ)
- Left lower quadrant (LLQ)

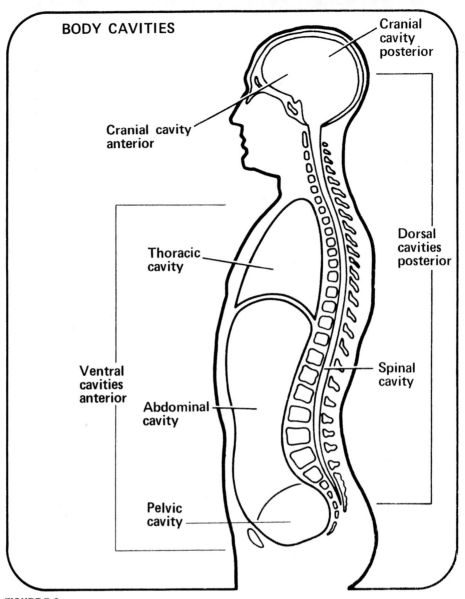

BODY CAVITIES

Cranial cavity posterior

Cranial cavity anterior

Dorsal cavities posterior

Thoracic cavity

Ventral cavities anterior

Spinal cavity

Abdominal cavity

Pelvic cavity

FIGURE 5.3

*T*HE BODY'S ORGANIZATION: REVIEW

Complete the following.

1. The determination of the nature and cause of a disease is the _____ _____.

2. The determination of the outcome of a disease or disorder is the _____ _____.

3. Write the word that describes each of the following body positions.
   (a) Closer to the head _____
   (b) Closer to the feet _____
   (c) Toward the back _____
   (d) Toward the front _____
   (e) Toward the side _____
   (f) Toward the middle _____

(g)   Closer to the point of attachment _____

(h)   Farther from the point of attachment _____

4. Circle the correct answer.
   (a)   The wrist is proximal/distal to the fingers.
   (b)   The nose is lateral/medial to the ears.
   (c)   The knee is proximal/distal to the ankle.
   (d)   The spinal canal is dorsal/ventral to the heart.
   (e)   The ribs are lateral/medial to the sternum (breastbone).

5. Name the two body cavities.
   (a)   _____
   (b)   _____

6. The sheet of muscle that separates the thoracic cavity from the abdominal cavity is the _____.

7. Circle the correct answer.
   (a)   The plane that divides the body into right and left halves is the frontal plane/sagittal plane/transverse plane.
   (b)   The plane that divides the body into a top and bottom is the frontal plane/sagittal plane/transverse plane.

8. Another name for the frontal plane is the _____ plane.

9. Another name for the transverse plane is the _____ plane.

10. The _____ plane divides the body exactly in half.

11. The abdomen is divided into _____ regions.

12. List the four abdominal quadrants and give the abbreviation for each.
   (a)   _____   (c)   _____
   (b)   _____   (d)   _____

*T*HE CELL

The cell is the fundamental building block of all living matter. Cells are **microscopic** in size and are the living parts of organisms. The human body is made up of millions of cells of different types. Each one has a special task within the body, but all living cells have many things in common:

- They contain a jellylike substance made of water, protein, fats, sugar, acids, and some minerals.
- They come from preexisting cells.
- They use food for energy.
- They use oxygen to break down the food.
- They use water to transport **water-soluble** substances such as sodium.
- They grow and repair themselves.
- They reproduce themselves.

Structure of the Cell

Cells consist of three main parts:

- **Nucleus**—which directs cellular activities
- **Cytoplasm**—where the activities of the cell take place

■ **Cell membrane**—which keeps the living substance of the cell, called the protoplasm, within bounds and allows certain materials to pass into and out of the cell

Cells are made up of two main compartments: a nucleus, which contains the chromosomes (the hereditary material), and a surrounding mass of cytoplasm. The nucleus is important to the process of heredity, growth, and cell division. There are 23 pairs of *chromosomes,* threadlike structures containing several thousand genes each. Each gene is made of the chemical deoxyribonucleic acid (*DNA*), which controls inheritance (Fig. 5.4).

DNA molecules produce messenger **RNA** molecules, which are partial copies of the DNA. Each RNA passes into the cytoplasm and directs the formation of protein molecules necessary to maintain life. Through the RNA the nucleus controls the kinds of chemical reactions carried out by the cell.

Cells reproduce by division. In any cell preparing for division, the nucleus exactly duplicates its chromosomes. As the cell divides, the pairs of chromosomes pull apart and move to opposite sides of the nucleus. When division is complete the new cells are identical.

Cytoplasm is enclosed in the cell membranes. It is all the material outside the nucleus. Within the cytoplasm are structural and functional bodies called **organelles.** These include **mitochondria** where nutrients are burned and energy is released, and **endoplasmic reticulum,** which is a network of tubes and plates within the cytoplasm. Rough-textured endoplasmic reticulum has **ribosomes** bound to its surface. Together, the rough-textured endoplasmic reticulum and the ribosomes produce proteins. Smooth endoplasmic reticulum contains enzymes that synthesize **lipids** (fats). Other

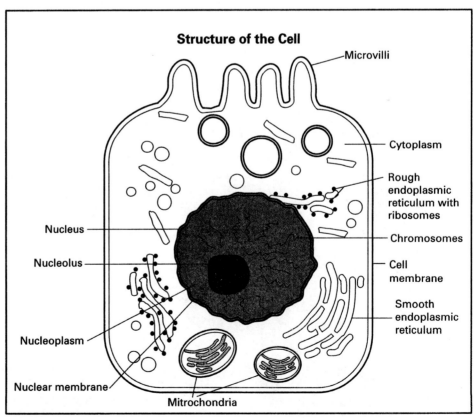

FIGURE 5.4

organelles include **Golgi apparatus, centrioles,** and minute amounts of glycogen and lipids.

The process of building from simple to complex materials is called **anabolism.** During this phase the body uses materials to grow and repair and builds up complex protein from more simple substances. **Catabolism** is the breaking down of complex materials into more simple substances, generally with the release of energy. Catabolism is thus the opposite of anabolism. **Metabolism** involves both anabolism and catabolism and is the sum of all chemical and physical changes that occur within the body.

$\mathcal{T}$ ISSUES

Cells usually do not work alone. They are organized through the process of **differentiation** into collections of cells that perform specific functions. Groups of cells of the same type that do a particular kind of work are called **tissues.**

Some of the primary kinds of tissues in the human body are:

- **Epithelial tissue**—The function of this tissue is to protect (skin), control permeability (control what enters and leaves the body), secrete (hormones, milk, mucus, perspiration), and receive sensations.
- **Connective tissue**—The function of this tissue is to connect (tendons), to support (bones), and to cover, ensheath, or line (the thin and sometimes fatty layer of connective tissue under the skin, the tough sheet of fibrous tissue over the limbs), and to pad or protect (bursal sacs).
- **Muscle tissue**—The function of this tissue is movement. Striated tissue is found in voluntary muscles, those you can move consciously. Smooth tissue is found in the involuntary muscles such as those that push food and water through the gastrointestinal tract. Smooth muscle allows such action as a dilation and contraction of the pupil of the eye and of blood vessels (Fig. 5.5).
- **Nerve tissue**—The function of this tissue is to carry nervous impulses from a portion of the brain or spinal cord to all parts of the body. Generally the body cannot renew nervous tissue.
- **Blood and lymph tissue**—The function of this type of tissue is transportation. The cells are singular and move within a fluid to every part of the body.

Body Systems

Tissues are grouped together to form **organs,** such as the heart, lungs, and liver. Each organ has a specific job. Organs that work together to perform similar tasks make up **systems.** It is easier to study anatomy and physiology by systems. Always remember that a system cannot work by itself; systems are interdependent (Table 5.1; Fig. 5.6).

FIGURE 5.5

TABLE 5.1	*T*HE BODY SYSTEMS	
System	**Function**	**Organs**
Integumentary	Provides first line of defense against infection, maintains body temperature, provides fluids and gets rid of wastes.	Skin; hair; nails; sweat and oil glands
Skeletal	Supports and protects the body	Bones; joints
Muscular	Gives movement to the body	Muscles; tendons; ligaments
Nervous	Controls activities of the body	Brain; spinal cord; nerves
Endocrine	Secretes hormones directly into the blood and regulates body function	Thyroid and parathyroid glands; pineal gland; adrenal glands; testes; ovaries; thymus gland; pancreatic islands of Langerhans; pituitary gland

(continued)

System	Function	Organs
TABLE 5-1 CONTINUED		
Circulatory	Carries food, oxygen, and water to the body cells and removes wastes	Heart; blood; arteries; veins; capillaries; spleen; lymph nodes; lymph vessels
Respiratory	Eliminates carbon dioxide and gives the body air to supply oxygen to the cells through the blood	Nose; pharynx; larynx; trachea; bronchi; lungs
Digestive	Takes and absorbs nutrition and eliminates wastes	Mouth; teeth; tongue; salivary glands; esophagus; stomach; small intestine; liver; gallbladder; pancreas; large intestine; rectum; anus
Urinary	Removes wastes from the blood, produces urine, and eliminates urine	Kidneys; ureters; bladder; urethra
Reproductive	To reproduce, allows a new human being to be born	Male: testes; scrotum; penis; bulbourethral glands; epididymis; vas deferens; ejaculatory duct; seminal vesicles; prostate Female: ovaries; uterus; breasts; uterine tubes (fallopian tubes or oviducts); vagina

Cells combine to form tissues, and tissues combine to form organs

FIGURE 5.6

CELLS, TISSUES, SYSTEMS: REVIEW

Complete the following.

1. List five things living cells have in common.

(a) _____

(b) _____

(c) _____

(d) _____

(e) _____

2. List the three main parts of cells.

(a) _____

(b) _____

(c) _____

3. Describe and state the function of each of the following cell parts.
   (a) Nucleus _____

   _____

   (b) Chromosomes _____

   _____

   (c) Rough-textured endoplasmic reticulum _____

   _____

   (d) Cell membrane _____

   _____

4. Define each of the following.
   (a) Anabolism _____
   (b) Catabolism _____
   (c) Metabolism _____

5. List the five types of tissue and state the function of each.
   (a) _____

   _____

   _____

   (b) _____

   _____

   _____

   (c) _____

   _____

   _____

   (d) _____

   _____

   _____

   (e) _____

   _____

   _____

6. Write the body system next to each definition.
   (a) Carries food, oxygen, and water to body cells and removes waste

   _____

   (b) Provides the first line of defense against infection

   _____

   (c) Supports and protects the body

   _____

   (d) Gives movement to the body

   _____

   (e) Secretes hormones directly into the bloodstream

   _____

   (f) Controls activities of the body

   _____

THE INTEGUMENTARY SYSTEM

The skin covers and protects underlying structures from injury or bacterial invasion. Skin also contains nerve endings from the nervous system, which aid the body in awareness of its environment.

The skin helps regulate the body temperature by controlling the loss of heat from the body. To increase heat loss, the blood vessels near the skin **dilate,** and the increased blood flow brings more heat to the skin. As the skin temperature rises more heat is lost from the hot skin to the cooler environment. Even more important in heat loss is the evaporation of perspiration (sweat). Perspiring carries heat away from the skin. When the body is conserving heat, sweating stops and blood vessels **contract.** This prevents the blood from carrying heat to the skin. The skin temperature falls, decreasing heat loss. In this way, the body temperature is kept almost constant.

Perspiration is produced by sweat glands, which are distributed over the entire skin surface, and released through ducts or pores. The body also rids itself of certain waste products through perspiration. Sebaceous glands in the skin secrete a thick oily substance through ducts. In this way, the skin is lubricated and kept soft and pliable. The oil also provides a protective film for the skin, which limits the absorption and evaporation of water from the surface. In elderly persons, these oil glands sometimes fail to function properly, and the skin becomes quite dry, scaly, and delicate.

The hair and the nails are called *skin derivatives* because they develop from the epidermis. Each hair has a root embedded in the skin, into which the oil glands open. Fingernails and toenails grow from a nail root in the skin. If the nail root is destroyed, the nail stops growing.

The skin covers the entire body. The outer layer of the skin (the layer you can see) is called the **epidermis.** Cells are constantly flaking off or being rubbed off this outer layer of skin. Beneath the epidermis is the **dermis.** In this layer of skin are the new cells that will replace the cells that are lost from the epidermis. **Pigment** is found in the epidermis and is responsible for the color of the skin. In sunlight, the production of pigment increases and a suntan results (Fig. 5.7).

Moisture on the skin can pick up dust and dirt from the air. Moisture can also mix with the skin particles being flaked off the epidermis. This process causes a condition that promotes the growth and spread of bacteria. This is the main reason for keeping the skin clean. The skin is where the battle for **asepsis** (being free of disease-causing organisms) begins.

The primary functions of the skin are:

■ To cover and protect underlying body structures from injury and bacterial invasion
■ To help regulate body temperature by controlling loss of heat from the body
■ To store energy in the form of fat and vitamins
■ To eliminate wastes by perspiration
■ To perceive heat, cold, pain, and pressure

MAGNIFIED CROSS SECTION OF THE SKIN

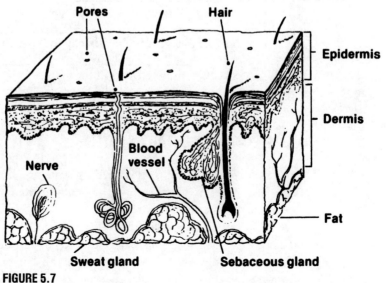

FIGURE 5.7

$\mathcal{T}$HE SKELETAL SYSTEM

The skeletal system is made up of 206 bones. The bones act as a framework for the body, giving it structure and support. They are also the passive organs of motion. They do not move by themselves; they must be moved by muscles, which shorten or contract. A muscle is stimulated to contract by a nerve impulse. This is an example of how systems interact. It is necessary to learn the names of the bones because they are like landmarks (Fig. 5.8).

There are four types of bones (Fig. 5.9):

- **Long bones,** such as the big bone in your thigh, the femur
- **Short bones,** like the bones in your fingers, the phalanges
- **Irregular bones,** such as the vertebrae that make up the spinal column
- **Flat bones,** like the bones of the rib cage

Bones are not inactive. They are dynamic and usually busy parts of the body. They store vital minerals that are necessary for many other body activities. The bones of the head are designed to protect the very delicate tissue of the brain. They are joined by sutures, similar to a zigzag embroidery pattern, and totally surround the brain and

SKELETON AND SURFACE MUSCLES

FIGURE 5.8

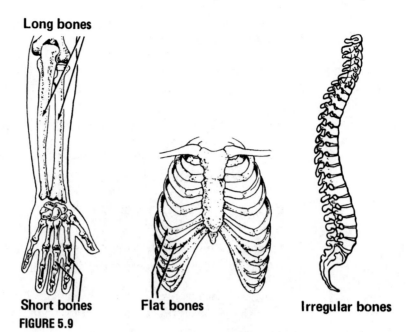

Long bones

Short bones   **Flat bones**   **Irregular bones**

FIGURE 5.9

cranial nerves. Some other bones that protect vital organs include the vertebrae of the spinal column, which protects the spinal nerve cord, and the rib cage, which guards the heart and lungs.

When the fetus is developing in the uterus, the entire skeleton is formed in cartilage by about 2½ months after conception. From this cartilage, bone is formed, much as if you replaced a wooden bridge, piece by piece, with steel. The bones of the head are formed from strong membranes. They do not completely undergo **ossification** (which means development of bone) until after the child is born. This is a great aid during childbirth, when the baby's bones can overlap a little.

Broken bones can mend solidly, but the process is slow and gradual. Bone cells grow and reproduce slowly. The hardening of the new bone is a gradual procedure of depositing calcium. Blood supply to bone tissue is poor, when compared with other areas of the body. Therefore, resistance to infection in the bone is relatively low.

Joints (Motion)

To keep a human body healthy, all the systems of the body must work together; no one system can stand alone. The skeletal system, muscular system, nervous system, and circulatory system all interact during each body movement. Movement of the body occurs at the joints. This is a perfect example of how several systems must work together.

Joints or articulations are areas in which one bone connects with one or more bones. They act as levers in all motion. Joints are made up of many structures. The tough white fibrous cord, the **ligament,** connects bone to bone. The **tendons** connect muscle to bone. Each of the joints—especially those in the shoulder, hip, and knee—is enclosed in a strong capsule. This capsule is lined with a membrane that secretes a fluid called **synovial fluid.** This fluid acts as a buffer, very much like a water bed, so the ends of the bones do not get worn out as they move. Other structures that protect the bone include the pad of cartilage at the end of the bone, a sac of synovial fluid (which is known as a **bursa**), and a disk of cartilage called the **meniscus.** Many such safeguards are built into the body. Injury to joints may cause a ligament or tendon to be strained, in what we call a sprain. Inflammation of the bursa causes **bursitis.**

SYNOVIAL (MOVABLE) JOINTS

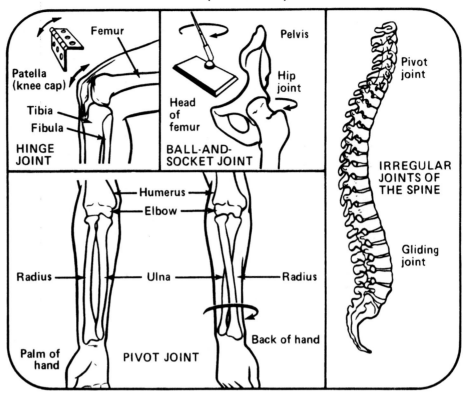

FIGURE 5.10

There are several kinds of joints in the human body. A hinge joint, such as in the knee, is freely movable. There are also less movable joints, such as those between the vertebrae. Some joints do not move at all, such as the joints between the bones of the skull (Fig. 5.10).

*T*HE MUSCULAR SYSTEM

The muscular system makes all motion possible, either that of the whole body or that which occurs inside the body (Fig. 5.10). Groups of muscles work together to perform a body motion. Other groups perform just the opposite motion. These two groups are called antagonistic groups. For example, flexing your arm, which means bending it at the elbow, causes your biceps to contract and the triceps to relax. Extending your arm, or straightening it, causes the biceps muscle to relax while the triceps contract. **Flexion** and **extension** are the two terms you should know that describe these motions, respectively. Two others are **abduction,** which means moving a part away from the body midline, and **adduction,** which means moving it toward the body (Figs. 5.11 and 5.12).

Muscle is the most infection-free of all the body's basic tissues. This is largely because of its exceptionally rich blood supply. Muscles not only move the body but also help keep it warm, especially during activity. If a muscle is kept inactive for too long, it tends to shrink and waste away. This is called **atrophy. Contracture** is a permanent muscle shortening. This is the reason that regular exercise is so important to good health. Range-of-motion exercises are often given to inactive patients to prevent these problems.

COORDINATION OF MUSCLES

FIGURE 5.11

FIGURE 5.12

*I*NTEGUMENTARY, SKELETAL, AND MUSCULAR SYSTEMS: REVIEW

1. List three functions of the skin.
   (a) _____
   (b) _____
   (c) _____

2. Complete the following.
    (a) The outer layer of the skin is the _____.
    (b) Beneath the epidermis is the _____.

3. Label the following diagram.

4. Complete the following.
    (a) There are _____ bones in the body.
    (b) Name the four types of bones.
        (1) _____
        (2) _____
        (3) _____
        (4) _____
    (c) List three functions of bones.
        (1) _____
        (2) _____
        (3) _____
    (d) The term for development of bone is _____.
    (e) Another term for a joint is _____.
    (f) A ligament connects _____.
    (g) A tendon connects _____.
    (h) The fluid secreted by the joint capsule is called _____ fluid.
    (i) The joint in the knee is called a _____ joint.
    (j) The joints between _____ do not move at all.
    (k) The function of the muscular system is _____.
    (l) Bending an extremity is called _____.
    (m) Straightening an extremity is called _____.
    (n) Moving a part away from the midline is called _____.
    (o) Moving a part toward the midline is called _____.
    (p) Shrinking and wasting of a muscle is _____.
    (q) A permanent shortening of a muscle is a _____.

5. Label the bones in the following diagram.

SKELETON AND SURFACE MUSCLES

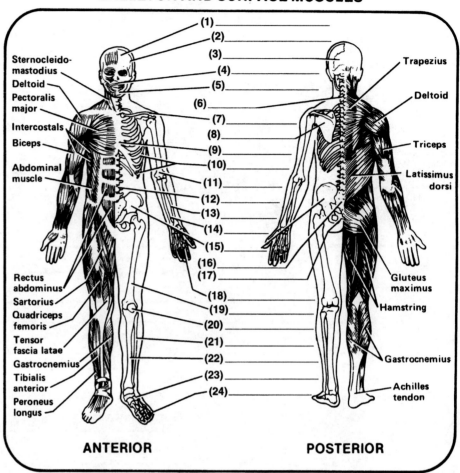

Sternocleido-mastodius
Deltoid
Pectoralis major
Intercostals
Biceps
Abdominal muscle

Rectus abdominus
Sartorius
Quadriceps femoris
Tensor fascia latae
Gastrocnemius
Tibialis anterior
Peroneus longus

(1) _____
(2) _____
(3) _____
(4) _____
(5) _____
(6) _____
(7) _____
(8) _____
(9) _____
(10) _____
(11) _____
(12) _____
(13) _____
(14) _____
(15) _____
(16) _____
(17) _____
(18) _____
(19) _____
(20) _____
(21) _____
(22) _____
(23) _____
(24) _____

Trapezius
Deltoid
Triceps
Latissimus dorsi
Gluteus maximus
Hamstring
Gastrocnemius
Achilles tendon

ANTERIOR   **POSTERIOR**

6. Label the muscles in the following diagram.

SKELETON AND SURFACE MUSCLES

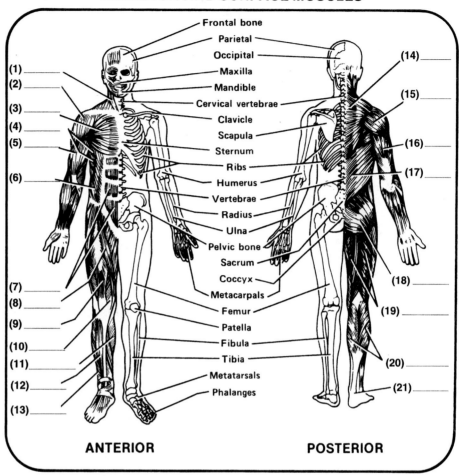

THE NERVOUS SYSTEM

The nervous system controls and organizes all body activity, both voluntary and involuntary. The nervous system is made up of the brain, the spinal cord, and the nerves. The nerves are spread throughout all areas of the body in an orderly way. Structurally the nervous system is divided into the **central nervous system (CNS),** which is made up of the brain and spinal cord and the **peripheral nervous system (PNS),** consisting of the cranial and spinal nerves. Functionally the PNS is divided into the **somatic nervous system (SNS),** made of nerve pathways that control motor response such as of the skeletal muscles and the **autonomic nervous system (ANS),** which maintains involuntary control of the body's systems. The ANS is further divided into the **sympathetic** and **parasympathetic nervous system.**

Nervous tissue is made up of cells called **neurons** and other supporting cells called **neuroglia.** A typical neuron is made up of a cell body, or soma, with one long column called the **axion** and many small outbranchings called **dendrites.** Nerve impulses move from the dendrites through the cell body along the axon. Our bodies contain structures called **receptor-end organs.** Any perceptible change in our external or internal environment sets up a nervous impulse in these receptor-end organs. This impulse is carried by sensory neurons to some part of the brain or spinal cord where it

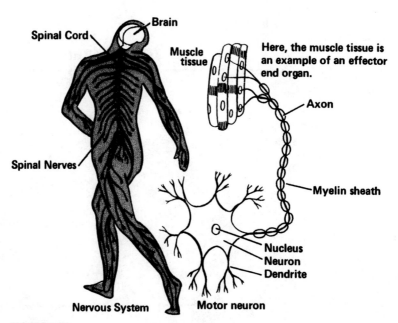

FIGURE 5.13

connects electrically with an interneuron at a site called a **synapse.** The 20 billion or so interneurons analyze the sensory inputs and coordinate the responses. Once that happens, the proper impulses are sent down motor neurons to the **effector-end organs,** those organs that are going to respond to the nerve impulse (Figs. 5.13 and 5.14).

Most nerve cells outside the brain and spinal cord have a protective covering known as the **myelin sheath.** The task of the myelin sheath is to insulate the nerve cell. The nerve cell can be compared with an electrical wire that requires insulation to keep the current in the correct pathway. This sheath helps prevent damage to the cells and often helps the nerve return to healthy function, or **regenerate,** if it has been injured. Nerve cells with a myelin sheath also carry an impulse faster than those without myelin. The neurons in the brain do not have this kind of protection. When they are injured, as they are by a stroke or **cerebral vascular accident (CVA),** it is necessary for another part of the brain to take over the function of the part that has been damaged. The rehabilitation department in your health care institution helps patients learn to do things again after such damage occurs.

The brain is well protected by bones, the **meninges** (membranes that cover the brain and spinal cord) and a cushion of fluid called **cerebral spinal fluid.** This fluid circulates outside and within the brain as well as around the spinal cord. The brain is a very complicated organ. It is made up of five portions. The **cerebrum** is divided into two halves, called hemispheres, that are connected by white matter known as **corpus callosum.** The right hemisphere controls most of the activity on the left side of the body, and the left hemisphere of the cerebrum controls the activity on the right side of the body. The cerebrum has many indentations known as **convolutions.** It is here that all learning, memory, and associations are stored so that thought is possible. Also, it is here that decisions are made for voluntary action. Certain areas of the cerebrum seem to perform special organizing activities. For example, the **occipital lobe** is the place where what we see is interpreted. The **frontal lobe** is the primary area of thought and reason. The **cerebellum** is the part of the brain that controls voluntary motion. It works with part of the inner ear, the semicircular canals, to enable us to walk and move smoothly through our world. The **midbrain, pons,** and **medulla** are primarily pathways through which nervous impulses reach the brain from the spinal cord (Fig. 5.15).

Motor message
from the brain

Sensory message
to the brain

FIGURE 5.14

Nerves throughout the body send messages into the tracts of white matter in the spinal cord, from which they rise to higher centers in the brain. There are 12 pairs of cranial nerves and 32 pairs of spinal nerves. These have many branches that go to all parts of the body.

One of the most important areas of the brain is an area called the **diencephalon.** It is here that small structures surround one of the ventricles of the brain. These structures help circulate cerebral spinal fluid and exercise an almost dictatorial control over the body's activities. They screen all nervous impulses going to the brain, either getting them there faster or slowing them down. One of these tiny structures is the **hypothalamus.** The hypothalamus and pituitary gland form a unit that *integrates* the nervous and endocrine systems. The hypothalamus functions to maintain a constant internal environment and patterns of behavior such as physical expression of emotion and sexual behavior. It seems to be the link between the mind and the body. It receives messages from the cerebrum, from the cerebellum, and from impulses coming up the spinal cord, and it has direct control over all the endocrine glands.

Much of the activity of the organs of the body is involuntary. In other words, we do not think about it, or, for the most part, we have no conscious control over this activity. The part of the nervous system that controls such things as digestion and the functions of other **visceral** (abdominal) organs is the autonomic nervous system. The

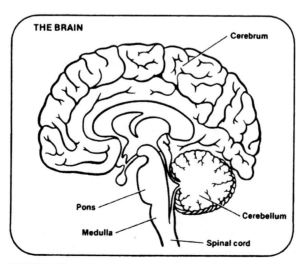

THE BRAIN

Cerebrum

Pons

Cerebellum

Medulla

Spinal cord

FIGURE 5.15

neurons that make up the autonomic nervous system use the same pathways as those neurons that control our voluntary actions; however, the two divisions of this part of the nervous system direct and control the activity of our internal organs. Each organ is supplied with neurons from each division of the autonomic nervous system.

One division is called the sympathetic division. The neurons that make up this division become active during stress, danger, excitement, or illness. These neurons cause the pupils of our eyes to become larger so we can see more clearly and can see better at a distance. These neurons also cause the heart to beat more strongly and to send more oxygen to the large muscles of the body in case it is necessary to fight or run. In today's fast-paced world, we are all subject to stress and sometimes we cannot run away from it or fight it. The action of the neurons from the sympathetic system then causes changes in the shape or activity of some of our organs. This action may also cause illness.

The parasympathetic division of the autonomic nervous system is in control when we are relaxed. It is known to conserve our energy. Fortunately, there is a checks-and-balances system between the two divisions. When one has been in action too long, the other automatically switches on. Most of us have had the experience of eating a large meal after being emotionally upset and feeling as if we had lead in our stomach. This is because the sympathetic division of the autonomic nervous system decreases **peristalsis** (which is movement of the gut), and digestion slows or stops.

The Sense Organs

The sense organs contain specialized endings of the sensory neurons. These are excited by sudden changes in the outside environment called **stimuli.**

- Eyes respond to visual stimuli (Fig. 5.16)
- Ears respond to sound stimuli (Fig. 5.17)
- Membranes of the nose respond to smells
- Taste buds, located chiefly on the tongue, respond to sweet and sour and other sensations
- Skin responds to touch, pressure, heat, cold, and pain

The Eye

The eye is the organ of sight. Light rays enter the eye through the **pupil,** the dark center of the eye, and pass through a series of structures that bend the light rays (**refraction**) so that they focus on the **retina,** the sensitive nerve layer of the eye that contains the **rods** and **cones,** the receptor cells of the retina. The light energy causes changes in the rods and cones so that nerve impulses are sent to the brain by way of the **optic nerve.** The parts of the eye that bend or refract the light are the **cornea,** a colorless, transparent structure that is a continuation of the **sclera** (the white of the eye); the **aqueous humor,** a fluid that is constantly produced and is contained in the eye in front of the lens; the **lens,** a circular, biconcave, transparent structure that changes shape and is thinned for distant vision and thickened for near vision by the **ciliary body;** and the **vitreous humor,** a jellylike substance that not only refracts the light but also maintains the shape of the eyeball.

The eye is made up of three layers. The outer layer is the sclera, and the middle layer is the **choroid,** the vascular layer between the sclera and the retina. The retina is the innermost layer of the eye. The front part of the choroid is made of the ciliary body, which contains the muscles that shape the lens; the **suspensory ligaments,** which hold

FIGURE 5.16

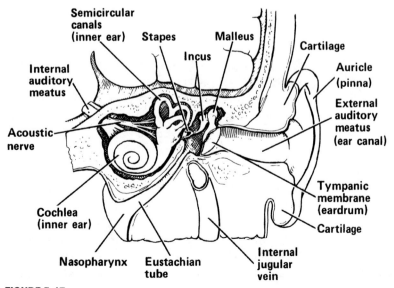

FIGURE 5.17

the lens in place; and the **iris,** the colored part of the eye that controls pupil size. The eye also contains two chambers, the **anterior chamber,** which lies between the cornea and the lens and iris and contains the aqueous humor, and the **posterior chamber,** which is behind the iris and contains the vitreous humor.

The **conjunctiva** is a membrane that lines the eyelid and covers the front of the sclera. Inflammation of the conjunctiva is called **conjunctivitis.** Pinkeye is a bacterial infection of the conjunctiva that is very contagious.

When the light rays that enter the eye are not properly bent, **errors of refraction** result because the light rays are not sufficiently focused on the retina. If a person is nearsighted (has **myopia**), the eyeball is too long, so the light rays are focused in front of the retina. If a person is farsighted (has **hyperopia**), the eyeball is too short from front to back, so the light rays are focused behind the retina. Persons with myopia have trouble seeing things that are far away. Persons with hyperopia have difficulty seeing things close up. Both conditions are improved by corrective lenses or surgery such as laser surgery.

Presbyopia is a condition in which there is a loss of elasticity of the lens of the eye that occurs after about the age of 40. Presbyopia also makes it difficult to see objects close up. **Cataracts** are a clouding of the lens of the eye that result in dimming of vision and are usually considered a consequence of aging. **Glaucoma** is a condition in which there is increased pressure inside the eyeball that, if untreated, can cause blindness because of damage to the retina and optic nerve. **Macular degeneration** is a progressive and usually untreatable deterioration of the **macula,** a small area on the retina.

The Ear

The ear governs both hearing and **equilibrium** (balance). It is divided into three parts, the outer ear, the middle ear, and the inner ear.

Sound waves enter the ear through the **external auditory meatus** (opening to the ear) and travel through the **auditory canal,** which is the tube that leads to the **tympanic membrane** or eardrum. The tympanic membrane vibrates as the sound waves hit it, causing the small bones of the middle ear or **ossicles** to vibrate and conduct the sound waves through the middle ear. The ossicles are the **malleus,** the **incus,** and the **stapes.** The stapes, as it vibrates, touches the **oval window,** a membrane that separates the middle from the inner ear.

The inner ear, called the **bony labyrinth,** has three parts. The **vestibule** lies next to the oval window, the **cochlea** is a bony, snail-like tube, and the **semicircular canals** are also bony tubes. The labyrinth contains fluids that conduct the vibrations to the **auditory nerves** (one of the pairs of cranial nerves), which transmit the information to the auditory center of the cerebrum in the brain, and hearing occurs. Another function of the inner ear is the maintenance of equilibrium. Through a relationship with the fluids and minute hairlike cells, the body relays messages to the brain so that balance is assured.

Hearing loss is a common disorder. There are three main types of deafness—**conduction deafness,** in which the sound waves fail to reach the inner ear because of some kind of obstruction; **nerve deafness** from damage to the inner ear or auditory nerve; and **mixed deafness,** which is a combination of the two.

Infection of the middle ear is called **otitis media** and is treated with antibiotics. **Tinnitus** is a ringing or buzzing sound in the ears often associated with **Ménière's disease,** a usually progressive disorder of the inner ear.

$\mathcal{T}$HE NERVOUS SYSTEM AND THE SENSE ORGANS: REVIEW

Complete the following.

1. Describe the function of the nervous system. _____

_____

2. List the components of the nervous system.
(a) _____
(b) _____
(c) _____

3. List the structural divisions of the nervous system.
(a) _____
(b) _____

4. List the parts of the central nervous system.
(a) _____
(b) _____

5. List the components of the peripheral nervous system.
(a) _____
(b) _____

6. List the functional divisions of the peripheral nervous system.
(a) _____
(b) _____

7. List the divisions of the autonomic nervous system.
(a) _____
(b) _____

8. A neuron is _____.

9. A synapse is _____

_____

_____.

10. To regenerate means _____.

11. The meninges are _____.

12. The cushion of fluid that protects the brain and spinal cord is called

_____.

13. Name two functions of the cerebrum.
(a) _____
(b) _____

14. The cerebellum controls_____.

15. There are _____ pairs of cranial nerves and _____ pairs of spinal nerves.

16. List two functions of the hypothalamus.
(a) _____
(b) _____

17. The part of the nervous system that controls the functions of visceral organs
is the _____ nervous system.

18. The division of the autonomic nervous system that becomes active during stress and prepares us for flight or fight is the _____ nervous system.

19. Label the following diagram of the brain.

20. List the parts of the eye that refract light.
    (a) _____
    (b) _____
    (c) _____
    (d) _____

21. The membrane that lines the eyelid and covers the front of the sclera is called the _____.

22. Write the correct term for each of the following.
    (a) Farsightedness: _____
    (b) Nearsightedness: _____
    (c) Loss of lens elasticity: _____
    (d) Clouding of the lens: _____
    (e) Increased pressure in the eye: _____

23. Label the following diagrams of the eye.

24. List two functions of the ear.
(a) _____
(b) _____

25. List the three divisions of the ear.
(a) _____
(b) _____
(c) _____

26. The eardrum is also called the _____.

27. List the three ossicles.
(a) _____
(b) _____
(c) _____

28. The inner ear is also called the _____.

29. The cranial nerve that conducts sound impulses to the brain is the

_____.

30. Ringing in the ears is called _____.

31. Infection of the middle ear is called _____.

32. Label the following diagram of the ear.

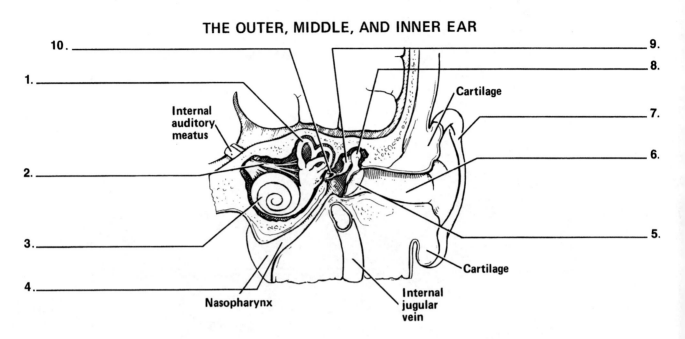

THE OUTER, MIDDLE, AND INNER EAR

*T*HE ENDOCRINE SYSTEM

The endocrine glands secrete substances called **hormones** (Fig. 5.18). These help the nervous system organize and direct the activities of the body. The hormones are secreted (flow) directly into the bloodstream. Exocrine glands, such as the salivary glands, deliver their products through ducts into a body cavity.

The hormones from the pituitary gland, both the anterior and posterior portions, regulate all metabolism of our billions of cells. The anterior portion manufactures and releases seven hormones.

The **pituitary gland** is the master gland. Its hormones directly affect the other endocrine glands, stimulating them to produce their hormones. Its hormones are especially important in reproduction and in all functions leading to puberty. This is the time at which a child takes on the physical characteristics of an adult man or woman. Hormones from the pituitary gland regulate the menstrual cycle in the female and sperm production in the male. Without these hormones, it would not be possible for us to reproduce. The pituitary gland and all these important hormones are under the direct control of the hypothalamus.

The **thyroid** gland produces hormones that regulate growth and general metabolism. The **thymus** gets smaller after puberty, but it plays an important part in the body's immune system. It is the system that prevents us from getting many diseases.

The **parathyroids** are located within the capsule of the thyroid. They produce a hormone that regulates, along with one of the hormones in the thyroid gland, the level of calcium and potassium in the blood. Calcium is important for many functions of our body, such as muscle contraction and conduction of nerve impulses.

The **pancreas** is both an endocrine gland and an exocrine gland, or a gland that has a duct. Its endocrine portion produces the hormone **insulin.** Insulin regulates the sugar content of the blood. If the body does not have enough insulin, the person becomes **diabetic.** He must be treated by reducing the carbohydrate or sugar intake and by regulating the balance between insulin and blood sugar.

ENDOCRINE GLANDS

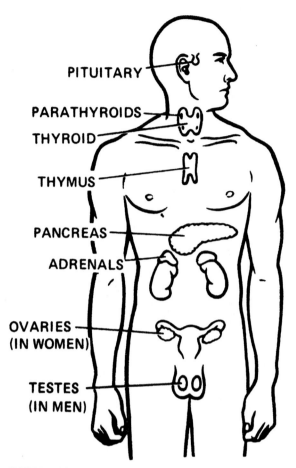

PITUITARY

PARATHYROIDS

THYROID

THYMUS

PANCREAS

ADRENALS

OVARIES
(IN WOMEN)

TESTES
(IN MEN)

FIGURE 5.18

The **adrenal glands** lie on top of the kidneys. They are very important in help-ing the body adapt to stress conditions, giving considerable aid to the autonomic ner-vous system.

The **ovaries** in the female are responsible for secreting the hormones estrogen and progesterone. The rise and fall of the levels of these hormones in the blood deter-mine the menstrual cycle. The hormones are also important in causing an ovum, or egg, to develop and in maintaining a pregnancy.

The **testes** in the male produce testosterone, the primary sex hormone of the male, which also causes the production of sperm.

*T*HE CIRCULATORY SYSTEM

The circulatory system is made up of the blood, the heart, and the blood vessels—**arteries, veins,** and **capillaries** and the **lymphatic system** (lymph vessels, lymph nodes, spleen, and thymus). The heart actually acts as a pump for the blood, which carries the nutrients, oxygen, and other elements needed by the cells. Important facts to know about blood include:

- The blood carries oxygen from the lungs to the cells.
- Carbon dioxide is carried by the blood from the cells to the lungs.

- Nutrients (food) are picked up (absorbed) by the blood from the duodenum (part of the small intestine) and brought to the cells.
- Waste products from the cells are carried by the blood to the kidneys to be eliminated in urine.
- The hormones from the endocrine glands are transported by the blood.
- Dilation (enlargement) and contraction (narrowing) of the blood vessels help regulate body temperature.
- The blood helps maintain the fluid balance of the body.
- The white blood cells defend the body against disease.

The heart is made up of four chambers—two **atria** and two **ventricles.** The atria are the two smaller chambers. The right ventricle sends the blood only as far as the lungs. Here, in the pulmonary circulation, the blood picks up oxygen and gets rid of carbon dioxide. This blood then returns to the heart, carrying its load of oxygen which is pushed into **systemic** circulation (to all parts of the body) by the left ventricle (Fig. 5.19).

The ventricles have thick muscle walls. When they contract, the left ventricle pushes the blood through the largest blood vessel, the **aorta,** to all parts of the body. The blood vessels that carry oxygen-rich blood are called **arteries.** The only exception is the **pulmonary artery,** which carries oxygen-poor blood to the lungs. Arteries

THE HEART

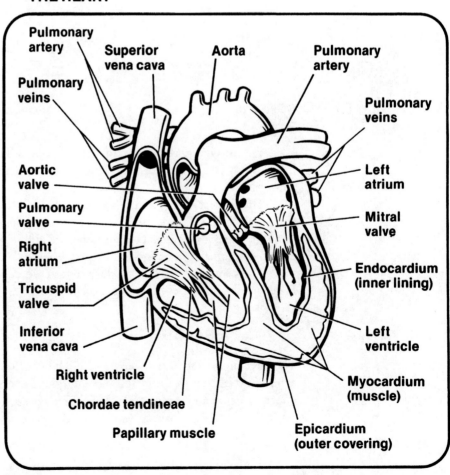

FIGURE 5.19

branch into a vast network throughout the body. As they branch, the blood vessels become smaller and smaller until finally they become thin vessels called **capillaries.** The walls of the capillaries are only one cell-layer thick. Through these walls, gases, nutrients, waste products, and other substances are exchanged among the blood in the capillaries, the tissue fluid, and the individual cell. After the blood has given up its oxygen, which is carried on the surface of the red blood cells, it is returned to the heart through the veins. In summary:

- All arteries carry blood away from the heart (Fig. 5.20).
- All veins carry blood back to the heart (Fig. 5.21).
- All arteries carry oxygenated blood except the pulmonary arteries.
- All veins carry deoxygenated blood except the pulmonary veins.

It is necessary that the heart muscle be supplied with blood carrying oxygen. The first branches of the aorta, which come from the heart's left ventricles, are the coronary arteries, which surround the heart. These carry needed oxygen to cardiac (heart) muscle tissue. If one of these branches of the coronary arteries becomes blocked by a blood clot, the patient has a heart attack (coronary thrombosis). This can result in the death of some heart tissue. The event is called a **myocardial infarction (MI).**

The liquid portion of the blood is called **plasma.** The cells are **red blood cells** (erythrocytes), which carry oxygen, and **white blood cells** (leukocytes), which fight

MAJOR ARTERIES

FIGURE 5.20

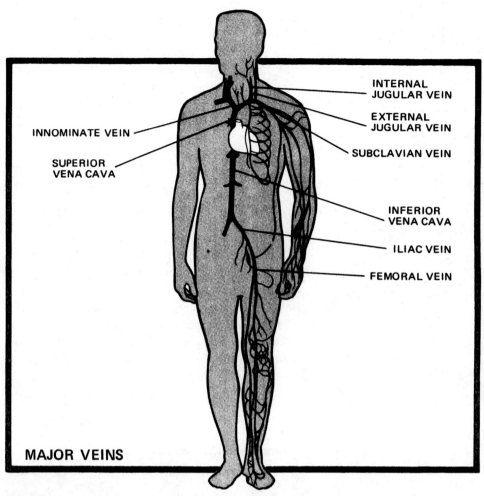

INTERNAL
JUGULAR VEIN

EXTERNAL
JUGULAR VEIN

SUBCLAVIAN VEIN

INNOMINATE VEIN

SUPERIOR
VENA CAVA

INFERIOR
VENA CAVA

ILIAC VEIN

FEMORAL VEIN

MAJOR VEINS

FIGURE 5.21

infection. If a patient has an inflammation in some area of the body, a physician often prescribes warm, moist compresses. These are applied to dilate (widen) the blood vessels in the area and to bring more of those important white blood cells to the place of infection to help fight it. People who have too few red blood cells have some type of anemia. People with too few white blood cells have a lowered resistance to disease. An increase in white blood cells in the blood may mean that an infection is present somewhere in the body.

The lymphatic system has several functions. It helps defend the body against disease-causing microorganisms by producing lymphocytes and monocytes (types of white blood cells) in the spleen and thymus gland and by producing antibodies. The lymphatic system also transports proteins and fluids that have leaked into the tissue fluid and the lipids (fats) from the small intestine back into the bloodstream.

The circulatory system is responsible for transporting all the necessary ingredients to a cell for its metabolism and for carrying away its products and waste material. The circulatory system works in close harmony with the respiratory system (Fig. 5.22).

*T*HE RESPIRATORY SYSTEM

The respiratory system provides a route or pathway for oxygen to get from the air into the lungs, where it can be picked up by the blood (Fig. 5.23). The organs that make up this system include the **nose** and **mouth, pharynx** (throat), **trachea** (windpipe),

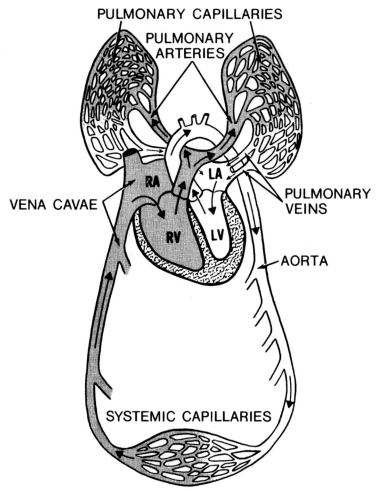

PULMONARY CAPILLARIES

PULMONARY ARTERIES

VENA CAVAE

PULMONARY VEINS

RA

LA

RV

LV

AORTA

SYSTEMIC CAPILLARIES

FIGURE 5.22

larynx (voicebox), **bronchi,** and **lungs.** Because we must have oxygen to live, it is necessary to keep this pathway open. The structures themselves help to do this. The trachea and bronchi are kept open by incomplete cartilage rings.

On top of the trachea, opening from the pharynx (the throat), is a structure known as the larynx. It is not only the opening to the trachea but also contains the vocal cords, which make it possible for us to talk. An important piece of cartilage, the **epiglottis,** covers the opening to the trachea when food is swallowed, preventing the food from going into the lungs.

As in the other body systems, the important work of the respiratory system is done at the level of the cell. The exchange of oxygen (O_2) and carbon dioxide (CO_2) occurs in an area of the lungs that is so small you must use a microscope to see it. The last branch of the bronchus is called the **alveolar duct.** At its end is a small sac, the **alveolus.** Many oxygen molecules fill this sac after you breathe in. The blood has less oxygen and therefore is able to pick up a great deal of oxygen from the alveolar sac. Carbon dioxide is exchanged so that it may be breathed out or exhaled. The blood containing fresh oxygen is then returned to the heart to be sent around the body starting in the largest artery, the aorta.

The respiratory system, then, is responsible for getting oxygen to the blood. **Internal respiration** occurs when cells exchange carbon dioxide, the gas waste product of cells, for oxygen. Internal respiration is "cell breathing." External respiration is "lung breathing" or the exchange of gases in the lungs. Both functions are equally important.

THE RESPIRATORY SYSTEM

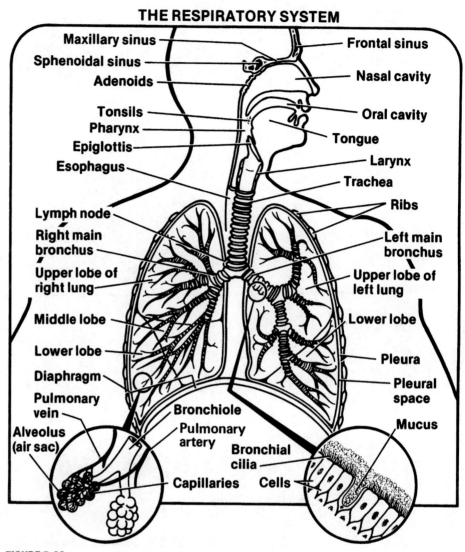

FIGURE 5.23

Breathing is regulated by a center in the **medulla,** a part of the brain. Often, especially after surgery, a patient must be encouraged to breathe deeply in order to keep all the air sacs open and inflated. In many of the larger health care institutions the Pulmonary Medicine Department (Respiratory Therapy) will, by a doctor's order, institute a treatment that will force the patient to breathe deeply and cough.

ENDOCRINE, CIRCULATORY, AND RESPIRATORY SYSTEMS: REVIEW

Complete the following.

1. Endocrine glands secrete _____ directly into the bloodstream.

2. Describe the function of the endocrine system. _____

_____

3. The _____ gland is called the master gland.

4. The _____ gland produces a hormone that regulates metabolism.

5. The _____ gland regulates the level of calcium and potassium in the blood.

6. The _____ is both an endocrine and exocrine gland.

7. The adrenal glands are located _____.

8. List the two hormones secreted by the ovaries.
   (a) _____
   (b) _____

9. The hormone secreted by the testes is _____.

10. Label the following diagram of the endocrine system.

ENDOCRINE GLANDS

11. List the components of the circulatory system.
   (a) _____
   (b) _____
   (c) _____
   (d) _____

12. List the three types of blood vessels.
   (a) _____
   (b) _____
   (c) _____

13. List five important facts to know about the blood.
   (a) _____
   (b) _____
   (c) _____
   (d) _____
   (e) _____

14. Describe the function of the heart. _____
   _____

15. Describe what happens in the pulmonary circulation. _____
   _____

16. The blood vessels that carry oxygen-rich blood are the _____.

17. There are four chambers in the heart—two _____ and
   two _____.

18. The largest blood vessel in the body is the _____.

19. The smallest blood vessels are called _____.

20. All veins carry deoxygenated blood except the _____ veins.

21. All arteries carry blood _____ from the heart, and all veins carry blood
   _____ the heart.

22. The liquid portion of the blood is called _____.

23. Erythrocytes carry _____.

24. Describe the function of leukocytes. _____.

25. People who have too few red blood cells have some type of _____.

26. List the organs included in the lymphatic system.
   (a) _____
   (b) _____
   (c) _____
   (d) _____

27. List two functions of the lymphatic system.
   (a) _____
   (b) _____

28. Label the following diagrams of the heart and the circulation.

THE HEART

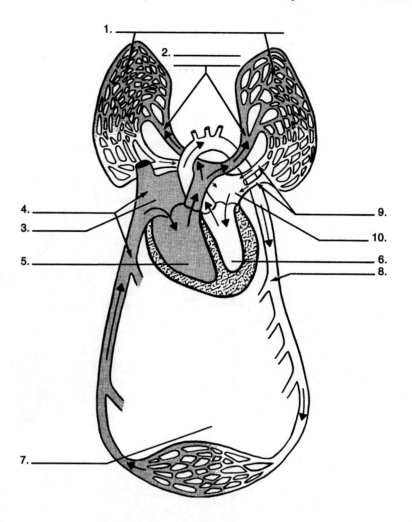

29. The respiratory system provides _____

_____.

30. The respiratory system brings air into the body through the nose and mouth. List the other organs that make up this system.

    (a) _____

    (b) _____

    (c) _____

    (d) _____

    (e) _____

31. What is internal respiration? _____

_____

32. What is external respiration? _____

_____

33. Which part of the brain regulates respiration?_____

34. Label the following diagram of the respiratory system.

THE RESPIRATORY SYSTEM

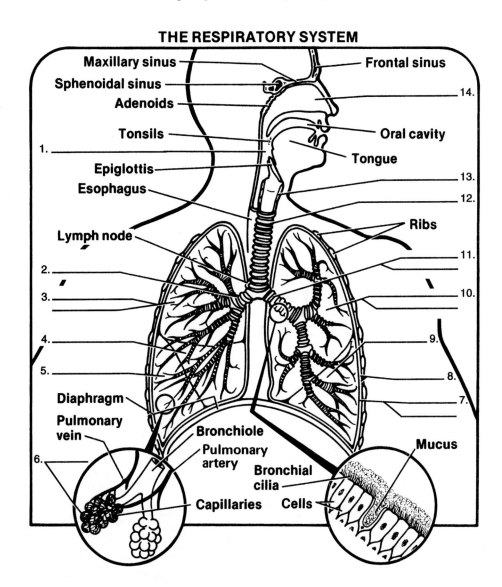

Maxillary sinus — Frontal sinus
Sphenoidal sinus — 14.
Adenoids —
Oral cavity
Tonsils —
1. _____
Tongue
Epiglottis —
13.
Esophagus —
12.
Ribs
Lymph node —
11.
2. _____
10.
3. _____
4. _____
9.
5. _____
8.
7.
Diaphragm —
Pulmonary
vein —
Bronchiole
Mucus
Pulmonary
artery
6. _____
Bronchial
cilia —
Capillaries   Cells —

𝒯HE DIGESTIVE SYSTEM

The three main functions of the digestive system are **digestion, absorption,** and **elimination.** The digestive system is responsible for breaking down the food that is eaten into a form that can be used by the body cells. This action is both chemical and mechanical. The **digestive** or gastrointestinal tract is about 30 feet long and extends from the mouth to the anus. All of it is important in reducing food to simple compounds (Fig. 5.24). The digestive system also includes the accessory organs—the salivary glands, the gallbladder, and pancreas.

Digestion begins in the mouth, where food is chewed and mixed with the substance called **saliva.** During swallowing, the food moves in a moistened ball down the esophagus to the stomach. The stomach churns and mixes the food at the same time it is being broken down chemically. The most important area of digestion is the **duodenum.** This is the first part of the **small intestine.** It is here that the digestive juices,

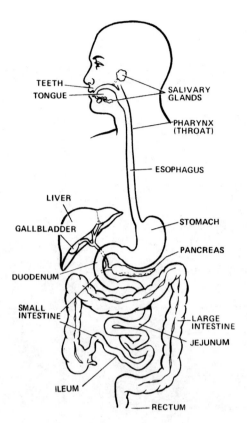

THE DIGESTIVE SYSTEM
FIGURE 5.24

not only from the duodenum itself but also from the pancreas, finish the job of breaking down food into usable parts. In addition, bile, which has been stored in the gallbladder after being manufactured in the liver, also enters the duodenum and helps the reduction process. The small intestine is about 21 feet long and 1 inch around. It has three parts, the duodenum, the jejunum, and the ileum.

Sufficient water is necessary for the chemical reduction of food into its end products. It is moved by the rhythmic contraction, called peristalsis, of the muscle walls of the organs of digestion.

Some of the final products of digestion are also absorbed in the area of the duodenum. These end products are:

- Amino acids, the building blocks for all growth and repair of body tissue, which come from dietary proteins
- Fatty acids and glycerols, from fat
- Simple sugars, such as glucose, from carbohydrates
- Water and vitamins

The lining of the duodenum is composed of thousands of tiny fingerlike projections called **villi.** Each villus is capable of absorbing these end products of digestion. The products are then moved into the bloodstream, where they are carried to individual cells (Fig. 5.25).

Some digestion continues to take place in other parts of the small intestine. What is left of the food moves through the **large intestine,** or **colon,** which is about 5 feet long and 2½ inches around. It is responsible for reabsorbing large amounts of water

INTERNAL VIEW OF STRUCTURE OF SMALL INTESTINE

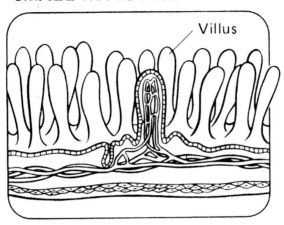

Villus

FIGURE 5.25

and for the elimination. The large intestine has three main parts, the ascending, transverse, and descending colon. The material that cannot be used by the body is excreted from the rectum through the anus as feces.

The lowest portion of the large intestine curves in an S-shape (the sigmoid portion) into the **rectum.** The rectum is made of very delicate tissue. It has an internal sphincter muscle and an external sphincter muscle. Sometimes blood vessels that supply this area become enlarged and filled with blood clots, causing hemorrhoids. The anus is the opening to the outside of the body (Fig. 5.26).

At the junction between the small intestine and the large intestine on the right side is a pouch with a projection of tissue called the **appendix.** Because there is very little peristalsis in this area, the appendix has a tendency to become infected, in a condition known as *appendicitis.* Surgery is usually performed to correct this condition.

THE LARGE INTESTINE

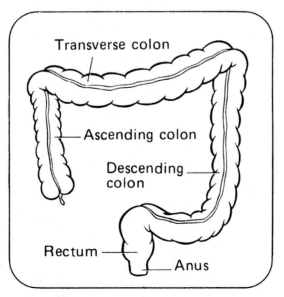

Transverse colon

Ascending colon

Descending colon

Rectum

Anus

FIGURE 5.26

The liver has important responsibilities aside from manufacturing bile. The liver is a storage area for glucose. This form of sugar is released in large amounts when the cells need it for energy to carry on their activities. The liver also is the place where toxins, or poisons, are removed from the blood. Damage to the liver can be caused by viruses, bacteria, drinking alcohol, or taking drugs that are harmful to its tissues. The liver is also responsible for production and storage of some proteins necessary for proper circulation of the blood and for blood clotting. Blood clots are not all bad. When a blood vessel has been injured, a clot may form that holds the blood within a closed tube (the blood vessel) until healing occurs.

THE URINARY SYSTEM

A body system vital in maintaining **homeostasis** (state of equilibrium or balance) is the urinary system, which gets rid of waste products. The organs that make up this system include (Fig. 5.27)

- The **kidneys**
- The **ureters** (tubes leading from the kidneys)
- The **urinary bladder**
- The **urethra** (which leads from the bladder to the outside of the body)

The functional unit of the kidneys is called a **nephron.** It is here that an exchange of substances takes place between the blood capillaries and a part of the nephron. A network of capillaries, called the **glomerulus,** lies within a cupping of a tube, known as **Bowman's capsule.** Materials from the blood that are not needed by the body are filtered into Bowman's capsule. They are then carried through a series of **tubules,** which help make up the nephron. As the filtered material flows through these tubules the blood vessels surrounding them reabsorb those materials still needed by the body,

THE URINARY SYSTEM

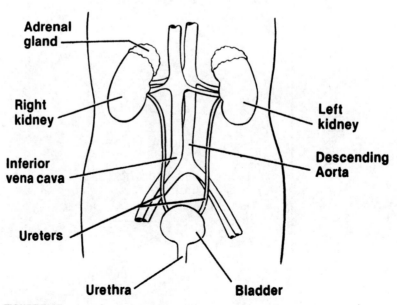

FIGURE 5.27

particularly water. Near the end of the winding tubules, substances from the blood, such as toxins and some drugs, pass into the urine. The filtrate that is left is collected in a larger tube. This tube joins those of all the other nephrons in a basinlike portion of the kidney. From here it drips steadily through the ureter, helped by a peristaltic motion very similar to that of the gastrointestinal tract, to the urinary bladder. There are stretch receptor-end organs in the muscular wall of the bladder. The bladder is capable of expanding greatly. When these receptors are stimulated by a full bladder, messages are sent to the brain that cause the person to urinate.

Because the urethra is open to the outside of the body, it may also provide a passageway for disease-causing organisms. These organisms may travel up to the bladder, infecting it and causing a disease known as *cystitis*. The infection may also spread through the ureters to the kidney, causing kidney damage.

The urinary system is perhaps the most important system for maintaining homeostasis, because this system determines the content of the blood. The blood content, in turn, determines the content of the tissue fluid, which is the immediate environment of the cells. Many changes in kidney function, some normal, can be found in urine samples. Such changes are also revealed in accurate measurement of **intake and output.** Sometimes in illness, especially after surgery, the patient is unable to void (urinate). An early sign of shock is a reduction in urine output because when the blood pressure drops, there is not enough blood passing through the kidneys to produce urine.

*T*HE REPRODUCTIVE SYSTEM

In the female the primary reproductive organs are the two **ovaries.** The main task of the ovary is the production of **ova** (eggs). These are specialized cells that are able to unite with a sperm cell released from the male during intercourse and then grow over a period of 40 weeks into a new human being. Developing ova lie in a lake of **estrogen,** a hormone that enters the blood stream during ovulation. **Ovulation** is the process whereby an ovum is released from one ovary into the opening of the oviduct (fallopian tube) and moves to the **uterus** (womb). This occurs once each month, usually 14 days before the onset of the next menstrual period. During this time, a woman is *fertile* (able to become pregnant). During ovulation, release of estrogen causes a buildup of the lining of the uterus (**endometrium**), preparing it for a possible pregnancy (Fig. 5.28).

Menstruation is the periodic (monthly) loss of some blood and a small part of the lining of the uterus, an organ that is full of blood vessels. The discharge flows out of the vagina for a period of 4 to 7 days (Fig. 5.29.) The process of ovulation is controlled by hormones from the pituitary gland, under the control of the hypothalamus. The hormones from the pituitary gland are involved in the development of the ovum and in maintaining pregnancy. **Menopause** is the normal cessation of menstruation.

In the human female there are three openings in the perineal area: (1) The external urinary **meatus,** the distal end of the urethra; (2) the **vagina,** which is not only the organ for intercourse but also the birth canal; and (3) the **anus,** the last portion of the gastrointestinal tract. (Fig. 5.30)

In the male the primary reproductive organs are the testes, which produce sperm. **Testicles,** or **testes,** are paired glands that lie in a sac called the **scrotum** outside the body, posterior to the **penis,** which is the primary male sex organ. During intercourse, sperm travel up the **vas deferens,** or sperm duct, to a point where they enter the urethra. Sperm are accompanied by secretions from other glands in the male reproductive system. These glands—the **seminal vesicles,** the **prostate gland,** and **bulbourethral glands** (Cowper's glands)—contribute water, nutrients, and vitamins, which, added to the sperm, make up the **semen,** a fluid that is ejaculated (expelled) at the same time

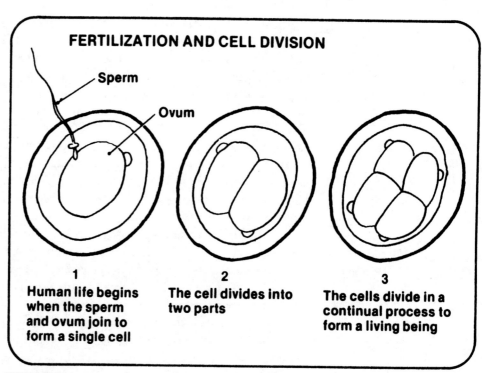

FIGURE 5.28

the male has an orgasm. There is only one duct in the penis. It is used for the flow of urine and for the ejaculation of sperm in its carrying medium, the semen. During intercourse, the internal sphincter of the male's urinary bladder closes tightly, so there is no chance for the urine to become mixed with the semen. The penis has three columns of spongy or cavernous tissue. During sexual excitement, blood rushes in through the penile artery, and the veins constrict, trapping the blood so it fills these spaces, causing the penis to become erect and **turgid.** All this activity occurs under the influence of **testosterone,** the primary male sex hormone, which is also manufactured in the testes. It is secreted into the blood through the influence of the hormones from the anterior pituitary, which is under the control of the hypothalamus.

FIGURE 5.29

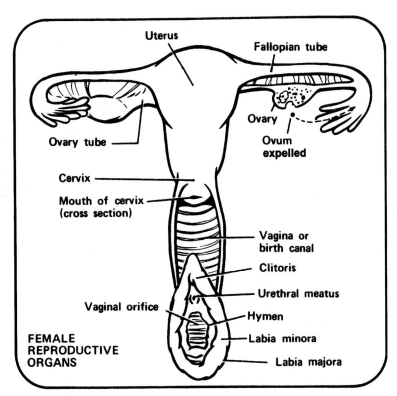

FIGURE 5.30

Sometimes during the aging process the **prostate gland,** which encircles the urethra like a doughnut, becomes enlarged. When the prostate expands, it squeezes the urethra, causing painful urination. Many men fear surgery on their prostate gland because they believe it will end their sex life. The amount of semen ejaculated will be less, but otherwise, men who have had a prostatectomy are often capable of having normal sexual relations. Vasectomy is the ligation or tying of the vas deferens to produce sterility (Fig. 5.31). The area between the thighs of both men and women that includes the external genitalia to the anus is the perineum.

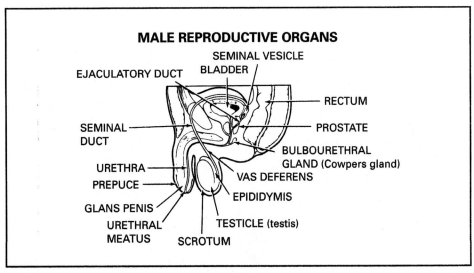

FIGURE 5.31

DIGESTIVE, URINARY, AND REPRODUCTIVE: REVIEW

Complete the following.

1. List the three main functions of the digestive system.
   (a) _____
   (b) _____
   (c) _____

2. The action of digestion is both _____ and _____.

3. Describe the difference between the digestive system and the digestive tract.
   _____
   _____
   _____
   _____

4. Another name for the digestive tract is the _____ tract.

5. Name the three parts of the small intestine.
   (a) _____
   (b) _____
   (c) _____

6. List the end products of digestion.
   (a) _____
   (b) _____
   (c) _____
   (d) _____

7. Describe villi and their function.
   _____

8. List the three main parts of the large intestine.
   (a) _____
   (b) _____
   (c) _____

9. Another name for the large intestine is the _____.

10. List two functions of the large intestine.
    (a) _____
    (b) _____

11. Label the following diagrams of the digestive system and the large intestine.

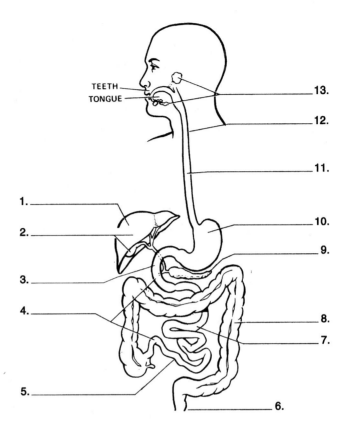

TEETH
TONGUE

1.
2.
3.
4.
5.

13.
12.
11.
10.
9.
8.
7.
6.

THE DIGESTIVE SYSTEM

THE LARGE INTESTINE

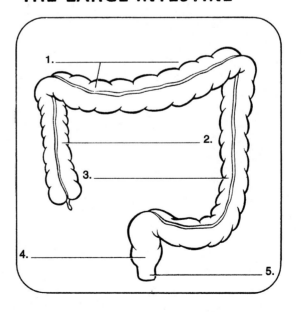

1.
2.
3.
4.
5.

12. List the organs that make up the urinary system.

(a) _____

(b) _____

(c) _____

(d) _____

13. The functional unit of the kidney is called a _____.

14. The glomerulus is a network of _____.

15. Tubules are _____.

16. Describe the function of the urinary system.

_____

_____

17. When the body is in homeostasis its internal environment is in _____.

18. The _____ leads from the bladder to the outside of the body.

19. Label the following diagram of the urinary system.

THE URINARY SYSTEM

20. The main task of the ovary is the production of _____.

21. Ova are _____.

22. The process in which an ovum is released from an ovary is called

_____

23. The process described in question 22 usually occurs _____

_____

24. The lining of the uterus is called the _____.

25. In the female, pituitary gland hormones are involved in:

(a) _____

(b) _____

26. The normal cessation of menstruation is called _____.

27. The male testicles lie in a sac called the _____.

28. The fluid that is ejaculated during the male orgasm is _____.

29. The primary male sex hormone is _____, which is manufactured in the _____.

30. The gland that encircles the male urethra is the _____ gland.

31. Removal of the prostate is called a _____.

32. Ligation of the vas deferens to produce sterility is called a _____.

33. Label the following diagrams of the female and male reproductive systems.

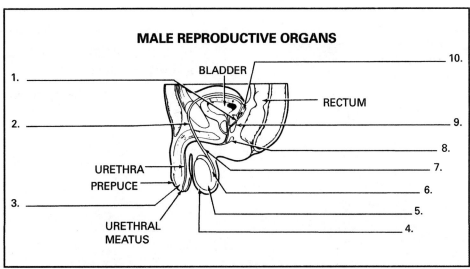

Summary

The cell is the basic unit of all living matter. The human body is made up of millions of cells. Cells reproduce by a process called cell division, which eventually produces groups of similar cells. When the cells that are similar in form and function become specialized, they are called tissues. When two or more tissues work together to perform a certain function, they form an organ, such as the heart. A system, such as the circulatory system, consists of a group of organs acting together to perform complex body functions. All cells, tissues, organs, and systems work in concert to keep a human being healthy.

Good reasons for studying human anatomy are to increase your knowledge of the science of medicine, to better communicate with the staff, and to become more efficient in the transcription of doctors' orders.

The best reason of all is that an appreciation of the design of the healthy human body and how it works will help you deliver good quality health care.

LEARNING ACTIVITIES

Choose the correct word from the following list to complete each statement.

| tissues | function | nucleus | cell membrane | structure |
| cytoplasm | systems | division | microscopic | organs |

1. Anatomy is the study of the _____ of the body.

2. Physiology is the study of the _____ of the body.

3. Cells are _____ in size.

4. Cells consist of three main parts: (1) _____, where the activities of the cell take place; (2) _____, which directs cellular activities; and (3)_____, which keeps the living substances of a cell, called the protoplasm, within bounds and allows materials to pass into and out of the cell.

5. Cells reproduce by _____.

6. Groups of cells of the same type that do a particular kind of work are called
_____.

7. Tissues are grouped together to form _____, such as the heart, lungs, and liver.

8. Organs that work together to perform similar tasks make up _____
_____.

Match the body location in Column A with its description in Column B.

Column A   **Column B**

(a) anterior   _____ Toward the back

(b) deep   _____ On or near the surface

(c) ventral   _____ Toward the front

(d) inferior   _____ Upper portion

(e) posterior   _____ On the back side

(f) superficial   _____ Lower portion

(g) superior   _____ On the belly side

(h) dorsal   _____ Distant from the surface

Complete the following.

1. The region of the body between the chest and the pelvis is called the

   _____.

2. The posterior opening in the body through which feces are excreted is the

   _____.

3. A membranous sac that serves as a container within the body to hold urine
   is known as the _____.

4. The fluid circulating through the heart, arteries, veins, and capillaries that
   carries nourishment and oxygen to the tissues and takes away waste matter
   and carbon dioxide is called _____.

5. The _____ extends from the small intestine to
   the anus.

6. A _____ is a part of the body where two bones
   come together.

7. The total of all the physical and chemical changes that take place in living
   organisms and cells is called _____.

8. The body area between the thighs which includes the area of the anus and
   the external genital organs is called the _____.

9. _____ is the movement of the intestines that
   pushes food along to the next part of the digestive system.

10. _____ refers to the lungs.

11. A substance that moistens food and helps in swallowing that also contains
    an enzyme (chemical) that helps digest starches is called _____.

12. The _____ is a pouch below the penis that con-
    tains the testicles.

13. The _____ is the part of the digestive tract be-
    tween the esophagus and the duodenum.

14. The tube leading from the urinary bladder to the outside of the body is
    called the _____.

15. Found in the female, the _____ is the birth
    canal leading from the vulva to the cervix of the uterus.

Match the body system in Column A with its description in Column B.

Column A	Column B
(a) Skeletal system	_____ Gives movement to the body
(b) Muscular system	_____ Takes in, absorbs food, converts it to energy
(c) Digestive system	
(d) Nervous system	_____ Supports and protects the body
(e) Urinary system	_____ Removes wastes
(f) Integumentary system	_____ Secretes hormones into the blood
(g) Endocrine system	_____ Controls the activities of the body
(h) Circulatory system	_____ Provides the first line of defense against infection
(i) Respiratory system	
(j) Reproductive system	_____ Carries food, oxygen, and water to body cells
	_____ Takes air into the body to supply oxygen to the cells
	_____ Allows a new human being to be born

CHAPTER 6

Diseases and Diagnoses

Aerobic bacteria	Microorganisms that require oxygen to live and grow
Anaerobic bacteria	Microorganisms that live and grow best without oxygen
Centers for Disease Control and Prevention (CDC)	A federal agency whose purpose is to promote health and quality of life by preventing and controlling disease, injury, and disability
Communicable disease	A disease that can be transmitted either directly or indirectly from one person to another
Contaminated	Made unclean
Epidemiology Department	Department responsible for infection control
Immunocompromised	Having the immune system impaired or weakened
Immunosuppression	The prevention of the body's natural immune response and ability to fight off infection as by drugs
Incontinent	Unable to control bowel or bladder
Isolation technique	Procedure to keep pathogens that cause the patient's illness inside the isolated patient's unit
Nosocomial infection	Hospital-acquired infection
Nurse epidemiologist	Nurse responsible for monitoring patient infections and for infection control
Occupational Safety and Health Administration (OSHA)	A federal agency responsible for assisting employers provide a safe working environment for their employees
Personal protective equipment (PPE)	Clothing and equipment such as gloves, masks, face shields, gowns, and protective eyewear that protects the health care worker from blood and other possibly infectious materials
Predispose	To make more likely to develop a disease or condition
Preexisting condition	A disease or disorder that is already present

When you have completed this chapter, you will be able to:

- Define the terms listed in the vocabulary.
- Define the terms related to disease.
- List the major disease categories.
- List the seven danger signs of cancer.
- Discuss AIDS and hepatitis and ways to prevent occupational exposure.
- Define medical asepsis and discuss its purposes.
- Compare regular and reverse isolation and discuss the health unit coordinator responsibilities in relation to isolation.

- Define Standard Precautions, and list the three types of transmission precautions as defined by the Centers for Disease Control and Prevention.
- Define communicable diseases and discuss methods to prevent spread.

A doctor makes a diagnosis through careful evaluation of the patient's history, physical examination, laboratory and other tests, x-rays, and the disease process. Doctors may compare symptoms of similar diseases to determine which disease the patient may have. This process is called a **differential diagnosis** (DD). They may establish a diagnosis by eliminating other possibilities. This process is called diagnosis by **exclusion.** The value of establishing a diagnosis is to provide a logical basis for treatment and prognosis.

The many diagnostic examinations ordered by the physician help him or her to make the correct diagnosis and to evaluate the course of the disease and the effects of the treatment prescribed. This is not a simple process, and the health unit coordinator can do a great deal to help the physician and the patient by performing the necessary duties to the best of his or her abilities.

$\mathcal{T}$ERMS RELATED TO DISEASE

The following list describes terms related to disease.

- **Disease**—a deviation from normal body structure or function that is harmful to the organism (person)
- **Acute disease**—a disorder of sudden onset and of short duration
- **Chronic disease**—a disorder usually having a slow onset and lasting for an extended period of time
- **Subacute disease**—a disorder not as severe as acute and of shorter duration than chronic
- **Functional disease**—a disorder of body function or performance without any observable change in the body tissues or structure
- **Organic disease**—a disorder resulting in structural change in body tissues or organs

$\mathcal{M}$AJOR DISEASE CATEGORIES

There are many ways to group diseases. The following list will help the health unit coordinator understand the general categories:

- **Allergic diseases.** An allergy is an abnormal reaction to a substance that is harmless to most people and may be caused by many substances including dust, pollens, and proteins.
- **Congenital diseases** are disorders present at birth. These may include a wide variety such as harelip, clubfoot, or congenital heart defects. A hereditary disease is passed on in the genes. Many congenital diseases are not hereditary but are acquired **in utero** (while the baby is forming in the uterus). A mother who contracts German measles or syphilis may produce a baby with congenital disease. Hemophilia is an example of a hereditary disease passed through the genes, usually by mother to son, resulting in an excessive tendency to bleed.
- **Nutritional diseases**—lack of essential nutrients or inability of body to absorb and utilize them.
- **Degenerative diseases** are disorders that result from "wear and tear" on body tissues. Diseases of the heart and blood vessels rank high on the list of degen-

erative diseases. Lifetime habits slow down or hasten the degenerative process, and all body tissues do not age at the same rate.

- **Infections or inflammatory diseases.** *Infection* is a reaction of the body to "germs" (pathogenic microorganisms) that multiply and cause symptoms. *Inflammation* is the reaction of the body to injury in the form of pain, swelling, heat, and the like. Inflammation and infection are not the same. There may be inflammation without the presence of infection.
- **Metabolic diseases** are diseases that disturb cellular activity. Diseases of the endocrine system fall in this category.
- **Trauma** means injury and includes accidents such as falls, burns, blows, cuts, stabbings, gunshot wounds, injuries caused by heat, electricity, radiation, poisoning, and snake and other bites.
- **Neoplastic disease.** A *neoplasm* is a new growth or tumor. **Benign neoplasms** generally do not invade surrounding tissue, are not malignant (cancerous), and do not metastasize (spread). **Malignant neoplasms** are cancerous tumors. They may likely invade surrounding tissue and frequently metastasize.

Cancers are classified through a process of **grading** and **staging.** Grading expresses the cancer's degree of differentiation. Benign (noncancerous) tumors are made up of well-organized and specialized (differentiated) cells that look very much like normal, mature tissue.

Staging is based on the size and spread (metastases) of the tumor. There are two main staging systems. The TNM system reports the size of the primary tumor, **T;** regional extension or nodes, **N;** and existence of metastases, **M.** Generally, the higher the number assigned to each letter, the more serious the prognosis (forecast of outcome)—e.g., T4, N4, M4. Another method of staging uses O to IV based on the size of the tumor and the extent of its spread. Cancer is a prevalent disease in our society and there is much to learn about the subject. As a preventive health measure, the health unit coordinator should acquaint his or herself with the following seven danger signs of cancer according to the American Cancer Society.

Know Cancer's Seven Warning Signals

- Change in bowel or bladder habits
- A sore that does not heal
- Unusual bleeding or discharge
- Thickening or lump in breast or elsewhere
- Indigestion or difficulty in swallowing
- Obvious change in wart or mole
- Nagging cough or hoarseness

A person noticing any of these symptoms should see a doctor at once.

PREDISPOSING CAUSES

Some conditions increase the likelihood of developing a disease. They include the following:

- Age—Certain age groups are more apt to contract certain diseases—for example, chickenpox in children and heart attacks in the elderly.
- Sex—Men are more likely to contract certain diseases than women, and vice versa.

- Occupation—Certain occupations **predispose** an individual to disease. Excessive exposure to asbestos has been linked to cancer, and coal mining to lung disease.
- Genetics—Some people inherit a tendency toward certain diseases such as diabetes, heart disease, and sickle-cell anemia.
- Environment—Poor, overcrowded, unhygienic living conditions can predispose to disease.
- Personal habits—The use of drugs and alcohol, smoking, poor diet, sexual habits, stress, and overwork can lead to illness.
- **Preexisting condition**—The presence of any disease can make it easier to contract others.
- Emotions—Certain diseases are linked with emotions and anxiety. Peptic ulcers and some hypertension are examples.
- **Immunosuppression** (e.g., due to AIDS, chemotherapy, or treatment with immunosuppresant drugs to improve the chances of successful organ transplants)
- Chronic illness (e.g., allergies, kidney failure, diabetes)
- Drug therapy (e.g., long-term use of antibiotics, birth control pills, corticosteroids)
- Pregnancy

$\mathcal{A}$SEPSIS

People who work in health care institutions must learn the importance of cleanliness. Everyone tries constantly in many ways to achieve ideal sanitary conditions. You, too, must take part in this team effort to keep everything absolutely clean. Cleanliness is a part of every health care institution's effort to control disease and keep **communicable diseases** from spreading (Fig. 6.1).

FIGURE 6.1

You will understand the importance of cleanliness in the health care institution if you know something about pathogens—the microorganisms that cause diseases. It may help to know what they are, how they spread, and how they can be destroyed (Fig. 6.2).

$\mathcal{T}$HE CAUSE OF DISEASE

People once believed that sickness was caused by evil spirits. About 500 years ago scientists began to suspect that some diseases were caused by very small living things they called *germs* (**pathogens**).

Microorganisms That Can Infect The Body and Common Portals Of Entry

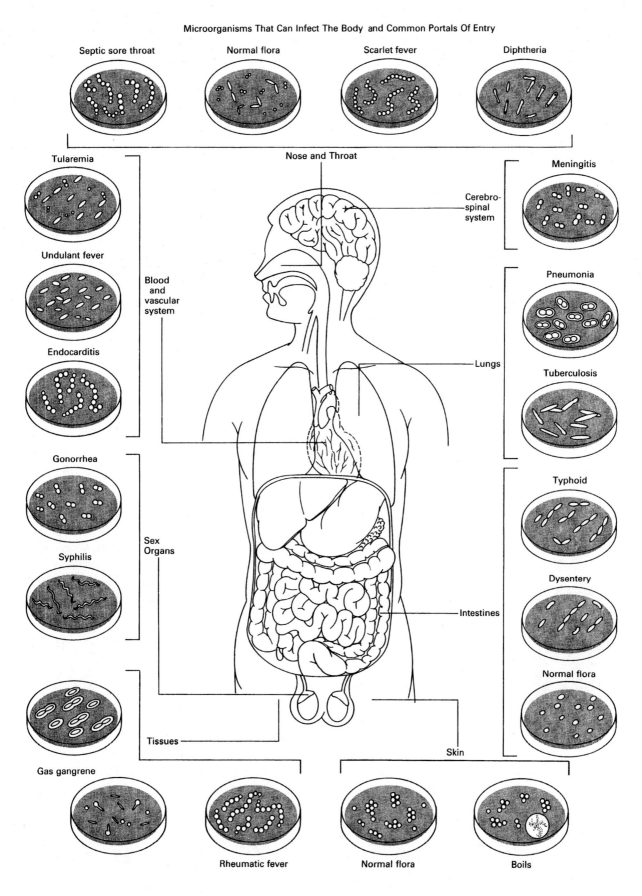

FIGURE 6.2

A pathogen is a disease-causing microorganism. However, very few microorganisms are pathogens. Only about 3% of all microorganisms are known to cause disease. *Micro* means very small. Microorganisms can be seen only under a microscope. *Organism* means a living thing. Different kinds of microorganisms (also called microbes) are:

Classifications of Disease-Causing Microorganisms

- Viruses
- Bacteria
- Rickettsiae
- Fungi
- Protozoa

The Nature of Microorganisms

Some microorganisms are helpful to people. For example, certain microbes cause a chemical change in food called **fermentation.** Fermentation is the change that produces cottage cheese from milk, beer from grains, cider from apples, and sauerkraut from cabbage. Other microorganisms in the human digestive system break down the foods not used by the body and turn them into waste products (feces).

There are other kinds of microorganisms, however, that are harmful to man. These are the microbes that cause disease and infection. Disease-producing microorganisms called pathogens grow best at body temperature, 98.6°F (37°C). Pathogens destroy human tissue by using it as food. They also give off waste products called **toxins.** These are absorbed into and poison the body.

Each organism has its own normal environment or home called its natural habitat. When organisms gain access to areas of the body in which they do not belong, that is, they move out of their normal habitat and into a foreign area, they become pathogens. For example, *E. coli* belongs in the colon, where it helps to digest food. When it gets into the bladder or into the bloodstream, it can cause a urinary infection or a blood infection called **septicemia** (Fig. 6.3).

Bacteria are single-celled organisms with the ability to reproduce by cell division about every 20 minutes. They are classified into two major groups based on their reaction to a staining process called Gram's stain—Gram negative or Gram positive. Bacteria are also classified according to their shape. A round bacterium is called a **coccus.** When these bacteria appear in clusters they are called **staphylocci,** when in chains, **streptococci,** and when in pairs, **diplococci.** Rod-shaped bacteria are called **bacilli.** Spiral-shaped bacteria that are rigid are called **spirilla,** flexible ones are called **spirochetes,** and curved, **vibrios.**

In the hospital you will often hear the words staph or staphylococcus and strep or streptococcus. **Staphylococcus** and **streptococcus** are two types of bacteria that are found in all health care institutions. They are commonly found on the human skin and mucous membranes of the gastrointestinal tract (**normal flora**). They enter the body through a portal of entry. When staphylococci get inside the skin, they may produce a local infection. There may be soreness, tenderness, redness, and/or pus. Sometimes staphylococcus infections can affect the whole body. When streptococci enter the body, they may cause a septic sore throat, a local infection, or rheumatic fever, a general infection.

There are many conditions that contribute to the growth of bacteria.

- Food—bacteria grow well in the remains of food left in a patient's room
- Moisture—bacteria grow in moist places

Bacteria may enter the body through skin breaks, or the nose and mouth, which are all portals of entry

FIGURE 6.3

- Temperature—High temperatures (170°F) kill most bacteria. At 50 to 110°F most disease-causing bacteria grow rapidly. The normal human body temperature of 98.6° enables bacteria to thrive easily. Low temperatures do not kill bacteria but retard their activity and growth rate.
- Oxygen—**aerobic bacteria** require oxygen to live; **anaerobic bacteria** can survive without oxygen
- Light—In darkness, bacteria become very active and multiply rapidly. Light is bacteria's worst enemy. When exposed to direct sunlight, they become sluggish and die rapidly.
- Dead and living matter—saprophytes are plants that live on dead matter or tissues; parasites are organisms that live on living matter or tissue.

A **virus** is another type of microorganism. Viruses are much smaller than bacteria and can survive only in living cells. Viruses can infect all living things—humans, animals, plants, and even bacteria. Some viruses can cause certain types of cancers. Many diseases are caused by viruses, including mumps, measles, influenza, cold sores, human warts, genital herpes, some respiratory and intestinal infections, rabies, hepatitis, and AIDS. Antibiotics are not effective against viral infections. Antiviral agents have been developed that are effective against some viruses.

AIDS

Two of the viral diseases mentioned, AIDS (acquired immunodeficiency syndrome) and hepatitis B are bloodborne diseases that pose the biggest threat to health care workers from occupational exposure. AIDS is caused by the human immunodeficiency virus (HIV), which is transmitted by exposure to contaminated blood and the exchange of sexual and perinatal fluids. It is not an easily transmitted virus, but the results of contracting the AIDS virus are very serious. This is why health care workers take great precautions to avoid coming in contact with the patient's blood or other body fluids.

HIV is not passed by casual contact, and there is no evidence that it is spread in the air. People who are infected with HIV may not have symptoms for years and can know if they are infected only if they have had a blood test and been told they are infected (**seropositive**). The screening test for HIV is the enzyme-linked immunosorbent assay (**ELISA**). If the ELISA test is positive, a confirmatory test called the **Western blot test** is performed.

It may take several months (generally 3–6 months, with the average being 25 days) from the time of exposure to HIV to the time when enough antibodies have built up in the blood to result in a positive blood test. The virus can still be transmitted to others during that time.

Within a month or two after infection with HIV there may be symptoms of illness such as sore throat, muscle and joint pain, sweating, diarrhea, and fever, and the person may think he or she has the flu. There also may be no symptoms at all. Then there is generally a long period of years during which no symptoms are present.

The first symptoms of illness may include night sweats, fatigue, mouth and genital sores, fevers, yeast infections, rashes, and persistent swollen lymph glands. Finally, with full-blown AIDS, the last stage of the cycle of infection that began with the HIV infection, the patient is unable to fight off infection and becomes very ill with **opportunistic infections** (infections from organisms in the environment that do not affect persons with normal immune systems) and certain cancers such as **Kaposi's sarcoma** (a cancer that produces multiple dark red or bluish red skin lesions and affects many body organs) and **lymphoma** (cancer of the lymph nodes). These conditions are known as AIDS-defining infection. Common opportunistic infections include *Pneumocystis carinii* pneumonia (PCP), cytomegalovirus infection (CMV), herpes simplex, toxoplasmosis, and mycobacterial disease.

AIDS is caused by a retrovirus that destroys certain lymphocytes in the body called T-cell helper lymphocytes and the immune system. A diagnosis of AIDS is made when the blood count shows 200 or fewer CD_4 or T-cells per cubic millimeter (cmm) of blood. The normal level is about 1000 per cmm of blood. Drug therapy includes the use of RT inhibitors and protease inhibitors in combinations that have greatly improved the treatment of AIDS.

Hepatitis

Viral hepatitis may be caused by a number of different viruses. However, in the United States acute hepatitis is usually caused by either hepatitis A virus (HAV), hepatitis B virus (HBV), or hepatitis C virus (HVC). Hepatitis A is generally a less serious type of disease that is transmitted by food and water contaminated with the virus by contact with infected feces. If a food handler, for example, has hepatitis A and does not properly wash the hands after using the toilet, the disease may be spread to others.

Hepatitis B is transmitted in the same way as HIV, through infected blood and body fluids. About one-third of all hepatitis is caused by HBV. Hepatitis C accounts for about 17% of the cases and is also transmitted by blood or blood products, but transmission as a result of sexual exchange of body fluids and perinatal fluid is unusual.

It is estimated that some 16,000 people die yearly as a result of liver damage after having chronic hepatitis. Hepatitis B and C are very serious diseases, and health-care workers must protect themselves from occupational exposure by using the Standard Precautions discussed later in this chapter.

Vaccines are available for HAV and HBV. Health-care workers who have the potential for being exposed to bloodborne pathogens receive a series of HBV vaccinations at the start of or during their employment.

Symptoms of hepatitis include fatigue, **anorexia** (lack of appetite), nausea, **arthralgia** (joint pain), and in more severe cases, **jaundice** (a yellow color to the skin and mucus membranes). Liver damage may occur, and serum enzymes will be elevated. (Fig. 6.4.)

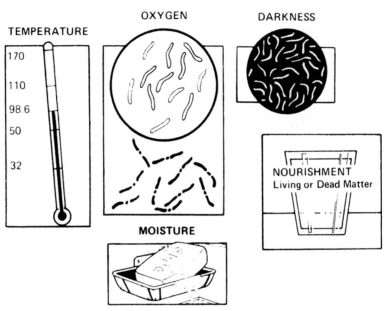

CONDITIONS THAT PROMOTE BACTERIAL GROWTH
FIGURE 6.4

*H*ISTORY OF INFECTION CONTROL

The germ theory of disease was not actually proven until a little over 100 years ago. The French scientist Louis Pasteur made two important discoveries about bacteria. First, he discovered that many diseases are caused by bacteria. Second, he discovered that bacteria could be killed by heat.

Pasteur's name has been used to refer to this method of killing bacteria. **Pasteurization** is the process of heating milk to about 140°F (60°C) and keeping it at that temperature for 30 minutes. Pasteurization kills harmful bacteria and makes milk safe for us to drink (Fig. 6.5).

FIGURE 6.5

A few years after Pasteur's discoveries, the British surgeon Joseph Lister found that many pathogens could also be killed by carbolic acid. Lister recognized that many deaths in hospitals seemed to be connected with unclean conditions. He was the first to require that surgical wounds be kept clean and the air in the operating room kept pure.

Lister changed things in hospitals by introducing the principles and methods of aseptic surgery. **Aseptic** means pathogen-free, without disease-producing organisms. Lister developed a technique for keeping pathogens out of open wounds or for destroying them. His method was to spray the skin around the wound with carbolic acid. Also, surgical instruments were made aseptic by being dipped in a carbolic acid solution. This technique was a major advance in the battle against disease.

People working in hospitals began to realize that some disease-producing microorganisms are everywhere. They are in the air, on the furniture, on and inside the patients' bodies, and on all the equipment. Doctors knew that pathogens multiply very rapidly. They also knew that if pathogens are not killed, they spread infection and disease from one person to another. Therefore, it was necessary to apply the principles of asepsis to the entire health care institution (Figs. 6.6 and 6.7).

MICROORGANISMS ARE EVERYWHERE

FIGURE 6.6

𝒯HE CHAIN OF INFECTION

For pathogens to survive and successfully produce a disease there must be a continuous chain of events. This is known as the **chain of infection.** If any link in the chain is broken, the pathogens are destroyed. The model that follows is useful in understanding the infection process cycle. Methods of preventing the spread of infection by breaking the various links of the chain are discussed later in the chapter.

WAYS THAT MICROORGANISMS ARE SPREAD

Direct contact	Touching the patient Secretions from the patient Urine from the patient Feces from the patient Blood from the patient
Indirect contact	Touching objects Dishes Bed linen Clothing Instruments Belongings
Droplet spread within three feet	Sneezing Coughing Talking
Vehicle	Contaminated Food Drugs Water or blood
Airborne transmission	Dust particles and moisture in the air

FIGURE 6.7   The chain of infection.

1. **RESERVOIR HOST** (animals and people who become infected)
The host provides nourishment for pathogens to multiply.
The host is also a source of transfer of the pathogens.

5. **SUSCEPTIBLE HOST** (an individual who, because of a low resistance to disease, is capable of being infected)

2. **MEANS OF EXIT** (a pathway through which the pathogens can leave the reservoir host such as the mouth, nose, eyes, ears, gastrointestinal, urinary, and reproductive tract, and open wounds)

4. **MEANS OF ENTRY** (a pathway through which the pathogen can get into the host) These are the same pathways as those listed under the means of exit.

3. **MEANS OF TRANSMISSION** (ways that the pathogens can be spread from one person to another) These include direct contact with the infected person or their infected discharge, and indirect transmission, which includes transfer through contaminated hands, equipment, food, water, the vapor created when a person coughs or sneezes, and insects.

DISINFECTION AND STERILIZATION

A continuous battle goes on in health care institutions to prevent the spread of pathogens. This battle is called **medical asepsis.** In spite of the best efforts of health care personnel, there are always some harmful microorganisms around us. They can be made harmless, however, by simple cleanliness procedures. We can keep ourselves clean by bathing and frequent handwashing. We can keep the institution and its equipment clean with soap, water, and solutions that assist in keeping down bacterial growth. Also, there are two very important methods for killing microorganisms or keeping them under control. These methods are:

- **Disinfection**—the process of destroying as many harmful organisms as possible. It also means slowing down the growth and activity of the organisms that cannot be destroyed.
- **Sterilization**—the process of killing all microorganisms, including spores, in a certain area.

Spores are dehydrated forms of some bacteria that serve as a defense for the bacteria and are very difficult to destroy. Some can even live in boiling water. Spores *can* be destroyed, however, by being exposed to pressurized steam at a high temperature. Machines called **autoclaves** (Fig. 6.8) can produce this high-temperature, pressurized steam. Autoclaves are used to kill spores and other disease-producing microorganisms. Spores may also be destroyed by chemicals called **sporicides.** Another method of sterilization uses a chemical gas instead of heat to destroy microorganisms. This method can be used to sterilize equipment made of plastics without melting them. These are both effective ways of sterilizing objects used in a health care institution. When an object is free of all microorganisms, it is called **sterile.**

AUTOCLAVE

FIGURE 6.8

Sterilization is necessary if the article comes in direct contact with a wound, as in the case of surgical instruments. Most supplies and equipment used in the care of patients can be disinfected to prevent them from spreading disease or infection. Disposable supplies must always be incinerated or burned.

Medical Asepsis

Medical asepsis means preventing the conditions that allow pathogens to live, multiply, and spread. As a health unit coordinator you will share the responsibility for preventing the spread of disease and infection.

The health unit coordinator should know that the main purposes for medical asepsis are:

- Protecting the patient against becoming infected a second time by the same microorganism. This is called **reinfection.**
- Protecting the patient against becoming infected by a new or different type of microorganism from another patient or a member of the hospital staff. This is called **cross infection.**
- Protecting all other patients and hospital staff against becoming infected by microorganisms passing from patient to patient, staff to patient, or patient to staff. This is called **infection control.**
- Protecting the patient against becoming infected with his own organisms. This is called **self-inoculation.**

Handwashing. In your work you will handle supplies and equipment used in the treatment and care of patients. Pathogens will get on your hands. They will come from the patient or from the things he or she has touched. Your hands could carry these microorganisms to other persons and places. The pathogens could also be transported to your own face and mouth. Handwashing is the most important measure a health worker can take to prevent the spread of disease (Fig. 6.9).

WASHING YOUR HANDS

REMEMBER . . .
As a health worker you must wash your hands frequently. This is the single most important way to prevent the spread of infection and disease.

FIGURE 6.9

*I*SOLATION

Communicable diseases spread very quickly and easily from one person to another. **Nosocomial infections** are hospital-acquired. To prevent the spread of communicable disease, hospitals employ two types of procedures:

1. **Aseptic procedures** such as handwashing and other clean techniques, as well as sterile practices that are used on certain patients as indicated.

2. **Special isolation procedures** that are used on patients who are diagnosed with or suspected of having communicable diseases.

The purpose of **isolation techniques** is to keep the pathogens that cause the disease inside the isolated patient's unit. As you know, these pathogens are everywhere in the sick room. They are on the floor, furniture, bedding, articles brought to the bedside, and on the patient himself. The area, the articles, and the patient are said to be **contaminated.** Isolation techniques, including the use of masks and gowns, keep pathogens away from equipment and personnel (Fig. 6.10).

When strict techniques, such as the use of sterile sheets and gowns, are used to protect the patient from outside pathogens, this is called **reverse** or **protective isolation** (Fig. 6.11).

FIGURE 6.10

Isolation procedures involve separating infected patients from other patients and from health care workers by using a variety of *barriers* such as gloves, masks, gowns or plastic aprons, and through actual *isolation* (the separation of the patient from other patients and personnel) in special private rooms. These decisions are made based on the patient's diagnosis or suspected diagnosis.

Protective isolation uses both Standard Precautions for all patients and Transmission-Based Precautions for specialized patients who are **immunocompromised** and at increased risk for bacterial, fungal, parasitic, and viral infections from other patients and the environment. Immunocompromised patients have a diminished ability to fight off disease.

In 1991 the **Occupational Safety and Health Administration (OSHA)** made available a set of regulations known as the OSHA Occupational Exposure to Bloodborne Pathogens Standards.

*I*SOLATION PRECAUTIONS

Early in 1996 the **Centers for Disease Control and Prevention (CDC)** and the Hospital Infection Control Practices Advisory Committee (HICPAC) published new guidelines for isolation precautions in hospitals.

The new guidelines contain two levels of precautions, *Standard Precautions* and *Transmission-Based Precautions*.

ISOLATION

PURPOSE OF ISOLATION

ISOLATION TECHNIQUES ARE USED WHEN PATIENTS HAVE INFECTIOUS OR COMMUNICABLE DISEASES THAT CAN BE SPREAD TO OTHERS. THE PURPOSE OF ISOLATION TECHNIQUES IS TO PREVENT THE SPREAD OF THESE DISEASES TO OTHER PATIENTS, STAFF, AND VISITORS.

REGULAR ISOLATION

OBJECTIVE OF REGULAR ISOLATION TECHNIQUES

PROTECTS OTHERS FROM CONTRACTING DISEASE FROM PATIENT

KEEPS INFECTIOUS ORGANISMS WITHIN BOUNDS WHERE THEY CAN BE DESTROYED OR SEPARATED

STAFF, OTHER PATIENTS, AND VISITORS

PATIENT WHO HAS INFECTIOUS COMMUNICABLE DISEASE

IN REGULAR ISOLATION, CONTAMINATION IS PREVENTED FROM SPREADING FROM THE ROOM.

REVERSE OR PROTECTIVE ISOLATION

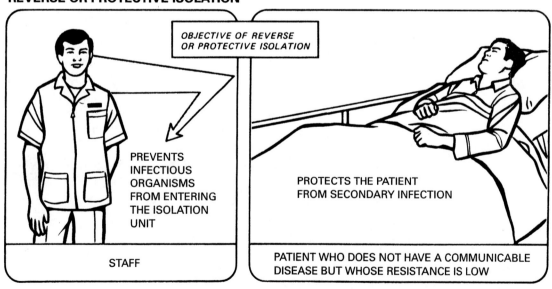

OBJECTIVE OF REVERSE OR PROTECTIVE ISOLATION

PREVENTS INFECTIOUS ORGANISMS FROM ENTERING THE ISOLATION UNIT

PROTECTS THE PATIENT FROM SECONDARY INFECTION

STAFF

PATIENT WHO DOES NOT HAVE A COMMUNICABLE DISEASE BUT WHOSE RESISTANCE IS LOW

SOMETIMES A PATIENT WHOSE RESISTANCE IS LOW AND WHO COULD EASILY CATCH A DISEASE IS ISOLATED FROM POSSIBLE INFECTIONS. THIS IS COMMONLY DONE FOR BURN PATIENTS OR FOR THOSE WHO ARE IMMUNOCOMPROMISED. IT IS CALLED *REVERSE* OR *PROTECTIVE* ISOLATION. IN PROTECTIVE ISOLATION, CONTAMINATION MUST BE PREVENTED FROM ENTERING THE ROOM.

FIGURE 6.11

Standard Precautions are designed for the care of all patients regardless of diagnosis or infection status. They were formerly known as Universal Precautions.

Standard Precautions integrate the characteristics of Universal Blood and Body Fluid Precautions and Body Substance Isolation Precautions.

Standard Precautions are used when any procedure is performed that may cause health care worker to come in contact with blood, body secretions (except perspiration), excretions, nonintact skin, or mucous membranes. The application of Standard Precautions includes:

- Proper handwashing technique
- Proper use of gloves
- Appropriate and correct use of **personal protective equipment (PPE)**
- Correct handling of used needles and other sharps
- Proper handling of used patient-care equipment, environment, and linen
- Careful consideration of patient placement (e.g., private room)

Transmission-Based Precautions are used for patients who are known or suspected to be infected with pathogenic microorganisms or communicable disease, or **colonized** (when a positive bacterial culture shows a developing infection even in the absence of symptoms) by pathogenic microorganisms.

These guidelines combine and revise the previous category and disease-specific isolation procedures into three types of precautions:

- Airborne precautions
- Droplet precautions
- Contact precautions

These may be used in combination with one another, because many diseases have several routes of transmission. They are used *in addition to* Standard Precautions.

Airborne Precautions

Airborne Precautions are used (in addition to Standard Precautions) when patients are known or suspected to have infections that can spread through the air and remain in the air for a long time. Examples of such diseases include varicella (chickenpox), tuberculosis (TB), and rubeola (measles).

Patients should be placed in a private negative-pressure isolation room with the door closed. If this is not possible, nursing will consult with the **epidemiology department** (department responsible for infection control).

Respiratory protection is worn when the room of a patient with known or suspected TB is entered. Respirators such as the HEPA-filter or the N95 filter air that is breathed in, thereby protecting the staff or visitor from inhaling the pathogens that may be present in tiny airborne droplets. Persons susceptible to varicella or rubeola should also wear respiratory protection.

If a patient must be moved from the room, the patient should wear a surgical mask that filters air that is breathed out.

Droplet Precautions

Droplet Precautions are used (in addition to Standard Precautions) when patients are infected with diseases that can be spread by coughing, sneezing, or talking. These diseases are transmitted by large-particle droplets through the air. Examples of such diseases include influenza (flu), some types of meningitis and pneumonia, pneumonic plague, diphtheria, rubella, and mumps.

Such patients should be placed in a private room or, if that is not available, with another patient with the same disease. Caregivers and visitors should wear a surgical mask when within 3 feet of the patient. Large-particle droplets generally travel no more than 3 feet before dropping from the air. If the patient must leave the room, he or she should wear a surgical mask.

Hospitals use special signs and symbols to let others know about the type of isolation that is being used. The accompanying chart shows the category-specific color-code labels for communication (Fig. 6.12).

CONTACT PRECAUTIONS

Contact Precautions are used (in addition to Standard Precautions) when patients are infected or colonized with microorganisms that can be spread by direct contact (touching the patient's skin) or indirect contact (touching contaminated articles in the patient's room). Many infections require the use of Contact Precautions. Some examples include wound, gastrointestinal, or respiratory infections or colonizations with multiple drug-resistant bacteria; certain enteric infections including hepatitis A, some *E. coli* and shigella for **incontinent** patients, and many highly infectious skin infections.

Patients requiring Contact Precautions should be placed in a private room or, if not available, with a patient with the same infection. Gloves must be worn when entering the room and removed before leaving, followed of course by careful handwashing. Gowns should also be worn for most patient care. If the patient is transported outside the room, the patient should wear a mask and other appropriate barriers to minimize the risk of transmission of microorganisms to others.

If unanticipated contact with these body substances occurs, washing must be done as soon as possible (handwashing, face washing, showering, etc.).

SPECIAL AREAS FOR PREVENTIVE MEASURES

Certain patient care areas in the health care institution need special attention to ensure cleanliness. Precautions to prevent communicable conditions from spreading are more strict than in other areas. This is because the patients in these areas may have a low resistance to disease, however, they do not have any communicable conditions. These areas include:

- Newborn nursery (Fig. 6.13)
- Premature care nursery
- Postpartum patient care unit
- Surgical patient care unit (operating room)
- Delivery room
- Cardiac care unit
- Intensive care unit
- Dialysis unit (Fig. 6.14)

EPIDEMIOLOGY

Many hospitals employ a **nurse epidemiologist.** This RN is responsible for the careful monitoring of all patient infections. Recall that infections contracted during the hospitalization are called nosocomial infections. Nurse epidemiologists conduct studies to

STANDARD PRECAUTIONS

WASH HANDS

- Before and after patient care.
- Before and after using gloves.
- Between patient contact.

WEAR GLOVES

- When touching blood, body fluids, secretions, excretions & contaminated items.
- Before touching mucous membranes and nonintact skin.

MASK/EYE PROTECTION

- To protect mucous membranes of the eyes, nose & mouth when procedures and activities are likely to generate splashes or sprays of blood and body fluids.

WEAR GOWN

- To protect skin and clothing during procedures and activities likely to generate splashes or sprays of blood & body fluids.
- Remove soiled gown immediately and wash hands.

TAKE CARE

- To prevent injuries when using needles, scalpels & other sharp instruments.
- When handling sharp instruments after procedures.
- When cleaning used instruments.
- When disposing of used needles.

©1996 *King Graphic Design, Dana Point, California*

AIRBORNE PRECAUTIONS
In addition to Standard Precautions

VISITORS: Report to Nurses' Station Before Entering Room

PATIENT PLACEMENT

- Private room.
- Negative pressure room.
- Door closed.

WEAR MASK

- Tuberculosis—N95 Respirator.
- Chickenpox (Varicella), Measles (Rubeola):
  - Immune persons, no mask required.
  - Susceptible persons, not to enter room.

PATIENT TRANSPORT

- Limit transport of patient to essential purposes only.
- Use surgical mask on patient during transport.
- Notify area receiving patient.

©1996 *King Graphic Design, Dana Point, California*

DROPLET PRECAUTIONS
In addition to Standard Precautions

VISITORS: Report to Nurses' Station Before Entering Room

PATIENT PLACEMENT

- Private room, if possible.
- If cohorting patients, maintain separation of three feet between patients.

WEAR MASK

- Wear regular mask if within three feet of patient.

PATIENT TRANSPORT

- Limit transport of patient to essential purposes only.
- Use surgical mask on patient during transport.
- Notify area receiving patient.

©1996 *King Graphic Design, Dana Point, California*

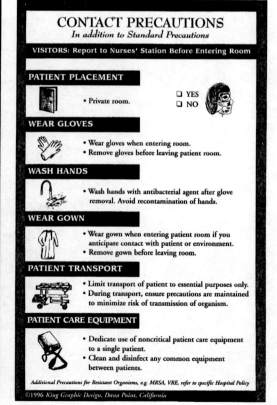

CONTACT PRECAUTIONS
In addition to Standard Precautions

VISITORS: Report to Nurses' Station Before Entering Room

PATIENT PLACEMENT

- Private room.

☐ YES
☐ NO

WEAR GLOVES

- Wear gloves when entering room.
- Remove gloves before leaving patient room.

WASH HANDS

- Wash hands with antibacterial agent after glove removal. Avoid recontamination of hands.

WEAR GOWN

- Wear gown when entering patient room if you anticipate contact with patient or environment.
- Remove gown before leaving room.

PATIENT TRANSPORT

- Limit transport of patient to essential purposes only.
- During transport, ensure precautions are maintained to minimize risk of transmission of organism.

PATIENT CARE EQUIPMENT

- Dedicate use of noncritical patient care equipment to a single patient.
- Clean and disinfect any common equipment between patients.

Additional Precautions for Resistant Organisms, e.g. MRSA, VRE, refer to specific Hospital Policy

©1996 *King Graphic Design, Dana Point, California*

FIGURE 6.12 (Courtesy King Graphic Design, Dana Point, CA. To order call Etna Communications, 3023 North Clark St., Suite 744 Chicago, IL 60657-5200 1-800-347-6893.)

FIGURE 6.13

FIGURE 6.14

determine if the hospital itself contributes to the disease, assists doctors in setting standards to prevent disease, assists nursing in the establishment and maintenance of isolation techniques, and compiles and delivers records to state health agencies as necessary.

*I*SOLATION AND THE HEALTH UNIT COORDINATOR

It is a nursing responsibility to see that all patients are isolated properly according to the CDC guidelines.

- The appropriate isolation precaution sign (Standard Precautions, Airborne Precautions, Droplet Precautions, or Contact Precautions) is placed on the patient's door. Sometimes more than one sign is necessary because some infections and conditions have multiple routes of transmission.
- All departments who will have contact with the patient are notified.
- Isolation supplies such as gloves, gowns, and masks are ordered for the patient's room.

- The physician is notified by nursing, and a written order for isolation is requested.
- The infection control officer or nurse epidemiologist is notified immediately.
- The word *isolation* and type of isolation is indicated on the patient's chart, Kardex, and other forms as explained by your instructor.
- Family and other visitors are directed to the nurse for an explanation of the isolation procedure.
- Isolation is indicated when requisitioning from other departments. Dietary will use disposable dishes and utensils. Other departments will take special precautions.
- Whenever possible, the use of noncritical patient care equipment is dedicated to a single patient.
- When a patient must be transported to an area outside the patient's room, personnel in the area to which the patient is being sent are informed of the transport and of the precautions that must be used.
- The Admitting Department is notified when isolation is discontinued (this may change the cost of the room to the patient) to allow them to schedule another patient for the room.
- Environmental Services are notified when isolation is discontinued so that special cleaning procedures may be employed before another patient is admitted to the room.

Special Considerations

Although the health unit coordinator does not perform direct patient care, he or she must be acutely aware of the necessary precautions to be taken by all health workers in preventing the contraction of disease.

- Wash your hands frequently. Scrub with plenty of soap and water as warm as you can tolerate. Use a lot of friction and be sure to get under nails and rings. FRICTION GETS RID OF PATHOGENS. Rinse thoroughly. Use a paper towel and dry your hands well. Use another dry paper towel to turn off the water. Do not touch the sink or area around it with your clean hands (Fig. 6.15).
- Protect yourself from body substances. When handling laboratory specimens destined for the lab, wear gloves. Bag these specimens in plastic for transportation. Always wash your hands after handling any specimen container.
- Remember that *any* health worker in danger of contamination must wear protective gear—masks, gowns, gloves, and so on.

A Hold hands lower than elbows.

B Interlace fingers and thumbs.

C Wash the wrists with a rotating motion.

FIGURE 6.15   Handwashing

D Turn the water off with a dry paper towel.

₤EARNING ACTIVITIES

1. Complete the following.
   (a) Prognosis _____
   (b) Disease _____
   (c) Acute disease _____
   (d) Chronic disease _____
   (e) Functional disease _____
   (f) Organic disease _____
   (g) Metastasis _____
   (h) Malignant _____

2. List the seven danger signs of cancer.
   (a) _____
   (b) _____
   (c) _____
   (d) _____

(e) _____
(f) _____
(g) _____

3. List the five types of microorganisms.
   (a) _____
   (b) _____
   (c) _____
   (d) _____
   (e) _____

4. Define the following.
   (a) Aseptic_____
   (b) Sterile_____
   (c) Medical asepsis_____
   (d) Isolation_____
   (e) Nurse epidemiologist_____
   (f) Nosocomial infection_____

5. List five patient care areas where extra precautions are taken to prevent the spread of communicable diseases.
   (a) _____
   (b) _____
   (c) _____
   (d) _____
   (e) _____

6. List the two levels of isolation precautions.
   (a) _____
   (b) _____

7. List the three types of transmission-based precautions.
   (a) _____
   (b) _____
   (c) _____

8. Standard Precautions should be used when _____
_____
_____
_____.

9. The purpose of isolation is _____
_____.

10. Regular isolation protects _____.

11. Reverse or protective isolation protects _____.

12. The single most important way to prevent the spread of infection and disease is to _____.

13. Discuss the health unit coordinator's responsibilities in regard to isolation. _____
_____
_____

Match the term in Column A with its description in Column B.

Column A

(a) Allergic disease
(b) Congenital disease
(c) Degenerative disease
(d) Neoplastic disease
(e) Trauma

Column B

_____ New growth of tissue
_____ Abnormal reaction to generally harmless substance
_____ Injuries
_____ "Wear and tear" disorders
_____ Disorder present at birth

14. List the two bloodborne diseases that present the greatest threat to health care workers.
    (a) _____
    (b) _____

15. Name the two tests used to diagnose HIV infection.
    (a) _____
    (b) _____

16. Define *opportunistic infections*._____

17. List the three types of hepatitis that account for most of the cases in the United States.
    (a) _____
    (b) _____
    (c) _____

18. For which of the bloodborne types of hepatitis is there a vaccine? _____

19. Describe how health care workers can protect themselves from bloodborne infections. _____

20. Why are Standard Precautions used with *all* patients regardless of their diagnosis or infection status? _____

_____

_____

_____

21. You are at the nurses' station and a patient walks up carrying a plastic cup and says, "Here's the urine specimen my nurse wants," and hands it to you. What should you do if no nurse is immediately available to take the specimen? _____

_____

_____

_____

22. What can you, as a health unit coordinator, do to prevent the spread of infection to yourself or to others? _____

_____

_____

_____

23. Mr. Emelio has just been placed in isolation with Contact Precautions. List the precautions that must be taken in addition to Standard Precautions.

(a) _____

(b) _____

(c) _____

(d) _____

(e) _____

(f) _____

24. Mr. Emelio is a very nice man and he has a big family to whom he is very close. How do you think being in isolation is going to affect him and his family? _____

_____

_____

25. What can you and the nurses do to make isolation easier for him and his family? _____

_____

_____

26. How do you think you would feel if you had to be put in isolation in a hospital? Please explain. _____

_____

_____

_____

_____

CHAPTER 7

Medical Law and Ethics

VOCABULARY

Abandonment	The withdrawal of a physician from the care of a patient without reasonable notice of such withdrawal or without discharge from the case by the patient
Advance Directive (AD)	A legal document in which an individual gives written instructions expressing his or her wishes regarding health care in the event a person can no longer make those decisions
Assault	An unlawful threat or attempt to do bodily injury to another
Battery	Unlawful touching of another person without their consent with or without resultant injury
Breach	Breaking of a law, promise, or duty
Civil law	A statute that enforces private rights and liabilities, as differentiated from criminal law
Consent	Permission granted by a person voluntarily and in his right mind
Contract	An agreement between two or more parties for the doing or not doing of some definite thing
Defamation	An attack on a person's reputation, called *libel* when written or *slander* when spoken
Defendant	A person sued; in criminal proceedings, also called the accused
Do-not-resuscitate (DNR)	An order by a physician not to administer cardiopulmonary resuscitation (CPR) if the patient goes into cardiac or respiratory arrest
Durable power of attorney	A legal document that allows an individual named in the document to act on behalf of another. A durable power of attorney for health care (DPAHC) allows the patient to express his or her health care decisions and the amount of authority he or she wishes his agent to assume
Duty of care	The obligation under law for a health care worker to perform services for a patient that meet the common standards of practice expected for a comparable worker; the *patient* is protected by recognition of the health worker's responsibility for duty of care
Emancipated minor	A person who is underage but has established through legal action that he or she is living apart from the parents and is financially responsible and able to consent to treatment
Ethics	A code of conduct that represents ideal behavior
Euthanasia	An act by an individual to assist a person to die when that person is suffering from an incurable condition
Expert witness	A person who offers testimony in court because he or she possesses special knowledge, training, or skill in an area that is important to the case
False imprisonment	Holding or detaining a person against his or her will
Felony	A major crime for which greater punishment is imposed than for a misdemeanor
Guardian	A court-appointed person whose duty it is to make decisions for and protect the interests of another person who cannot make his or her own decisions
Incompetent	Wanting in physical or mental fitness
Invasion of privacy	To make public knowledge any private or personal information without the individual's consent

Judgment	The final decision of a court in an action or suit
Libel	Written defamation
Licensure	Authorization by the state to practice one's profession or vocation; involves control of educational standards, licensing examinations, means for revocation of license, and prohibitions for the unlicensed
Litigation	A lawsuit
Living Will	A written agreement between the patient and physician to withhold heroic measures if the patient's condition is such that it cannot be reversed
Malpractice	Literally, "bad practice" by a professional; care below the expected community standard that has led to injury
Negligence	Failure to do something a reasonable person *would do* under ordinary circumstances, or doing something a reasonable person *would not do* under ordinary circumstances; negligence can work in two ways, by action or by omission
Plaintiff	One who institutes a lawsuit
Privileged communication	Information given by a patient to medical personnel that cannot be disclosed without consent of the person who gave it
Proximate	In a case where negligence has been claimed, the act must be immediately related to (or the *proximate* cause of) the injury
Reasonable care	The *health care worker* is protected by law if it can be determined that he or she acted reasonably as compared with fellow workers
Respondeat superior	Responsibility of an employer for the acts of an employee
Slander	Oral or spoke defamation
Statute	Law that has been enacted by a legislative branch of the government
Statute of limitations	The time established for filing lawsuits
Subpoena	A writ that commands a witness to appear at a trial or other proceeding and to give testimony
Tort	A private or civil wrong
Will	A document in a form prescribed by law and stating the orders of a person for the disposition of his property after his death

Note: The student should be aware that these definitions are simplified as an introductory study.

OBJECTIVES

When you have completed this chapter, you will be able to:

- Recognize the definitions of legal terms from the vocabulary.
- Discuss the purpose of licensing of medical personnel.
- Discuss the legal physician–patient relationship.
- Demonstrate your understanding of the terms *duty of care* and *reasonable care.*
- Demonstrate your knowledge of the rights of the individual under the law and how these rights might be violated.
- Discuss your knowledge of your responsibility in relation to legal records.
- List several basic rules to follow for the prevention of litigation.
- List and define the forms and elements of negligence.
- Define *ethics.*
- Define *advance directive.*

- Discuss the difference between legal aspects and ethical considerations.
- State the necessity for and utilization of ethics in hospital situations.
- Apply guidelines of ethical behavior in health-related situations.

The practice of medicine is carried on within a framework of laws. It is important that those in the medical field be familiar with the basic legal ground rules of the profession. Laws concerning patients and workers in health care institutions were written to protect both the patient and the worker. As a health unit coordinator you need to understand how the law affects you, the patients, and the health care institution. You will want to become aware of potential legal hazards and know how to avoid legal trouble as a result of your work.

*L*ICENSING

The principal way in which medicine is regulated by law in this country is by licensing. Every state in the nation requires that hospitals be licensed. A doctor must have a license to practice medicine; a nurse must have a license to practice nursing. Many other groups of health care workers must be licensed to practice their vocation (e.g., licensed radiology technicians, licensed physical therapists, and pharmacists).

The statutes dealing with licensing of physicians and nurses are commonly referred to as *medical practice* or *nurse practice acts.*

The laws that grant health workers licenses also have the power to take those licenses away.

*T*HE LEGAL SIDE OF THE PHYSICIAN/PATIENT RELATIONSHIP

In the legal sense, the relationship between the doctor and the patient is contractual. That is, each of the parties agrees to do something. In the case of many hospitalized patients, this contract was begun in the doctor's office prior to hospitalization. Although this contract is rarely written, the simple sequence of a person's asking for treatment and the doctor's undertaking to treat is sufficient to create a contract and set up certain obligations each has to the other.

The patient's obligation is to pay for the services received. The doctor's legal responsibility is more complicated. The law requires of every doctor the duty to apply knowledge and skill with reasonable care and to use his or her best judgment. The doctor is duty-bound by law to give that patient a standard of care equal to that provided by similar physicians. In the eyes of the law, all patients regardless of race, religion, or financial status are entitled to the same skillful care.

The legal duty of the doctor does not require that the patient be cured or even be improved. The test of legality is whether the quality of care is up to the legal standard. If a promise of cure is made that does not indeed occur, the failure to perform could result in a suit for breach of contract. The health unit coordinator should avoid comments that would lead a patient or his family to believe that treatment will definitely be successful.

*D*UTY OF CARE

In a hospital, the patient must be guaranteed safe care, and the conscientious health worker must be protected from lawsuits. The term **duty of care** refers to protection of the patient. The patient is entitled to and expects safe care. The law requires every health care worker to perform services for the patient in such a way that the health care worker meets the common or average standards of practice expected for a comparable worker. In other words, the patient can expect that the health unit coordinator will perform his or her duties in a manner that will be at least comparable to those of other health unit coordinators in the community under similar circumstances.

The health care worker is protected by the law if he or she uses what is termed **reasonable care.** Reasonable care describes the standard or level of care that is equal to the care given by a worker of comparable training and experience under similar circumstances. If the health care worker does not equal this standard of reasonable care, and harm comes to the patient as a result, he or she may be judged negligent.

NEGLIGENCE AND MALPRACTICE

Negligence is the failure to give reasonable care or the giving of unreasonable care. That is, the worker may do something wrong or may fail to do something she or he should have done under the circumstances, and the patient is harmed.

The Forms of Negligence

- **Malfeasance**—the performance of an unlawful or improper act
- **Misfeasance**—the performance of an act in an improper manner that results in injury to the person
- **Nonfeasance**—failure to perform an act when there is a duty to do so
- **Malpractice**—negligence by a professional
- **Criminal negligence**—reckless disregard for the safety of another person

THE FOUR ELEMENTS OF NEGLIGENCE

In order for a plaintiff to recover damages (usually money) for a claim of negligence, four elements of negligence must be proven. They are:

- **Duty of care** (It is clear that a duty to the patient existed.)
- **Breach of duty** (There was a failure to meet the duty of care.)
- **Injury** (An injury resulted.)
- **Causation** (The breach of duty was the proximate cause of the injury.)

The higher the educational level and requirements of the health care worker the greater the possibility that he or she may be held responsible for his or her actions.

Although the health unit coordinator works under the supervision of the registered nurses, you must exercise great care in the performance of your duties and keep in mind that the terms *duty of care* and *reasonable care* apply to all health care workers in the health care institution.

PATIENT'S BILL OF RIGHTS

The American Hospital Association publishes a document called *A Patient's Bill of Rights* with the hope that it will be posted in hospitals and given to patients on admission. The intent of this document is to make both patients and personnel aware of what the patient has a right to expect.

The law operates to protect the patient, but it also operates to protect the public. Certain diseases and conditions must be reported by physicians and hospitals. These include syphilis; trauma such as stabbings, gunshot wounds, or attempted suicide; child or elder abuse; births and deaths; and requests for plastic reconstruction to change the identity.

Patient's Bill of Rights

1. The patient has the right to considerate and respectful care.
2. Patients have the right to obtain from their physician complete current information concerning their diagnosis, treatment, and prognosis in terms they can be reasonably expected to understand.
3. An informed consent should include knowledge of the proposed procedure, along with its risks and probable duration of incapacitation. In addition, the patient has a right to information regarding medically significant alternatives.
4. The patient has the right to refuse treatment to the extent permitted by law, and to be informed of the medical consequences of his action.
5. Case discussion, consultation, examination, and treatment should be conducted discretely. Those not directly involved must have the patient's permission to be present.
6. The patient has the right to expect that all communication and records pertaining to his care should be treated as confidential.
7. The patient has the right to expect the hospital to make a reasonable response to his request for services. The hospital must provide evaluation, service, and referral as indicated by the urgency of the case.
8. The patient has the right to obtain information as to any relationship of his hospital to other health care and educational institutions, insofar as his care is concerned. The patient has the right to obtain information as to the existence of any professional relationships among individuals, by name, who are treating him.
9. The patient has the right to be advised if the hospital proposes to engage in or perform human experimentation affecting his care or treatment. The patient has the right to refuse to participate in such research projects.
10. The patient has the right to expect reasonable continuity of care.
11. The patient has the right to examine and receive an explanation of his bill regardless of the source of payment.
12. The patient has the right to know what hospital rules and regulations apply to his conduct as a patient.

Advance Directives

The Patient Self-Determination Act of 1991 is a federal law that requires hospitals to inform their patients about the advance directive laws in their state. Advance directives give adult patients the opportunity to formulate decisions and give instructions about the health care they wish to receive (or not receive) should they become incompetent. Forms are made available to the patient on admission, and the completed form is placed in the medical record. If the advance directive is not completed when the patient is admitted, it can be done later, revised, or not done at all.

AIDS

AIDS is an incurable but preventable disease that has reached epidemic proportions in the United States. As a result of the widespread prevalence of the disease and the availability of blood testing for exposure to the virus, a number of laws dealing with AIDS and AIDS-related issues have been passed. These laws vary widely among the states. Keep in mind as you read the statements that follow (from California guidelines) that you must be aware of the laws that apply to your state and that these are simply representative of the areas of concern.

1. Mandatory Testing by Blood Banks and Plasma Centers:
   (a) Required testing of blood and blood components before use: Generally blood or blood components may not be used for humans unless they have been tested and found nonreactive for the probable causative agents of AIDS and to detect viral hepatitis.
   (b) Reporting for donor referral register: If donor blood tests positive, blood banks or plasma centers must provide the information to the Department of Health Services for inclusion on the Donor Referral Register.

2. Provision of Testing Sites for Free Testing to Detect Antibodies to HIV, which is the probable causative agent of AIDS.

3. Mandatory Reporting of Diagnosis of AIDS:
   (a) Duty of physicians and hospitals to report: This includes the reporting to county or state health officers of all transfusion-associated AIDS cases and all hospitalized patients with a confirmed diagnosis of AIDS.
   (b) Follow-up contact: Health officials must contact persons with confirmed AIDS diagnosis to instruct them not to donate blood and suggest treatment sources and to conduct follow-up studies.

4. Testing by Health Care Providers:
   (a) Written consent prior to testing: Before a person's blood is tested to detect antibodies to the probable cause of AIDS (HIV virus), a written consent must be obtained. Some exceptions to this may apply (Fig. 7.1).
   (b) Confidentiality of test results:
      (1) Generally no disclosure of test results may occur without the written permission of the patient that includes to whom the disclosure will be made. Written authorization may be required for each separate disclosure of test results (Fig. 7.2).

      Note: These guidelines indicate there is no mandatory reporting requirement for HIV antibody test results, but a *diagnosis* of AIDS must be reported by the physician.
      (2) Penalties for unauthorized disclosure: Penalties are provided for the disclosure of the results of a blood test to detect antibodies to the probable causative agent of AIDS to anyone without the written authorization of the patient. Penalties may vary based on whether the disclosure is negligent or willful. It can result in fines and even imprisonment.
      (3) Limitations of use of test results: Much controversy exists regarding employment and insurance decisions and AIDS. The results of a blood test to detect antibodies to HIV may not be used to determine insurability or employability. However, a diagnosis of AIDS, established by other means, may not be expressly forbidden by law.

$\mathcal{D}$NR ORDERS

Under certain circumstances a patient's condition is such that a decision has been made not to perform CPR (cardiopulmonary resuscitation) and/or ACLS (advanced cardiac life support). These decisions should be made with the agreement of the physician, patient's family, and whenever possible, the patient, and then clearly communicated to the staff.

JCAHO requires that hospitals have policies in place regarding DNR (do not resuscitate) orders. JCAHO guidelines say that a DNR order must be written on the chart and should state exactly the treatment that will *not* be given. The guidelines also require that the patient's wishes be documented and that the patient's caregivers be involved in the discussion to withhold CPR and ACLS.

A sticker is usually placed on or inside the patient's chart indicating the DNR, and the notation is made on the patient's Kardex.

CONSENTS

The underlying relationship between the hospital and the patient is contractual, and the law holds that a person has the exclusive right to determine what shall be done with his or her body. Therefore, it is essential that this contractual relationship be clearly defined and that the patient's understanding be expressed in a written agreement signed by him or his personal representative.

Consider the following information as guidelines when dealing with consents. Consult your policy manual or ask your head nurse/nurse manager for specific information relative to your hospital.

1. The patient should first read, or have read to him or to her, the consent in order that he or she knows what he or she is signing. The law requires that to be legally valid the consent must be an *informed consent;* that is, the procedures and risks involved should be fully explained in terms understandable to the patient.

2. The patient must be of sound mind and not sign under duress (be forced to sign). The mental competency of the patient is important. Patients may not sign when they are under the influence of drugs or alcohol.

3. The signature on a consent must match the signature on the conditions of admission. The Conditions of Admission form is signed on entering the hospital.

4. All signatures must be in ink. Full legal names must be used. A married woman may sign Mary K. Jones or Mrs. John H. Jones.

5. All dates, times, signatures, including the signature of witnesses, must be legible, and the witness must be over 21 (18 in some states).

6. No abbreviations may be used. All words must be spelled out.

7. Witnesses, in the number indicated, must always sign in the space so allocated in the form as witness to the signature of the person signing the permit.

8. All signatures must be witnessed and dated.

9. The patient may indicate an X if unable to write and there are two witnesses.

Who May Sign States vary on their laws regarding consents. Each state will have laws regarding special consideration for people in custody, married minors, and unmarried minors. Generally:

1. All adults, male or female, 18 years of age and over must sign their own consents with two possible exceptions:

   (a) An actual emergency when two physicians sign a statement, incorporated in the consent. "The immediate treatment of the patient is necessary because _____."

   (b) When the patient has been declared incompetent and has a guardian.

Patient's Name: _____

I am consenting to be tested to see whether I have been infected with the Human Immunodeficiency Virus (HIV), which is the probable causative agent of Acquired Deficiency Syndrome (AIDS).

THE MEANING OF THE TEST

This test is not a test for AIDS but only for the presence of HIV. Being infected with HIV does not mean that I have AIDS or that I will have AIDS or other related illnesses. Other factors must be reviewed to determine whether I have AIDS.

Most test results are accurate, but sometimes the results are wrong or uncertain. In some cases the test results may indicate that the person is infected with HIV when the person is not (false positive). In other cases the test may fail to detect that a person is infected with HIV when the person really is (false negative). Sometimes, the test cannot tell whether or not a person is infected at all. If I have been recently infected with HIV, it may take some time before a test will show the infection. For these reasons, I may have to repeat the test.

CONFIDENTIALITY

California law limits the disclosure of my HIV test results. Under the law, no one but my doctor and other care givers are told about the test results unless I give specific written consent to let other people know. Additionally, doctors may inform my spouse, any sexual partner(s) or needle-sharing partner(s), or the county health officer if a doctor thinks that is necessary. All information relating to this test is kept in my medical record.

BENEFITS AND RISKS OF THE TEST

The test results can help me make better decisions about my health care and my personal life. The test results can help me and my doctor make decisions concerning medical treatment. If the results are positive, I know that I can infect others and I can act to prevent this.

Potential risks of the test include psychological stress while awaiting the results and distress if the results are positive. Some persons have had trouble with jobs, housing, education or insurance when their tests results have been made known.

MORE INFORMATION

I understand that before I decide to take this test I should be sure that I have had the chance to ask my doctor any questions I may have about the test, its meaning, its risks and benefits, and any alternatives to the test.

By my signature below, I acknowledge that I have read and understood the information in this form, that I have been given all of the information I desire concerning the HIV test, its meaning, expected benefits, possible risks, and any alternatives to the tests, and that I have had my questions answered. Further, I acknowledge that I have given consent for the performance of a test to detect HIV.

Signature: _____   _____
                    (patient / parent / conservator / guardian)   *If signed by other than patient, indicate relationship   Date and Time

Witness:_____

   *This consent may be signed by a person other than the patient only under the following circumstances:
   1. The patient is under twelve (12) years of age or, as a result of his/her physical condition, is incompetent to consent to the HIV antibody blood test; and
   2. The person who consents to the test on the patient's behalf is lawfully authorized to make health care decisions for the patient, e.g., an attorney-in-fact appointed by the patient under the Durable Power of Attorney for Health Care; the parent or guardian of a minor; an appropriately authorized conservator; or, under appropriate circumstances, the patient's closest available relative (see chapters 2 and 20);
   3. It is necessary to obtain the patient's HIV antibody test results in order to render appropriate care to the patient or to practice preventative measures. Health and Safety Code section 199.27.

CONSENT FOR THE HIV TEST

FIGURE 7.1

Authorization for Disclosure of the Results of the HIV Antibody Blood Test

A. EXPLANATION

This authorization for use or disclosure of the results of a blood test to detect antibodies to the HIV virus, the probable causative agent of Acquired Immune Deficiency Syndrome (AIDS), is being _____
requested of you to comply with the terms of the Confidentiality of Medical Information Act, Civil Code Section 56 et seq. and Health and Safety Code Section 199.21(g).

B. AUTHORIZATION

I hereby authorize _____
                         (Name of Physician, Hospital or Health Care Provider)

to furnish to _____
                (Name or Title of Persons Who Is to Receive Results)
the results of the blood test for antibodies to the HIV virus.

C. USES

The requester may use the information for any purpose, subject only to the following limitations: _____
_____

D. DURATION

This authorization shall become effective immediately and shall remain in effect indefinitely or until _____ , 2 ____ , whichever is shorter.

E. RESTRICTIONS

I understand that the requestor may not further use or disclose the medical information unless another authorization is obtained from me or unless such use or disclosure is specifically required or permitted by law.

F. ADDITIONAL COPY

I further understand that I have a right to receive a copy of this authorization upon my request.
Copy requested and received: _____Yes _____No Initial _____

Date: _____ , 2 ___ _____
                                      Signature

                                 _____
                                      Printed name

FIGURE 7.2

2. All persons in custody of the law must give their consent for treatment.

3. Married minors are freed from parental authority and may sign their consent, including a divorced minor.

4. Unmarried minors must have their consent signed by one parent or legally appointed guardian. Consent of both parents is recommended. A stepparent may not consent unless the child has been legally adopted.

5. **Emancipated minors** who through legal action have established that they are living away from home and are financially responsible may sign their own consents.

6. An executor of the patient's estate does not have the legal right to consent to treatment. Only in the case of legal guardianship determined by the court may a member of the family consent (such as a son consenting to treatment of his mother).

Consent to Operation

Purpose: Any procedure that breaks the skin may be interpreted as an *operation*. The patient's valid surgical consent is necessary to preclude liability for battery, unless the patient needs immediate care to save his life (Fig. 7.3).

Any invasive procedure requiring entrance into a body cavity such as the various endoscopies, many diagnostic procedures using injections of radiopaque substances, insertion of catheters into vessels, and procedures requiring general, local, or regional anesthesia requires consent.

Consent to Sterilization

1. A Consent to Sterilization is to be completed in addition to the Consent to Operation whenever it is anticipated that a particular operation will possibly render the patient, either male or female, sterile (unable to reproduce).

2. In most states, the signature of the spouse is desirable for married persons to avoid a charge of conspiracy between physician and the spouse, if available. If not available, the patient possesses full power to consent (Fig. 7.4).

$\mathcal{T}$ELEPHONE CONSENTS

Telephone consents may be obtained in an emergency situation in which a delay of treatment would jeopardize the life or health of the patient. Generally:

1. Two people must listen to a consent by telephone. Both people must witness the consent noting time and date.

2. Confirmation by written letter or telegram must follow immediately, which is to be attached to the consent and remains a part of the permanent record.

Length of Consents

Consents are considered valid for a reasonable time after signing, as long as no changes in the anticipated surgery occur as a result of further tests and study of the patient, and as long as the patient is not discharged.

$\mathcal{T}$ERMINATION OF PATIENT CONTRACT

The legal aspects of terminating a contract with a patient are as important as those involved in establishing the relationship. A doctor cannot lawfully abandon a case. The law says that once a doctor has entered into a contractual relationship with a patient he/she is obligated to continue to care for that patient until there is no need for further treatment, the patient dismisses the doctor, or the doctor withdraws from the case. If the doctor does withdraw, he or she legally must advise the patient of any further need for treatment and give him sufficient time to obtain the services of another physician.

AUTHORIZATION FOR AND CONSENT TO SURGERY OR SPECIAL DIAGNOSTIC OR THERAPEUTIC PROCEDURES

To_____
Name of Patient

Your/the patient's attending physician is_____, M.D.

Your/the patient's supervising physician or surgeon is _____ , M.D.

1. The hospital maintains personnel and facilities to assist your/the patient's physicians and surgeons in their performance of various surgical operations and other special diagnostic or therapeutic procedures. These operations and procedures may all involve risks of unsuccessful results, complications, injury, or even death, from both known and unforeseen causes, and no warranty or guarantee is made as to result or cure.

    You have the right to be informed of such risks as well as the nature of the operation or procedure; the expected benefits or effects of such operation or procedure; and the available alternative methods of treatment and their risks and benefits.

    You also have the right to be informed whether your physician has any independent medical research or economic interests related to the performance of the proposed operation or procedure. Except in cases of emergency, operations or procedures are not performed until you have had the opportunity to receive this information and have given your consent. You have the right to consent or to refuse any proposed operation or procedure any time prior to its performance.

2. Your/the patient's physicians and surgeons have recommended the operations or procedures set forth below. Upon your authorization and consent, the operations or procedures set forth below, together with any different or further procedures which in the opinion of the supervising physician or surgeon may be indicated due to any emergency, will be performed on you/the patient. The operations or procedures will be performed by the supervising physician or surgeon named above (or in the event of any emergency causing his or her inability to complete the procedure, a qualified substitute supervising physician or surgeon), together with associates and assistants, including anesthesiologists, pathologists and radiologists from the medical staff of   whom the supervising physician or surgeon may assign designated responsibilities. The persons in attendance for the purpose of performing specialized medical services such as anesthesia, radiology or pathology are not agents, servants or employees of the hospital or your/the patient's supervising physician or surgeon but are independent contractors, and therefore your agents, servants, or employees.

3. If your physician determines that there is a reasonable possibility that you may need a blood transfusion as a result of the surgery or procedure to which you are consenting, your physician will inform you of this and will provide you with a brochure regarding blood transfusions. This brochure contains information concerning the benefits and risks of the various options for blood transfusions, including predonation by yourself or others. You also have the right to have adequate time before your procedure to arrange for predonation, but you can waive this right if you do not wish to wait. You should understand that transfusions of blood or blood products involve certain risks, including the transmission of disease such as hepatitis or Human Immunodeficiency Virus (HIV) and that you have a right to consent or refuse consent to any transfusion. You should discuss any questions that you may have about transfusions with your physician.

4. The pathologist is hereby authorized to use his or her discretion in disposing any member, organ, or other tissue removed from your/the patient's person during the operation(s) or procedure(s) set forth below.

5. To make sure that you fully understand the operation or procedure, your physician will fully explain the operation or procedure to you before you decide whether or not to give consent. If you have any questions, you are encouraged and expected to ask them.

6. Your signature below constitutes your acknowledgment (1) that you have read and agree to the foregoing; (2) that the operation or procedure set forth below has been adequately explained to you by the above-named physician or surgeon and by your/the patient's anesthesiologist and that you have received all of the information you desire concerning such operation or procedure; (3) that you have had a chance to ask questions; and (4) that you authorize and consent to the performance of the operation or procedure.

Operation or Procedure _____

_____

_____

_____
Date

_____
Time

_____
Witness

Signature _____
(Patient / Parent / Conservator / Guardian)

If signed by other than patient, indicate relationship:

_____

AUTHORIZATION FOR AND CONSENT TO SURGERY OR SPECIAL DIAGNOSTIC OR THERAPEUTIC PROCEDURES

FIGURE 7.3

**MEMORIAL HOSPITAL
STERILIZATION PERMIT**

Date _____ Hour _____.M.

I hereby authorize and direct Doctor _____
and assistants of his choice to perform the following operation upon me at the above
named hospital: _____ and to
do any other procedure that his (their) judgment may dictate during the above
operation. It has been explained to me that I may (or will probably) be sterile as a
result of this operation but no such result has been warranted. I understand that the
word "sterility" means that I may be unable to conceive or bear children and in giving
my consent to the operation have in mind the possibility (probability) of such a result.
I absolve said doctor, his assistants and the hospital from all responsibility for my
present condition or any condition that may result from said operation.

Signed _____

Signature Witnessed:

By _____ By _____

I have read the foregoing matter and, as the spouse of the above named patient, do
hereby join in authorizing the performance of the surgery under the terms set forth
and consented to above.

Signed _____

Signature Witnessed:

By _____ By _____

FIGURE 7.4

*D*OCTOR AVAILABILITY

A doctor must be reasonably available to her patients. If a doctor is ill or out of town, she will have to make arrangements for another qualified physician to take care of her patients. The health unit coordinator should make every effort to assist the doctor and her office staff in the communication of messages so that the doctor can be made available to her patients with a minimum of delay.

*T*HE PATIENT'S RECORDS

The patient's chart is a legal document and is the property of the hospital. It must be accepted as evidence of truth in a court of law. The patient's chart should be used only by health workers authorized to do so. To meet the standards of the law the patient's chart must be:

- Complete
- Accurate

- Neat
- Honest
- Legible
- Signed
- In ink

Careful documentation is essential. In a court of law the usual rule is: If it wasn't charted, it didn't happen.

Corrections

If corrections are necessary, the proper technique is to line out the original entry so that it can still be read, make the correction, and initial and date it. **DO NOT ERASE.** Any chart with erasures will not be admitted as legal evidence (Fig. 7.5).

FIGURE 7.5

AVOIDING LITIGATION

Legal actions against health care workers are more common today than ever before. Although legal problems do arise, you as a health unit coordinator should be able to work with confidence after you realize legal problems can often be prevented. Remember:

- Stay within the limits of your training. Do not attempt to give nursing care when you have been trained to work as a health unit coordinator.
- Do not recommend treatment, make a diagnosis, or give a prognosis.
- Consistently practice with conscientious care and with an understanding of the terms *duty of care* and *reasonable care*.
- Obtain written consents.
- Always consider human rights.
- Keep up-to-date, comprehensive, and accurate records.

Sexual Harassment

Sexual harassment can occur in any workplace. According to the U.S. Equal Employment Opportunity Commission (EEOC), it is a form of sex discrimination, and prevention is the best way to eliminate it. Employers should have a process in place so that they can take immediate steps when they receive a complaint from an employee.

Sexual harassment includes actions by another of the opposite or same sex that are unwelcome and can affect a person's employment and work environment. It is a violation of the Civil Rights Act of 1964.

Your hospital will have a policy regarding this issue. Should you be the victim of unwelcome sexual advances or other forms of behavior of an offensive sexual nature, you should, if possible, tell the harasser to stop the behavior immediately. You should also use the complaint and grievance procedure available in your place of employment.

ℰTHICS

Ethics is a code of behavior that represents ideal conduct for a particular group. Each group of health care professionals requiring a license has a code of ethics that has been adopted by its membership. Codes of ethics for different groups have many things in common. They are based on good judgment, reason, and an understanding of the difference between right and wrong.

The National Association of Health Unit Coordinators has adopted the following code of ethics (Fig. 7.6):

National Association of Health Unit Coordinators Code of Ethics

This code of ethics is to serve as a guide by which Health Unit Coordinators may evaluate their professional conduct as it relates to patients, colleagues, and other members of the health care profession. This code of ethics shall be subject to monitoring, interpretation, and periodical revision by the association's Board of Directors.

Therefore, in the practice of our profession, we the members of the National Association of Health Unit Coordinators accept the following principles:

- **Principle One:** Each member shall conduct themselves in such a manner as to gain the respect and confidence of the patients, health care personnel, and the community, as well as respecting the human dignity of each individual.
- **Principle Two:** Each member shall protect the patients' rights, including the right to privacy.
- **Principle Three:** Each member shall strive to achieve and maintain a high level of competency.
- **Principle Four:** Each member shall strive to improve their knowledge and skills by participating in educational and professional activities and sharing the benefits of their attainments with their colleagues.
- **Principle Five:** Unethical and illegal professional activities shall be reported to the appropriate authorities.

FIGURE 7.6 (Printed courtesy of NAHUC)

Ethics deal with moral responsibility. Unethical behavior is not always illegal, but it may reflect unfavorably on the hospital and can result in discipline or even loss of employment.

Legal requirements are set by society. Violation of these requirements can result in legal discipline. Many times the line between ethical behavior and legal requirements is not entirely clear. For example, it would be unethical for a health unit coordinator to ask a nurse to *give* her some of the patients' medications. If she *took* the medications, it would be stealing, which is, of course, illegal.

If a health unit coordinator went to another unit, saw the chart of a neighbor, and read it, this would be unethical. If she talked about the contents of the chart, this would be illegal.

The health worker who consistently practices ethical behavior should not have to worry about meeting the requirements of the law.

Confidentiality

Information acquired in a doctor–patient relationship is considered a confidential or privileged communication. Employees are obligated to safeguard information regarding patients and the hospital.

As a health unit coordinator, you have access to certain clinical and personal patient information. You must be thoroughly aware of the grave responsibility you have of maintaining the confidentiality of all matters relating to patients (Fig. 7.7).

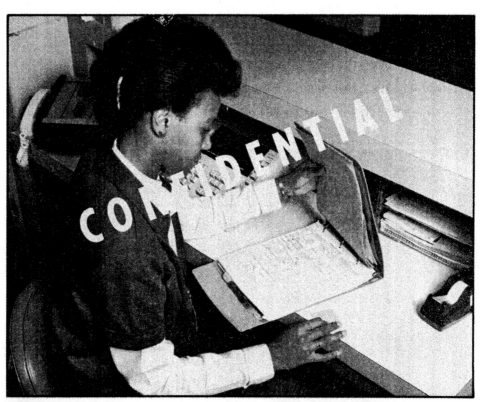

FIGURE 7.7

Ethical behavior means keeping your promises and doing what you ought to do. As a health unit coordinator, you should observe the following code of ethical behavior:

- Be conscientious in the performance of your duties. This means do the best you can.
- Be generous in helping your patients and your fellow workers.
- Carry out faithfully the instructions you are given by the nurse in charge.
- Respect the right of all patients to have beliefs and opinions that might be different from yours.
- Let the patient know that it is your pleasure, not your job, to assist him or her.

LEARNING ACTIVITIES

Match the legal term in Column A with its definition in Column B.

Column A

(a)   Duty of care

(b)   Consent

(c)   Invasion of privacy

(d)   Slander

(e)   Ethics

(f)   Assault

(g)   Negligence

(h)   Privileged
        communication

(i)   Libel

(j)   Battery

(k)   Tort

(l)   Litigation

(m)   Misdemeanor

(n)   Incompetent

(o)   Malpractice

(p)   Felony

Column B

_____ To threaten to injure another person

_____ "Bad practice" by a professional

_____ The highest concept of right and wrong

_____ Information kept in trust by medical
        personnel

_____ Meeting expected standards

_____ Written defamation

_____ Verbal defamation

_____ To make public knowledge any private
        or personal information without
        the individual's consent

_____ A lawsuit

_____ Permission granted by a person
        voluntarily and in his right mind

_____ Private or civil wrong

_____ Unlawful touching of another person
        without his or her consent

_____ Failure to give reasonable care

_____ Major crime

_____ Less serious crime

_____ Want of physical or mental fitness

Complete the following.

1. The principal way in which medicine is regulated by law is through
_____.

2. In a legal sense, the relationship between the doctor and the patient and the
hospital and the patient is _____.

3. The person protected by the law by "reasonable care" is the _____.

4. The person protected by the legal term "duty of care" is the _____.

5. To meet standards of the law the patient's chart must be:
(a) _____
(b) _____
(c) _____

(d) _____
(e) _____
(f) _____
(g) _____

6. The document published by the American Hospital Association with the intent of making both patients and personnel aware of what the patient should be able to expect is called _____.

7. An advance directive is _____.

8. List five ways to prevent involvement with lawsuits.
(a) _____
(b) _____
(c) _____
(d) _____
(e) _____

9. List the four elements of negligence.
(a) _____
(b) _____
(c) _____
(d) _____

True or False. Circle T if the statement is true and F if it is false.
(a) T F To be legal a consent must be an informed consent.
(b) T F Abbreviations may be used on a consent.
(c) T F All persons in the custody of the law must give their consent for treatment.
(d) T F Emancipated minors may give their own consent for medical or surgical treatment.
(e) T F Consents must be in ink.

Choose and circle the one best answer.

1. Health unit coordinators may be said to have acted with reasonable care if they:
(a) Have been a unit manager
(b) Have taken college classes
(c) Have been health unit coordinators for 10 years
(d) Did what other health unit coordinators of similar background would have done under similar circumstances

2. A health unit coordinator decided that since she was not busy she would help the nurses by giving a patient a bedpan. The patient had undergone surgery that morning and was injured when the health unit coordinator turned him improperly. The unit coordinator could have avoided this tragedy if she had:
(a) Obtained a written consent
(b) Asked another unit coordinator to help her
(c) Stayed within the limits of training
(d) Had the patient walk to the bathroom

3. A consent is not valid if the patient, when signing it, can be proven to have been:
(a) Under the influence of sleeping pills
(b) Not mentally competent
(c) Forced to sign
(d) All of these

4. A health care worker read the history on a neighbor's chart and then talked about it at a party. The neighbor accused him of defamation of character. The health care worker was most likely guilty of:
   (a) Assault
   (b) Slander
   (c) Libel
   (d) Abandonment

5. Your child is ill, and you ask the medication nurse to give you some of a patient's medications. This is:
   (a) Malpractice
   (b) Negligence
   (c) Unethical
   (d) Illegal

6. If a health worker were to take the medication, this would be:
   (a) Assault
   (b) Unethical
   (c) Illegal
   (d) (b) and (c)

Consider the following situations. Using the principles of law and ethics, state how you would respond to each.

1. A patient comes to the desk and asks you to come into her room. She says she wants to thank you for being so nice and hands you a $20 bill.

2. You observe a nursing assistant helping herself to a discharged patient's medication that was supposed to have been returned to the pharmacy.

3. You overhear a patient's family members talking in the hall. They say they have retained an attorney and are going to sue the hospital, the patient's doctors, and all the staff who took care of their dad.

4. During change of shift, while you are giving reports to the oncoming unit coordinator, you smell alcohol on her breath *again*.

5. It is Friday and you are scheduled to work the weekend. Friends have just invited you to go with them to their fabulous vacation home for the weekend.

6. A well-known member of your community was admitted to your nursing unit today. Her husband had beaten her up. The police were called and the whole town is talking about it. Your friends know you work at the hospital and are pressuring you to tell them "everything."

7. A relief team leader who works 2 days a week is feeling harassed. She asks you if you will please just go into Mr. Jacobs room and help the old gentleman swallow his meds because she is so behind in her work.

8. The same nurse asks you to call Dr. O'Hearns's office and get the admitting orders on the new patient in room 12B, Mr. Priest.

9. A man who is unknown to you comes up to the desk, says he is a doctor on Mrs. Haxton's case, and asks to see her chart.

10. While delivering some reports to the unit coordinator on the next floor you see a chart with your neighbor's name on it. You are *very* curious about what is wrong with her.

11. A visitor asks you what the diagnosis is of the patient who is in isolation across the hall from his wife.

Communications

Accusatory	Charging someone with fault or blame
Active listening	To hear both the words and the meaning behind the words that are being spoken
Aggressive behavior	Quarrelsome, hostile, offensive actions
Assertive behavior	The use of techniques that require that others recognize one's rights while maintaining a positive atmosphere
Body language	The use of nonverbal expressions such as facial expressions, posture, and gestures in communication
Burnout	A condition that results from chronic stress and characterized by feelings of frustration and an inability to cope
Component	Element or part
Conscientious	To be careful, thorough, dependable; to be led by one's conscience
Divulge	To make known; to tell or reveal a secret
Empathy	To try to put oneself in another's place to try to understand what that person is feeling
Feedback	The repeating of messages or parts of messages to assure understanding of the message
Impede	To get in the way of something
Medical jargon	The technical or specialized language used by a particular group
Negativism	An attitude that resists suggestion and development or improvement
Objective	Goal or what is aimed for
Obstreperous	Unruly and uncontrollably noisy and resisting advice or control
Positive personality	The use of healthy methods of coping with life and relating to others
Selective listening	Hearing only what one wants to hear
Stress	Any change to which one must react
Trivial	Something little or small
Value system	A set of beliefs that one holds to be desirable and correct

When you have completed this chapter, you will be able to:

- Define the terms listed in the vocabulary.
- Define the elements and the components of communication.
- Discuss the responsibilities of both the sender and the receiver in the communication process. List some barriers to communication.
- Define kinesics and the importance of body language in the process of communication.
- Describe the proper use of the telephone and the intercom system.
- Discuss the importance of effective communication.

- Describe the several types of paging systems.
- Discuss written communication and accepted techniques for message taking and composition.
- Compare ways we are alike and different.
- List the possible concerns of the hospitalized patient.
- Discuss various methods of intra- and interdepartmental communication.
- Stress the importance of confidentiality.
- Discuss the importance of effective communication with the patient's family and visitors and rules for dealing with visitors.
- Contrast negative and positive personalities; assertive and aggressive responses.
- Define stress and ways to reduce stress.
- Discuss Maslow's hierarchy of needs.

Communication is one of the fundamental functions you will perform. More than ever in today's busy world of information systems it is essential that you, as the human communication link of your unit, become an expert communicator.

It has been estimated that health unit coordinators communicate with someone at least once every 60 seconds and at the hectic, often heavily populated nurse's station, the health unit coordinator is often challenged to use his or her skills of communication effectively.

We do not all possess the same level of communication skills, but we can learn and practice speaking, listening, and writing. It can be both fun and satisfying to become capable of handling each situation so pleasantly and efficiently that you are recognized for your outstanding reception techniques.

The health unit coordinator is a vital link between the patients and staff of the nursing unit and between the unit, the rest of the hospital, and the outside world (Fig. 8.1).

Communication is defined as the **sending and receiving of a message.** Messages are a very important part of the health unit coordinator's job. It is essential to understand the various means of communication you will use, the type of information you will transmit, and the appropriate procedure in each case because a patient's welfare, or perhaps even his life, may depend on your ability to communicate a message.

$\mathcal{P}$RINCIPLES OF COMMUNICATION

Recall the definition of communication—the sending and receiving of a message. In order for effective communication to take place, both the sender and the receiver must share the responsibility (Fig. 8.2).

1. **Sender**—transmits the message
2. **Symbols**—the writing or words we use to convey a message
3. **Receiver**—receives and interprets the message
4. **Feedback**—the receiver repeats the message to the sender (i.e., interprets) to establish accuracy

Therefore, when a message is sent, the sender turns his ideas into words (symbols) and transmits these words to the receiver. The receiver then must change his words back into ideas. If effective communication has taken place, both ideas will be the same.

FIGURE 8.1 The health unit coordinator serves as a vital link between the nursing unit and the rest of the hospital, doctors' offices, the patients' family and friends, and the community.

FIGURE 8.2

$\mathcal{T}$HE SENDER

As the sender of a message, there are things you can do to make the communication more effective. First, an effective message must have three **objectives** (what it is to achieve) and three **components** (what it is to contain). It must also be conveyed in a manner that will make it easy for the receiver to listen and to understand.

Objectives of an Effective Message

1. **To be understood**—Construct your message in a logical manner and speak or write clearly.

2. **To result in the action that you want**—Your message was ineffective if this does not occur.

3. **To maintain good feelings**—Speak with courtesy and in a pleasant tone of voice at all times.

Components of an Effective Message

1. An effective message must contain all the necessary information.

2. The information must be meaningful to the receiver. Do not use unfamiliar **medical jargon** the receiver may not understand.

3. The message should be simple and should get to the point.

When your responsibility is the sending of verbal messages, practice your skills of communication.

1. Avoid distractions. If you are communicating face-to-face, do not fidget or use distracting hand movements.

2. Look the receiver in the eye.

3. Think about your body language. It is often effective to lean forward when talking to another.

4. Use your personality, and whenever it is appropriate, smile!

$\mathcal{T}$HE RECEIVER

As the receiver of a message, you also have a responsibility to see that effective and satisfying communication takes place. There are many reasons why you may shut out a message:

- The message does not seem important.
- The sender is a poor communicator.
- You are preoccupied with something else.
- You feel defensive or hostile toward the sender.
- The physical environment distracts you.
- Your emotional or physical state may interfere.

Since inadequate or inaccurate communication may directly affect a patient's welfare, you must learn the skills of receiving as well as of sending messages.

1. Really listen to what the sender is saying. To be an **active listener** you must concentrate and not think of other things at that moment.

2. Keep an open mind and don't prejudge.

3. Avoid **selective listening,** which means hearing just what you want to hear.

4. Think about what the message means.

5. Repeat the message as you understand it. *Always* repeat numbers such as telephone numbers and laboratory results.

6. Give **feedback.** Ask questions and get actively involved in the exchange.

7. If the communication is face-to-face, look at the sender. Through your body language, indicate your interest in the message and your willingness to participate in the communication.

BODY LANGUAGE

There are two main avenues of communication—*verbal* and *nonverbal.* Verbal is the use of words in speaking and writing. **Nonverbal communication** is unspoken and includes facial expressions, movements, posture, and gestures. This is called **body language.** Probably the greatest part of communication is nonverbal. Our gestures and expressions are often the truest indicator of our inner feelings no matter what specific words we use.

Kinesics, the study of body language, can be fascinating. You, as the health unit coordinator, as the constant communicator, must be aware of the implications of body language. A smile, a frown, or the way that you sit or stand can reflect such feelings as acceptance, hospitality, or hostility and can enhance or **impede** your ability to communicate effectively.

If your posture is erect when you sit at your desk, if you seem alert, and if you look at others straight in the eye when you talk with them, leaning forward and smiling, your body language is saying, "I like my job. I'm happy to be here, and I want to communicate with you." If you slouch, look away, or use other body gestures that indicate **negativism,** your body language is saying something else.

Integrate your understanding of kinesics with your new information on verbal communication and practice your skills to become the most effective communicator you can be.

METHODS OF COMMUNICATION
THE TELEPHONE

There will be a telephone on each health unit coordinator's desk which is an extension of the hospital's central switchboard. There are similar extensions in all other units and in all the various departments of the hospital, such as the laboratory, radiology, and pharmacy. The **multibutton key telephone** is the most common telephone set used in the hospital because it allows the user to handle several incoming and outgoing calls simultaneously. The buttons at the bottom of the telephone glow intermittently—a steady light indicating lines are in use, or a flashing light indicating a line is on hold. A hold button provides complete privacy by closing off all other extensions and should always be used so that the caller will not overhear conversation at the nurses' station while waiting. This telephone operates as follows:

1. **To place a call:**
   - Choose a line that is not in use—the button will be unlighted.
   - Push down the button (key), pick up the receiver, and dial the number. (*Note:* Your instructor will explain exactly how the telephone works in

your hospital. If you are calling outside the hospital, it is often necessary to dial one or several numbers to get an outside line.)

- If you accidentally choose a line that is on hold, depress the hold key to reestablish the hold.

2. **To answer a call:**
   - Determine the line to be answered by the ring and/or by the lighting of the button at the bottom of the telephone.
   - Before removing the receiver, depress the key for the line to be answered, and speak.

3. **To hold a call:**
   - After picking up the receiver, ask the caller if he or she will please hold the line and wait for a reply.
   - Depress the hold key for 2–3 seconds until you are sure the line is holding. When the call is on hold, both the line and hold key will return to normal positions with the light on.
   - You may now place or answer another call on a different line.

The **Touch-A-Matic Touch Tone telephone** is a multibutton memory telephone that can be programmed to reach frequently called numbers (such as other hospital departments) automatically simply by depressing a single button.

Many hospitals use a system in which outside callers hear a menu of options, giving the button to press for various departments or services, when to dial their party's extension, and to otherwise stay on the line for operator assistance (Fig. 8.3).

FIGURE 8.3

Rules of Telephone Courtesy

One of your most important duties is using the telephone. You will constantly be answering and placing telephone calls and must learn to use the telephone skillfully and courteously. Make a special effort to become expert at using the telephone. Ask yourself how you feel when someone is nice to you on the telephone—when they are helpful and efficient and when their voice is clear and pleasant.

Efficiency and courtesy go hand in hand. If you follow these simple rules and use your common sense, you will find that your work will be done more smoothly and easily.

- Answer all calls promptly.
- Keep a pencil and pad handy so that you can take down messages immediately and avoid omissions and inaccuracies.
- Always be polite. Use courteous terms such as "please" and "thank you." Avoid the use of slang such as "OK" and "bye bye." If someone says "Thank you," say "You're welcome" rather than "No problem," which is less polite.
- Use a pleasant voice at all times. Speak distinctly but do not shout. Hold the mouthpiece about 1 inch from your lips.
- Never answer anger with anger. Be calm, listen, and determine what action can be taken. Smile—it will show in your voice (Fig. 8.4).
- Do not leave the phone untended. If you must leave your station, arrange for someone else to take your calls. Leave word where you can be located and when you will return.

FIGURE 8.4

Answering Incoming Calls

- Answer the telephone by giving your location and your title, "2E Unit Coordinator." If your hospital also wishes you to use your name, you will be so instructed.
- If the caller does not identify himself, always ask "To whom am I speaking?" Then repeat the name as soon as possible.
- If the caller asks for information that you do not immediately have, say, "Will you please hold the line while I get the information?" and wait for a reply. When you return to the phone, thank him for waiting. If it will take you some time to get the information, offer to call back.
- If the call is for someone who is not immediately available, ask the caller whether she prefers to hold the line, to call back, or to leave a message. If she

chooses to wait, return to the line at frequent intervals to give her a chance to leave a message.

■ Never give out information about a patient. Never **divulge** medical orders pertaining to a patient. This rule applies to members of the hospital staff as well as to the patient's family. It is the nurse's responsibility to observe and describe accurately a patient's condition. When information about a patient is requested, say pleasantly but firmly, "Let me get the nurse for you, Dr. Jones," or "I don't know sir, but I will get Miss Smith, the nurse manager. Perhaps she can help you."

■ If you are asked to take a message, or if the caller has some complex instructions for you, write them down promptly.

■ Hospital policy usually states that personal telephone numbers of hospital staff are not to be given out. You should refer such calls to the nurse in charge or hospital supervisor.

Placing Outgoing Calls

■ Keep a list of the other hospital extensions and frequently called outside numbers at your desk. Do not ask information for a number unless you cannot find it yourself.

■ Plan your conversation before you make a call. Know the points you want to cover. Have any records or other materials you may need in front of you.

■ Give the person you are calling ample time to answer before you hang up—about 10 rings. However, do not tie up the line indefinitely hoping someone will answer. If the line is busy, hang up immediately.

■ When the person answers, identify yourself. "This is Miss Brown, Unit Coordinator from 2E." If you are calling outside the hospital, give the name of the hospital rather than the floor.

■ If the person who answers is not the one you want or does not identify himself, ask pleasantly for that person: "May I speak to Dr. Jones, please? This is Miss Brown, Unit Coordinator on 2E."

■ If you want to leave a message for someone, state your name and why you are calling: "This is Miss Brown, Unit Coordinator on 2E. I'd like to leave a message for Dr. Jones." Be sure to state the message clearly. Repeat any part of the message that is lengthy or might be confusing.

Transferring Calls

Do not transfer a call if you can handle it properly yourself. Otherwise:

■ Offer to transfer the caller to someone who can handle the call: "That is handled by our admissions department. If you wish, I can have your call transferred."

■ Be sure that the person knows what you are doing so that she does not think you have disconnected her.

■ If your hospital's telephone system requires that you reach the switchboard operator for the transfer, say: "Will you please transfer this call to the admissions department?"

It is common practice for nursing personnel to carry telephones while on duty. These may be checked out to the individual nurses each shift or kept on the medication and treatment carts. This saves many steps, as calls may quickly be transferred to the nurse who can then pick up calls on the land lines that have been strategically placed on the unit.

PAGING

If asked by the nurse to page a doctor who is elsewhere in the hospital, follow standard procedures for your hospital. Here is one type of paging system:

- Dial "0" to reach the switchboard operator.
- Tell the operator the name of the doctor to be paged and your location. "Please page Dr. Jones for extension 275." The operator will then page the doctor over a public address system.
- Keep the line free until the doctor has called back.

To call departments within the hospital there will be a list of extensions at your desk. To call physicians and other numbers outside the hospital you will use a roster, Rolodex®, or other list that has been compiled for that purpose. You may need to add frequently called numbers to that list.

Another popular system utilizes **individual pocket pagers** worn by physicians and key hospital personnel. To page a person with this system you would call the hospital operator and ask that the doctor or other individual be paged for the unit extension. You may also use the hospital's internal paging system and place the page yourself.

The operator will call the person being paged by dialing a preassigned number that will cause the pocket pager to buzz or beep; your page request will follow. You may punch in the message or the person will dial your extension to receive the message.

The **light system of paging** utilizes a light panel installed at intervals in the hallways of the hospital. Again, doctors and key personnel will have assigned numbers. When the hospital operator receives a message, he or she will light a number in the panel. The person assigned that number will respond by calling the switchboard.

MESSAGE RECORDING AND DELIVERY

An important part of correct telephone procedure is to record messages *accurately*. If possible, always relay any message directly to the person concerned. If the person is not in the nurses' station, take down the message in detail and see that it is delivered as soon as possible.

- Use the hospital message pad.
- Write the date, time, and name of the person for whom the message is intended.
- Be sure your recorded message answers the following five questions: who, what, when, where, and why.
- Listen carefully and repeat all messages to assure accuracy. Always repeat numbers (feedback) because it is common to transpose (switch) them by mistake when writing them down (Fig. 8.5).
- Always ask for the spelling of names when you are in doubt.
- Sign the message with your name and title (Fig. 8.6).

THE INTERCOMMUNICATIONS SYSTEM (INTERCOM)

An intercom system is located at each nurses' station. This system enables the health unit coordinator to have direct communication between the patient's room and the nurses' station. When the patient has a request, the patient signals from the room by

FIGURE 8.5

Date _____ Time _____

To _____
☐ **You were called by**   ☐ **You were visited by**

_____

Phone No. _____
☐ **Please call**   ☐ **Will call you**
☐ **Returning your call** ☐ **Waiting to see you**
MESSAGE:

_____

_____

Call taken by _____*J. Brown HUC*_____

FIGURE 8.6

depressing a button by the bed. When this is done, a light flashes over the room number on the intercom at your desk, and it makes a buzzing sound.

Answering the Intercom

■ Respond promptly by depressing the appropriate key (you will be shown your hospital's system) and say "Unit Coordinator, may I help you?" As in the answering of the telephone, your hospital may wish that you also state your name—"Miss Brown, Unit Coordinator, may I help you?"
■ Listen to the patient's reply.

- Always be courteous. The same general rules apply to the intercom as to the telephone, but remember that this device may be unfamiliar to a patient and he or she may not be accustomed to hearing a voice come out of "the wall."
- Write down the message using the technique for message recording.
- Relay the patient's request to the appropriate personnel.

The Pneumatic Tube

The pneumatic tube is a system in which air pressure sends tubes carrying messages, requisitions, or sometimes supplies from one hospital department to another. You will be instructed in the operation of the pneumatic tube if your hospital utilizes this system.

The Computer

Today computer use in hospitals is universal. The degree to which computers are used varies. Vital information about the patient is entered by the admitting department and added to by other hospital departments during the patient's hospitalization. This information can be retrieved at any time, and hospitals have strict guidelines regarding who has access to the information.

The computer is discussed in Chapter 11.

The Fax

A fax or facsimile is the transmission of a printed document through a telephone line. Both the party sending the fax and the receiver must have a fax machine. Faxes are a quick and efficient way of sending information and are used to transmit documents both within and outside the hospital. Your hospital will have strict guidelines on the use of faxes because of the issue of confidentiality.

To use the fax, place the document face down in the fax machine, dial the number of the receiver, and press the start or send button. The document passes through the sender machine and prints out on the recipient's machine. For this reason, be sure to keep plenty of paper in your machine so it is always ready to receive messages.

Communication within the Nursing Unit

Within the nursing unit some of the most important forms of communication other than the telephone and intercom include:

- **Kardex.** The patient care record card is a consolidated record of all procedures, treatments, medications, and tests for each patient. It is a unit worksheet used by the nursing staff, kept during every patient's stay, and discarded on discharge. The record card may be kept in a Kardex holder, but computerized Kardexes are widely used. A common practice is to print out patient care information on each patient at the beginning of the shift. Nurses keep this information on clipboards or in notebooks, and the paper Kardex is fast becoming obsolete (Fig. 8.7).
- **Assignment sheet.** The use of the assignment sheet was explained in Chapter 2. The assignment sheet tells you which nurse is caring for which patient.
- **Unit chalkboard or other erasable board.** Some nursing units utilize a chalkboard as a method of intradepartmental communication. The chalkboards may either reflect patient care assignments or indicate special information regarding patient care such as patients' schedules for surgery, x-ray, laboratory or other tests, or treatments. Because of the issue of patient confidentiality, this information must not be seen by other patients or by visitors.
- **Unit bulletin board.** Current memos, work schedules, and other appropriate materials are posted on the unit bulletin board. It is usually the health unit coordinator's responsibility to maintain the bulletin board in a neat and attractive manner and to keep the information current (Fig. 8.8).

```
                                        KARDEX          Pg. 1 of 3

  41001   EXAMPLE, IMA         1234567890 66 F ADM-04219   053097 16:49 4MS
  DX ADM BRONCHITIS            ADM  000022 GOODDOCTOR, GEO. AL1 pcn
  DX CUR pneumonia             ATT  000022 GOODDOCTOR, GEO. AL2 asa
    DX1 ARDS                   CON1 000023 ALSOGOOD, ALVIN  AL3 codeine
    DX2                        CON2 000024                  AL4
    DX3                        CON3 000026                  AL5
    DX4                        CON4 000027                  AL6
    SUR1 lobectomy 1995        CON5 000000                  HT 64
    SUR2                       CON6 000000                  WT 150
    SUR3                       CON7 000000
    SUR4                       INVS LNE
  HIST1                        DIAB
  HIST2                                                     IV
  HIST3                        IS TY                        OXYGEN
  HIST4                        COMM                         MRN-00219218

  ----- SKIN ASSESSMENT -----------------!----- ALLERGY/HT/WT -----------------
  ___ Assess skin q shift.               ! ___ Allergies/Ht/Wt entered in Merlin.
                                         !     (If ht/wt/allergies do not show in
  ___ Begin Pressure Ulcer Protocol.     !     upper right hand corner of this
                                         !     Kardex, then they still need to be
                                         !     entered.)
  ----- LABORATORY ----------------------!----- NUTRITION SERVICES -------------
  483 053097 ROUTINE URINE, CREATI-      ! 186 042197 CAFFEINE,BLAND,RESIDUE
      NINE RANDOM COLLECT BY NURSE       !     OR FIBER CONT BLAND LOW RESIDUE
  717 053097 ROUTINE TYPE & SCREEN       ! 296 042197 ORAL NUTRITION /
      COLLECT BY LAB                     !     SUPPLEMENTS - SUSTACAL PLUS
  718 053097 ROUTINE TYPE AND            !     FLUID RESTRICTION
      CROSSMATCH PACKED RBCS             ! 385 042197 STANDARD TUBE FEEDING
  719 053097 STAT CSF PANEL (INCL.       !     FORMULA T.F.PRO CONTINUOUS 40CC/
      CELL CT., GLUC, T.P)               !     HR
  720 053097 STAT CSF IMMUNOSUPPRE-      ! 387 042197 STANDARD PROTOCOL: REG.
      SSED PANEL                         !     DIETITIAN TUBE FEEDING CONSULT
  737 053097 STAT INDIA INK PREP (CSF)!  !1057 051497 STANDARD TUBE FEEDING
  738 053097 STAT CRYPTOCOCCUS           !     FORMULA T.F.PRO CONTINUOUS 40CC/
      ANTIGEN (CSF)                      !     HR
  739 053097 STAT CULTURE/GM. STAIN      !1058 051497 STANDARD PROTOCOL: REG.
      (CSF)                              !     DIETITIAN TUBE FEEDING CONSULT
      053097 STAT CULTURE, FUNGUS        !     TESTING SORT SORTING TEST
      (CSF)                              ! 313 052897 STANDARD TUBE FEEDING
      053097 ROUTINE CULTURE, BLOOD -    !     FORMULA T.F.PRO CONTINUOUS 60CC/
      MUNOSUP (HIV) COLLECT BY NURSE!    !     HR
      053097 ROUTINE CULTURE,            ! 315 052897 STANDARD PROTOCOL: REG.
      SPIRATORY (BRONCH-IMMUNOS)         !     DIETITIAN TUBE FEEDING CONSULT
      ECT BY NURSE                       ! 484 053097 PROTEIN CONTROLLED DIET-
      7 COLLECTION OF AUTOLOGOUS         !     RENAL,HEPATIC 35 GM PRO 2.5 GM
                                         !     K+ FLUID RESTRICTION 700 CC
```

JONES, MARY   0-35721   Rm. 126

FIGURE 8.7

FIGURE 8.8

𝒰NDERSTANDING HUMAN BEHAVIOR

Before we can understand others, it is helpful if we can understand ourselves. Self-understanding is not easy to achieve, however, it is useful to take a good look at ourselves and attempt to assess both our strong and our weak points. In order to improve, we must honestly appraise our personal traits. Before we can be more punctual, we must recognize that we are often late. Before we can benefit from constructive criticism, we must eliminate hostility toward the evaluator.

People are alike in many ways with basic physical and psychological needs, but each person develops his or her own behavior patterns for meeting these needs. Many factors influence our behavior and make us unique individuals, such as hereditary traits; our rate of development; prenatal influences including our mother's general health and habits (drugs, tobacco, and alcohol can cause birth defects); our home conditions and social environment; our interests; and our **value systems.**

Value systems strongly influence a person's behavior and consist of character traits such as honesty and loyalty, beliefs about love, sex, religion, family, and work. Along with this are our internal rules—our OKs and not OKs that are part of the way we view the world. Values and standards of behavior are learned early and modified throughout our lives. It is important to realize that there are vast differences among individuals as a result of these influences on behavior.

In the sense that all of us *share* certain basic needs and have inner pressures that drive us to fulfill these needs, we are alike. In the ways that we strive to *satisfy* these needs, we are all different. We also differ greatly in our expectations and ambitions.

There have been many studies of human behavior, and one of the most famous and useful is a model created by Professor Abraham Maslow. His model is known as Maslow's Hierarchy of Needs and ranks human needs in levels of priority (Fig. 8.9).

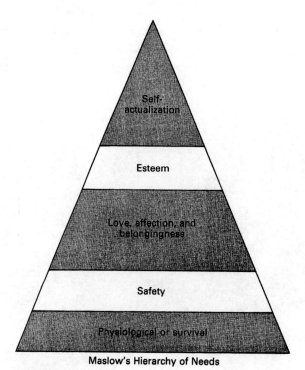

Maslow's Hierarchy of Needs

FIGURE 8.9

In this model, physical or survival needs are most basic; then the need for safety; then love, affection, and belonging; then self-esteem; and finally, self-actualization or the full development of one's potential or talents.

Dr. Maslow believed that each level of need had to be satisfied before an individual could attempt to satisfy the next. A person must be fed, clothed, and safe before he or she can deal successfully with goal-setting, social, and professional needs.

Emotions and Behavior

All of us have emotions—inner feelings that are responses to life situations. They are natural responses that vary in intensity according to what is happening and how we feel about what is happening. They can affect us both physically and mentally, and over a period of time emotions inadequately dealt with can actually make us ill.

Built into our bodies is a reaction to alarm called the *fight or flight* response designed to allow the body to deal with emergencies. The heart and respiration speed up, adrenalin is produced in large amounts, and muscles are prepared for extra activity. This syndrome usually disappears when the emergency passes.

There is another generalized reaction (both physical and emotional) that occurs in response to exciting, frustrating, confusing, demanding, irritating, and pressured outside influences. These influences may be either positive or negative, but the body's reaction does not go away quickly, does not serve a useful purpose, and if allowed to continue, can result in interference with our health. Both these demands on the body and its reaction to them are called **stress.**

For example, improper diet, long and hectic working hours, lack of exercise and recreation and/or a personal support system, alone or in combination, can produce stress. Although some stress is good because it motivates us to accomplish and achieve, too much stress can result in serious physical and psychological problems.

Some physical reactions to stress can include hypertension, gastrointestinal problems, headaches, and reduced resistance to infection. Emotional reactions can include nervousness, tearfulness, depression, anxiety, withdrawal and inability to function, anger, and alcohol and drug abuse.

Burnout is a term often used to describe a state in which a person no longer feels able to cope with his or her circumstances and may suffer decreased energy and productivity.

It is imperative that you learn to combat stress and burnout and use your emotional responses constructively. Eat properly, get plenty of rest and physical exercise, develop hobbies you enjoy, learn to relax, and develop techniques to reduce mental and physical pressures.

Positive versus Negative Personality

A **positive personality** is one that has developed healthy methods of coping with life. All of us are faced with difficulties at one time or another in our lives—financial, family, social, health, and so on. All of us are faced with making decisions and we must constantly analyze our problems and choose paths that we hope will lead us to successful solutions.

Positive people cultivate emotions that make them feel good. They like themselves and others. They try to see the bright side of the situation and they know that there are solutions to problems, and work to make things better.

Positive people don't let others drag them down. They surround themselves with people who are interested in growing and enjoying rather than by negative people who obstruct and complain.

Positive people are assertive. They can communicate with others in a way that declares confidence and strength without being unpleasant. They can disagree without being disagreeable but can stand up for their rights when they feel threatened. **Assertive behavior** is a positive approach to a situation. **Aggressive behavior** is negative and generally offensive.

When you are being assertive, try to use "I" statements to describe how you feel about the situation, and try to avoid "you" statements which may seem accusatory to the receiver.

Example:	Mary, an HUC, works the day shift and is very conscientious. Tom works 3–11:30 and for the last two weeks has been 10 to 15 minutes late, causing Mary to have to work overtime.
Assertive	"Tom—I don't intend to stay late to cover for you when you're late to work. I have to be home on time to pick up my child from the baby-sitter and I won't be late again."
Note	Tom isn't late again. You get treated the way you teach people to treat you.
Aggressive	"Tom—You are always late and you are really a terrible employee," and so on.
Example:	Jim is in an HUC on ICU. A respiratory therapy technician persistently asks him to place her telephone calls to other departments rather than dialing the telephone herself.
Assertive	"Janet—I would prefer not to place your telephone calls for you. I have my own work to do and I know we'll both be more efficient if you make the calls yourself."
Aggressive	"No way! You are asking me to do your work! Forget that!"
Remember	Be assertive and you won't be a victim. But choose your responses carefully. In general, work with a cooperative spirit.

COMMUNICATING WITH THE HOSPITAL STAFF

You have learned a great deal about the art of communications. The relations between yourself and your fellow workers depend on your approach to them. If you have a kind, courteous, tactful, sympathetic, and open manner you will find it easier to form positive relationships.

As a health unit coordinator you will be working with all other members of the hospital staff for one main purpose—to help care for the patients. You should perform all your duties in a spirit of cooperation and follow orders willingly. You should always maintain a professional attitude toward the other members of the staff no matter how well you may come to know them (Fig. 8.10).

Behaving courteously means putting the needs of another person before your own. It means cooperating, sharing, and giving. Being polite and considerate of others shows them that you care about them. Give your fellow workers support and work as a team.

Sometimes another staff member can upset you so much you get angry. You may feel like making a rude remark. *Don't* do it. Stop and think! Your fellow worker may be under stress because of a problem at work or at home. Try to be understanding and let the anger fade.

Learn to take criticism and accept suggestions without feeling you are being attacked. Try to avoid being defensive. Your supervisor may criticize you or tell you to do something. You may feel like saying "That's not my job" or "Why do you pick on me?" Stop, think, and examine your attitude. Calm down. Go ahead and do the right

FIGURE 8.10

thing. Develop a positive, mature attitude. Don't allow yourself to be caught up in the negative attitudes of others. Enjoy your job! (Fig. 8.11).

You will find your fellow workers and other health care personnel more agreeable and helpful if you treat them properly. The following are some good practices:

- Report to the nurse manager or charge nurse whenever you leave the nurses' station or the unit for any purpose and again when you return.
- Take all questions you may have about your work to your head or charge nurse.
- Tell the head or charge nurse about personal problems that you feel might be interfering with your work.

FIGURE 8.11

- Do not talk about your personal problems with other staff members.
- Do not discuss your personal problems with patients or their visitors.
- Follow all instructions you receive from your head or charge nurse.
- Report all complaints from patients and visitors to the head or charge nurse. Never ignore complaints, no matter how insignificant they may seem to you.
- Perform all your duties in the spirit of cooperation, and follow orders willingly.
- Accept tasks assigned to you without complaint.
- Follow the advice of your supervisors.
- Show a willingness to learn.

COMMUNICATING WITH THE PHYSICIAN

As a health unit coordinator you are in a position that requires frequent communication with the various physicians who visit the nursing unit.

Doctors are highly educated, dedicated, and busy individuals who come to the nursing units to visit their patients and to prescribe examinations and treatments to aid in the patient's recovery.

The health unit coordinator who learns the doctors' names, and their desire for speed and accuracy, and is willing and able to assist each doctor as efficiently and courteously as possible will do much to preserve or improve communication between the medical and nursing staffs (Fig. 8.12).

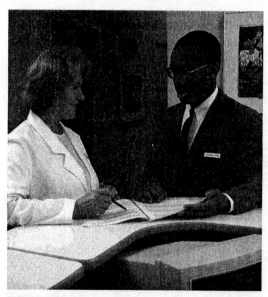

FIGURE 8.12

PATIENT RELATIONSHIPS

Relating to people means making a connection between yourself and another human being; putting yourself in another's place—**using empathy.**

Many things make a difference in a patient's behavior and attitude during an illness. The patient may be frightened, angry, or sad. Some factors are the diagnosis, seriousness of the illness, age, culture, previous illnesses, past experience in hospitals, and the patient's mental condition. Other things that can make a difference are the patient's personality and disposition and perhaps his financial condition.

Each patient is different in her reaction to pain, treatment, annoya
kindness. Always treat each patient as an individual—a person who ne
Practice the special kind of consideration that all patients need on an in
(Fig. 8.13).

What
a patient
worries
about...

Diagnosis

Being
uncertain
of the
future

Family
problems

Money

Medical
treatment

Job

Pain
from
illness

Sharing
intimate
details
of his
life

FIGURE 8.13

Although you will not have as much direct contact with patients as the nursing
personnel do, you will, however, greet newly admitted patients, speak with them frequently over their intercom, and perhaps enter their rooms to deliver mail or perform
some other occasional nonnursing task.

You represent the entire hospital: the patient's reaction to you may influence his
opinion of the whole hospital (Fig. 8.14).

Remember:

- Always be courteous.
- Greet patients pleasantly and address them by name. Do not use first names
(except those of children) unless you are asked to do so.
- Introduce yourself to patients and explain your position and how you may be
of service.
- Do not disturb patients by being noisy. Keep your voice down and avoid slam-
ming drawers and doors.
- Be friendly but avoid becoming too familiar with the patients. This means that
you do not discuss your personal life with the patients.
- Never ignore a patient who speaks to you about a problem, whether it concerns
her own condition or another member of the staff. All complaints must be relayed to the nurse, no matter how **trivial** or unreasonable they may seem to you.
- Relay all requests from patients for equipment or care to the nurse. You are
not authorized to handle such requests yourself.

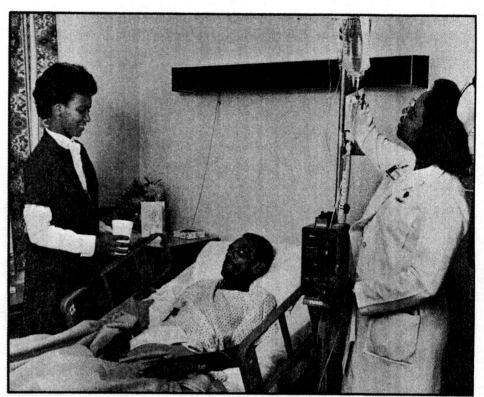

FIGURE 8.14

- Relay questions regarding hospital charges to the business office.
- There are certain privileges and restrictions that apply to particular patients, for example, VIPs, or someone on police hold.
- Keep all information about a patient confidential.

𝒫ATIENT REQUESTS

In handling patient requests, you must distinguish between those that are **medical** and must be referred to the nurse, and those that are **nonmedical** that you will be able to handle yourself. If you are in any doubt, ask the nurse.

There are many things that a patient may ask for that seem to you to be totally unrelated to his treatment (e.g., raising or lowering the bed, opening or closing the window, getting a drink of water or an additional pillow). There may, however, be good medical reasons for denying these requests. Explain to the patient that you are the health unit coordinator and that you will relay his request to a nurse who will help him. **Remember that if as a health unit coordinator you attempt to give nursing care, you are functioning outside your scope of training.**

Be sure to keep your word and deliver the message as quickly as possible to the appropriate nursing personnel.

𝓡ELATIONSHIPS WITH VISITORS

Your direct contact with not only patients but with their visitors requires complete dedication to the rules of courtesy and kindness. Remember that they are often worried and uncomfortable. The hospital environment is unfamiliar, and the staff are probably unknown to them.

Visiting hours are often the highlight of the day for patients. Knowing her family and friends are interested and concerned about her can do a lot to relax her tensions, ease her feelings of loneliness or isolation, relieve her fears, and cheer her spirit.

Visitors may be worried and upset over the illness of a member of the family. They need your kindness and patience. Pleasant comments about flowers or gifts brought by visitors for the patient may be helpful. Make all visitors feel welcome in the hospital.

If the patient is seriously ill or is an obstetrical patient, visiting hours may be different. Your instructor will tell you about the visiting hours and any rules for visitors in your health care institution. These rules, of course, must be followed. Three main rules usually apply to visitors in all health care institutions:

1. Visitors are not allowed to take institutional property away with them.

2. Visitors are not allowed to give nursing or medical care to a patient (they may help with care with the doctor's or nurse's permission).

3. Visitors may not bring food or drink to the patient unless permission has been given by the nurse.

Actions Helpful in Visitor Contacts

■ Listen to the family member. Whether it is a suggestion, a complaint, or "passing the time of day," listen to the person. Some suggestions by visitors can be very helpful. Some complaints may be valid, others not. When a complaint is first presented, you probably need to get more information. You might ask, "Where did this happen?" or "What did you do?" Say to the person, "I will tell the nurse manager about this," and then report it to the nurse in charge.

■ If the visitor asks for a patient's room number, check to be sure there have been no changes. Give the visitor the room number and directions to help find it.

■ Do not get involved in the family's private affairs and feelings. Never take sides in family quarrels. Never give information or opinions to someone about other family members.

■ When a visitor comes to the desk, stop whatever you are doing, direct your attention to the visitor, and answer his questions. Always let the visitor know he is welcome in the hospital; do not give the impression that he has interrupted you.

■ Be prepared to give information to visitors. Tell them under what circumstances family members are allowed to eat in the employee cafeteria. Mention where the coffee shop is and what hours it is open. Tell them where the public telephone is. Direct them to other places in the institution (e.g., the public restrooms, business office, gift shop, or chapel) (Fig. 8.15).

■ Avoid assuming familial relationships until you know who the visitor is. It is best to say, "Mr. Brown is in room 200" rather than "Your husband is in room 200."

■ Remember that a "significant other" may be the most important member of a patient's family.

Visitor Situations

Situations will arise occasionally that you cannot handle alone. Sometimes visitors, in their concern for the patient, will be very critical and complain about the care being given, the quality of the meals, the room location, and so on. If a polite answer from you does not seem to suffice, call the nurse in charge.

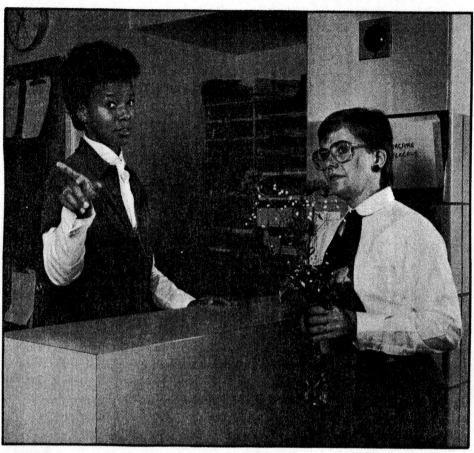

FIGURE 8.15

If you feel that a particular visitor upsets the patient in any way, report it to the head nurse. Certain visitors must sometimes be restricted from seeing the patient.

Drunken or **obstreperous** visitors may disturb patients. Notify your head nurse or, when necessary, call the hospital security guard to remove the visitor.

If a visitor falls or is injured on hospital property, get a nurse immediately to help her. In such cases, there are additional procedures you must follow; these will be explained on page 225.

RELATIONSHIPS WITH CHILDREN AND THEIR PARENTS

Several important things need to be considered and remembered with the pediatric patient (Fig. 8.16):

- Parents need to be with their children, and children need their parents.
- Parents are normally concerned and often are worried, frightened people.
- Most children first learn about the world from their parents.
- The younger the child, the more he needs his parents.

There are several things the unit coordinator can do to help:

- Do the best possible job of caring for the child. This is usually reassuring to the parents.

FIGURE 8.16

- Show interest and concern about the parents' welfare. Ask, "Is there anything we can do for you?"
- Do not make judgments about the parents' attitudes or behavior, even if they seem strange to you.
- Sometimes parents seem to be worried about something concerning their child in the hospital and are afraid to talk about it. If you suspect this, tell the nurse in charge.
- Help provide for children's safety at all times (Fig. 8.17).

FIGURE 8.17

*L*EARNING ACTIVITIES

Complete the following.

1. Define communication. _____

2. List the four elements of communication.
   (a) _____
   (b) _____
   (c) _____
   (d) _____

3. In order to be an effective listener you must first _____

   _____.

4. List the three components of an effective message.
   (a) _____
   (b) _____
   (c) _____

5. List eight general rules of telephone courtesy.
   (a) _____
   (b) _____
   (c) _____
   (d) _____
   (e) _____
   (f) _____
   (g) _____
   (h) _____

6. List three rules for answering the telephone.
   (a) _____
   (b) _____
   (c) _____

7. List three rules for placing a call.
   (a) _____
   (b) _____
   (c) _____

8. When answering the telephone or placing a call, you must always _____ yourself.

9. When placing a call outside of the hospital, you always state the _____ first.

10. The device that allows direct communication between the nurses' station and the patient's room is the _____.

11. When you take a message, you must always _____ numbers.

12. The health unit coordinator may never discuss a patient with _____

    _____

13. The health unit coordinator may discuss a patient only with _____

    _____

14. List five concerns a patient may have while in the hospital.
    (a) _____
    (b) _____
    (c) _____
    (d) _____
    (e) _____

15. List two rules that apply to all visitors.
    (a) _____
    (b) _____

Determining Responses to Hospital Situations

Discuss how you would handle each of the following situations.

1. A visitor lights a cigarette and smokes it in the hallway of the nursing unit.

2. The doctor reprimands you because the lab results for his patient are not on the chart.

3. You call the laboratory and they swear they never received the order.

4. A patient calls on the intercom and says he has asked for pain medication three times and still hasn't received it and he is really angry!

5. The hospital supervisor asks you to "float" to another floor for the rest of your shift because the regular unit coordinator got sick and went home.

6. A nursing assistant asks you to help one of her patients to the bathroom.

7. A patient's visitor comes to the desk holding an empty water pitcher.

8. A patient's daughter asks you if you think her mother is going to die.

9. Another unit coordinator tells you that she overheard the nurses saying they were going to be cutting back on staff.

10. The hospital calls you at home and tells you not to come in to work because the census is low.

11. You can't read a doctor's writing on the chart and she is just walking down the hall on the way to the elevator.

12. A visitor asks you where the gift shop is located.

13. Friends of Joe Doyle (in room 342) walk in carrying a large pizza.

14. A patient complains to you because his roommate is playing the radio too loud.

15. A visitor loudly complains to you about the care she is getting "at this hospital."

Telephone Practice

Pretend that you are the health unit coordinator and handle the following telephone situations:

1. A friend of a patient calls to ask about her condition. She also wants to know what is wrong with the patient and whether she is going to have to have surgery.

2. Dr. Know calls and wants to talk to the nurse caring for his patient in 212. The nurse is at lunch.

3. The laboratory calls with stat results on your patient, Mr. Behncke. The doctor left instructions that her office was to be called immediately with the results.

4. Radiology calls and wants to know whether Mrs. Pothier's prep for the barium enema was successful.

5. The head nurse asks you to call Acme Ambulance Company. They are to transport your patient, Mr. Blackstone, to Riversweet Convalescent Hospital today.

6. Mr. O'Hearn, the husband of a patient from your floor who is in surgery, calls to find out what time she is expected back from the recovery room.

7. Dr. Merryweather calls to find out how his patient, Mr. Gomez, is doing.

8. Mr. Goldstein calls to find out what time visiting hours are so that he can visit his wife. He asks if it is all right to bring in a hot water bottle.

9. Dr. Chino calls and starts to give you admitting orders on his new patient.

10. OR calls and says they are ready to pick up Mrs. Henry, and they say that she should have her on-call medicine.

11. The nurse asks you to call dietary and order a low-salt 1500-calorie diet for Miss Strong in room 440.

12. Dr. Amada asks you to call Dr. Morgan at her office and arrange for a consultation. The patient is Linda Bowman, age 48, room 610, diagnosis—acute pyelonephritis. Dr. Morgan is a urologist.

13. Admitting calls and says they have a new patient coming to the floor stat and you will have to move two men together to open up a room for a female.

14. Dr. Petrillo asks you to get the "old charts" on his new admit, Ida Aiken, in room 4A.

15. Mr. Teacher, the Education Director, calls and says that the staff meeting for this afternoon has been rescheduled for next Tuesday in the cafeteria at 4:30 P.M.

16. Mary, the health unit coordinator, listens carefully to Dr. Phillips, the tired and hurried doctor. She gives Dr. Phillips her full attention by concentrating and listening not only to the words but to the feeling behind the words. Mary is using _____ listening.

17. To repeat messages or parts of messages is to use _____.

18. Nonverbal communication such as facial expressions and gestures is called

_____.

19. Hearing only what we want to hear is called _____ listening.

20. The specialized language used among people in the health care industry is called _____.

21. Rank the five basic human needs according to Maslow, beginning with the most basic.
   (a) _____
   (b) _____
   (c) _____
   (d) _____
   (e) _____

22. Any change to which we must react is called _____.

23. A state of stress in which a person can no longer cope with his or her circumstances is called _____.

24. Stating your needs using "I" statements pleasantly but with confidence and strength is using _____ behavior.

25. Using "you" statements in an offensive and accusatory way is _____ behavior.

26. List six ways to work cooperatively with your coworkers.
   (a) _____
   (b) _____
   (c) _____
   (d) _____
   (e) _____
   (f) _____

27. List three ways to preserve or improve communication with a physician.
   (a) _____
   (b) _____
   (c) _____

28. Define empathy. _____

29. List six ways to work well with patients.
   (a) _____
   (b) _____
   (c) _____
   (d) _____
   (e) _____
   (f) _____

30. List three ways the health unit coordinator can help in working with children and their parents.
   (a) _____
   (b) _____
   (c) _____

31. Think of someone you know who has a positive personality. What kinds of behavior does he or she exhibit? Do you like to be around that person and why? _____

_____

_____

_____

_____

_____

32. Now, think of someone you know who has a negative personality. What is it about his or her behavior that makes you think of him or her? Do you like to be around that person?

_____

_____

_____

_____

_____

_____

33. What can one do to develop a more positive personality? List as many things as you can think of. Why is this important in terms of your job?

_____

_____

_____

_____

_____

_____

_____

_____

_____

_____

Hospital Safety and Emergencies

Cardiac arrest The sudden stopping of the heart and therefore the circulation

Code blue Term used to indicate a cardiac or respiratory arrest

Combustible Easily capable of burning

Crash cart An emergency cart kept on nursing units and in other patient care areas that contains emergency equipment and supplies to be used only in emergency situations

Defibrillator A device that is used to shock the heart into a more normal rhythm in the event that the heart goes into certain dangerous arrhythmias

Ergonomics The science of fitting the job to the worker

Incident In the hospital, an unusual occurrence

OSHA Occupational Safety and Health Administration

Quality occurrence report An incident report; a written report of an unusual occurrence

Repetitive Something done over and over

Respiratory arrest The stopping of breathing

Resuscitate To revive or bring back

WMSD Work-related musculoskeletal disorder

OBJECTIVES

When you have completed this chapter, you will be able to:

- Define the terms listed in the vocabulary.
- State the purpose of OSHA and list three OSHA-required programs.
- List the general rules of hospital safety.
- State the general rules of good body mechanics.
- Explain what you can do to prevent fires.
- Explain what to do in case of fire.
- Define PASS and RACE.
- Discuss your responsibilities during a medical emergency.
- Define and discuss the International Code.

OSHA

The **Occupational Safety and Health Administration (OSHA)** is a part of the U.S. Department of Labor. OSHA's stated mission is to save lives, prevent injuries, and protect the health of America's workers. To that end OSHA has established guidelines so that employers can provide a safe working environment for their employees. OSHA is concerned with every aspect of employee safety in the workplace. OSHA requires hospitals to maintain an Exposure Control Program designed to reduce the possibility of exposure to bloodborne pathogens (see Chapter 6); a Hazard Communication Program that mandates that employees be informed of chemical hazards in the environment and how they can be protected from them; and an Injury and Illness Prevention Program that includes the information necessary for the employee to protect him- or herself from the hazards in the workplace. All these programs have reporting, record-keeping, and employee-training components.

GENERAL SAFETY REGULATIONS

In hospitals, as everywhere, it is easier to take precautions against accidents than to handle them after they occur. By constantly being on the alert for potentially dangerous situations, you can do a great deal toward maintaining safe conditions for the patients, visitors, and the entire hospital staff (Figs. 9.1 to 9.3).

SAFE MOVEMENT WITHIN THE HOSPITAL

- Walk! Never run in the hallways. Running in the halls may cause injury to yourself or others or may create panic in the hospital.
- Walk on the right side of the hall—not more than two abreast. Be cautious of intersections. In doing this you should avoid traffic jams, collisions, and injury to yourself or others.
- Use handrails when using the stairs so that you won't fall and injure yourself.
- Watch out for swinging doors that can hit you or someone else and cause injury.

USE CAUTION AT INTERSECTIONS

FIGURE 9.1

BE SAFETY CONSCIOUS AT ALL TIMES

FIGURE 9.2

WATCH OUT FOR SWINGING DOORS

FIGURE 9.3

*O*THER SAFETY MEASURES

- Keep stairs and halls clear of equipment and obstructions. An apparatus that has been used for patient care should be returned to its proper place as soon as possible. Housecleaning equipment must not be left where people might trip over it.
- Wipe up spilled liquids or have wet floors mopped dry as necessary (Fig. 9.4).
- Do not leave rubber bands, paper clips, or other objects lying on the floor.
- Have burned-out light bulbs replaced immediately.
- Never try to repair or adjust any electrical equipment yourself. Call the maintenance department. Stand away from light fixtures while they are being repaired or while bulbs are being changed.
- If an electric extension cord must be used, never suspend or drape the cord so that it hangs over steam pipes or sharp metal hooks. Lay it where it will not be pinched off by a closed door. Make sure it does not become a tripping hazard.
- Sweep up broken glass immediately; do not pick it up with your fingers. Wrap glass particles in heavy paper and label for disposal. Glass that shatters into fine pieces can be blotted up with damp toweling (Fig. 9.4).

FIGURE 9.4

- Do not use electrical cords that are frayed or damaged. Disconnect the cord and report it to the maintenance department immediately.
- Do not sit on the edge of, or too far back in, your chair.
- Keep desk and file drawers closed when not in use.
- Do not tolerate roughhousing. Report any observed to the nurse in charge.
- Report immediately any unsafe conditions you may notice.
- If there are children on your nursing unit, be especially alert to potential hazards.
- If you must transport a patient by wheelchair, be sure to set the brakes on the wheels when moving the patient into or out of the wheelchair.
- If you are injured, even slightly, report the injury to the nurse in charge. In most cases you will be asked to visit the emergency department, be examined by a doctor, and complete an employee accident report. This is very important to the hospital's safety program and for the employment compensation claims.

BODY MECHANICS

Body mechanics refers to ways of standing and moving one's body to make the best use of strength and avoid injury and fatigue. It is important to understand the rules of good body mechanics and to learn to apply them in your work. You will be less tired at the end of the day and will avoid injury to your body. According to the Bureau of Labor Statistics more than 1 million workers injure their backs every year.

So, before you lift, *think*. Plan every step before you lift physically:

1. Size up the load. Does it weigh more than would be safe for you to lift?

2. Check the pathways. Look for obstacles and choose a clear, safe route.

3. Solve repetitive problems. Think through your job tasks and find a smarter way. Try to lift less and save your back.

4. Find a better way. Get help from someone else or arrange for mechanical help.

RULES TO FOLLOW FOR GOOD BODY MECHANICS

- Use good posture. Keep your body aligned properly. Stand with your feet about 6 to 8 inches apart to increase your base of support. Keep your head erect, pull your shoulders back, and tuck in your abdomen and buttocks. This will tilt the pelvis forward, help straighten the curve of the back, and decrease muscle strain.

- When an action requires physical effort, try to use as many muscles or groups of muscles as possible. For example, use both hands rather than one hand to pick up a heavy object.

- Try to place the thing to be lifted between the area of the knees and shoulders. Lifting something above the shoulders or below the knees is harder on the back.

- When you have to move a heavy object, it is better to push it, pull it, or roll it rather than to lift and carry it.

- When you must bend, widen your base of support by putting your feet 6 to 8 inches apart and one foot slightly forward. Bend at the knees, keep your back straight, and balance your weight evenly on both feet. When you use this technique you will provide yourself with the stability to keep your balance. This technique makes use of the stronger thigh and leg muscles rather than weaker back muscles that are used if you bend at the waist.

- When you lift an object:
  Squat close to the load
  Keep your back straight
  Grip the object firmly
  Hold the load close to your body
  Lift smoothly by pushing up with your strong leg muscles
  If you think you may not be able to lift the load, get help.
  When in doubt—don't! (Fig. 9.5).

- When you want to change the direction of movement:
  Pivot (turn) with your feet
  Turn with short steps
  Turn your whole body without twisting your back or neck (Fig. 9.6).

FIGURE 9.5

FIGURE 9.6

Good Posture Tips

Sitting: Try to avoid prolonged positions that put stress on your back. At your desk adjust your chair height so that you feel comfortable and aren't reaching or slouching. Your knees should be level with your hips. Support your back so you can sit up straight, and every so often get up and walk around. Sitting is one and a half times harder on the back than walking or standing.

Do some isometric exercises at your desk. Begin at your toes, tighten your muscles for a couple of seconds, and then relax. Repeat this exercise until you've worked your way up to your head. Even tighten your face and relax. Done several times a day, this is hardly noticeable and is an excellent stress reducer.

Standing: Adjust your posture by placing your head and back against a wall. Move your pelvis forward and bend your knees a little so that your back touches the wall. Tighten your abdominal muscles. This is the posture you should assume when standing.

*E*RGONOMICS

Ergonomics is the science of fitting the work to the worker. Workers who must perform repetitive motions or do their work in an uncomfortable position are among those most likely to develop **work-related musculoskeletal disorders (WMSDS)**.

Often, simple changes in the work environment such as adjusting the height of the work or varying duties and encouraging breaks from **repetitive** action can reduce ergonomic-related problems.

*F*IRE SAFETY AND PREVENTION

The common causes of fire are smoking and matches, heating and cooking equipment, electrical equipment and appliances, rubbish, trash, and flammable liquids. Each member of the hospital staff has a responsibility to see that proper care is taken in the use of equipment or materials that could cause fires (Fig. 9.7).

IT TAKES THREE THINGS
TO START A FIRE ...

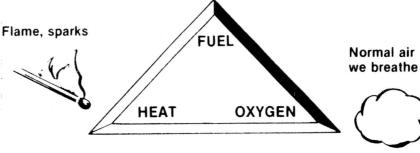

FIGURE 9.7

Fire safety means two things:

- Preventing fires
- Doing the right things if a fire breaks out.

*G*ENERAL FIRE SAFETY RULES

- Hospital smoking regulations should be strictly observed and enforced. Smoking is permitted only in designated places; never when oxygen is in use. Never empty ashtrays into plastic bags or containers of rubbish that can burn. *Smoking is the number one cause of fires in health care institutions.* Most hospitals have a strict nonsmoking policy (Fig. 9.8).

FIGURE 9.8

■ Report any electrical equipment that does not seem to be functioning properly to the maintenance department. A small spark, dimming or flickering lights, the smell of smoke, or the sense of extreme heat are all warning signals that should not go unheeded (Fig. 9.9).

FIGURE 9.9

■ Be sure flammable liquids are stored in the proper place with all caps or lids on tight. Keep all **combustibles** away from a potential source of heat.
■ See that rubbish and trash are removed frequently. A small spark landing on an accumulation of paper, rags, or other combustible trash can start a fire immediately.
■ Be familiar with your institution's fire plan (Fig. 9.10).

*I*N CASE OF FIRE

Fire strikes with a suddenness that demands immediate action. Part of your orientation program as a new employee will include information on what to do if a fire starts. You must know *what* to do and *how* to do it. Familiarize yourself with your hospital's fire policy so that in the event of a fire you will be confident of your ability to meet the crisis.

Alarm Boxes

At least one fire alarm box is located on the wall in your nursing unit. When the alarm is activated, it may sound automatically throughout the hospital or at a specific alarm control center. Know the location of your fire alarms and how to use them.

Extinguishers

Fire extinguishers are located at intervals throughout the hospital. Most hospitals have fire extinguishers that are rated A, B, and C, or ABC, depending on the type of fire to be extinguished.

FIRE SAFETY PLANNING

- **Know the floor plan of your department and the hospital as a whole**
- **Pay particular attention to exit routes**

FIRE

- **Know the exact location of fire alarms and fire extinguishing devices**
- **Know how to report a fire**
- **Know the emergency plan of your hospital and what you should do according to this plan**

FIGURE 9.10

Type A—Wood, paper, and cloth fires

Type B—Burning liquids

Type C—Electrical fires

Type ABC extinguishers may be used on all types of fires.

The acronym PASS is used to help personnel remember the steps to take in using a fire extinguisher.

P   Pull the pin on the upper handle.

A   Aim low. The nozzle should be pointed at the base of the fire.

S   Squeeze the handle of the extinguisher to release the fire retardant.

S   Sweep the nozzle from side to side while aiming at the base of the fire.

Fire Doors

Fire doors are specially constructed doors to separate one unit from another and one floor from another, to contain a fire and prevent its spread. Fire doors are designed to close automatically, and although they are used in normal passageways, they should never be wedged open.

FIGURE 9.11

Exit Routes

Somewhere on your unit, there will be a hospital map indicating the correct exit routes from your nursing unit in case it becomes necessary to evacuate the building or area. Learn these directions *thoroughly*.

*Y*OUR PRIORITIES IN CASE OF A FIRE

Another acronym, RACE, can be used to help staff remember what steps to take in a fire.

R   Remove the patient from the area of the fire.
A   Activate the alarm and Alert other staff about the fire.
C   Confine or Contain the fire by closing doors in the area of the fire.
E   Extinguish the fire if you can do so safely.

Also:

- Follow the instructions of the nurse in charge. These may include checking the fire doors to be sure they are closed, and closing the doors to patients' rooms.
- Return to the desk and remain alert for the signal to evacuate the patients from the unit.
- Keep the telephone lines open.
- Follow the fire emergency procedure for your hospital.
- Do not panic—lives could depend on your actions in an emergency.

MEDICAL EMERGENCIES

If a patient undergoes a sudden crisis such as hemorrhage, shock, prolonged convulsions, or severe trauma you may be asked to reach the doctor immediately. Follow the instructions of the nurse in charge. Keep the intercom open between your desk and the patient's room and prepare for emergency orders.

CARDIAC ARREST

Hospitals are equipped to handle cardiac arrest emergencies. When a patient's heart stops beating, it is called a **cardiac arrest.** When a patient stops breathing, it is called a **respiratory arrest.**

When a cardiac or respiratory arrest occurs in your nursing unit, you will be told to notify the switchboard to page the cardiac arrest team. Many hospitals have a special number you will dial (a hot line to the switchboard especially designated for cardiac arrests only); you will say "**code blue,**" then the room and the number—i.e., "code blue, Room 100." The nursing staff may say the patient has "coded."

When this message is broadcast, a team of specially trained doctors, nurses, respiratory therapists, and other predesignated personnel will hasten to your unit. Within a short time the necessary equipment will be assembled, and the cardiac arrest team will start to work to save the patient's life.

A **crash cart** (an emergency cart) (Fig. 9.12) containing emergency supplies such as drugs, portable oxygen, resuscitation bags, and boards for external cardiac massage will be brought to the bedside. A machine called a **defibrillator,** designed to produce an electrical shock to restart the patient's heart, will be on the emergency cart and is frequently used in these emergencies. Special forms are used to document the event (Fig. 9.13).

The health unit coordinator must remain at the desk, keep the intercom to the patient's room open for direction, be prepared for rapid emergency orders, and possibly direct visitors from the room in which the emergency is occurring. If the patient survives the cardiac arrest and is successfully **resuscitated,** the health unit coordinator should anticipate that the patient may be transferred to the coronary care unit.

CARDIOPULMONARY RESUSCITATION (CPR)

The American Red Cross and the American Heart Association offer classes on CPR—a method of saving lives. Most health care institutions require their employees to take these classes, which are often available at the hospital. This is valuable training that may some day enable you, on or off the job, to save a life.

FIGURE 9.12

*I*NTERNATIONAL HOSPITAL CODE SYSTEM

The International Hospital Code System is used to alert the staff to four major emergency situations. This system is used all over the world to report these emergencies. The four codes are:

1. **Code Red** means that there is a fire in the hospital.

2. **Code Blue** means that someone has stopped breathing (respiratory arrest), the heart has stopped beating (cardiac arrest), or both have happened.

3. **Code Yellow** means there is an uncontrolled individual or a threatening situation.

4. **Code Green** means that a specially designated team of people in the hospital should report to the *triage area*. Each hospital has picked a particular area to use when a disaster occurs. Patients are sorted out for treatment according to the severity of their injury in the triage area.

The health unit coordinator must know the meaning of the International Codes and how to report the codes according to individual hospital policy.

"CODE" REPORT AND CPR FLOW SHEET

Date _____

Est. Time of arrest

Arrest observed: Yes   No

Cardiac Arrest: Yes   No

Pulmonary Arrest: Yes   No

Resuscitation Successful   Yes   No

Disposition of Pt. _____   Place _____   Time _____

CPR Started within one minute _____

CPR Stopped _____

Physician in charge _____

Medication Nurse/Title _____

Recording Nurse/Title _____

Respiratory Therapist _____

Intubation   Yes   No   Et tube No. _____   Time _____   Intubation By: _____

Time	Pulse	BP	Rhythm	ABG Sent	Defibrillation watts secs	NA HCO3 - 1meq /cc IV Push - 50 cc	Epinephrine 1:10,000 IV Push Amp 10cc	Epi 1:1000 or 1:10,000 ET/c/SL ___cc	Lidocaine 100 mg 10cc IV Push	Calcium Chloride 10% / 10cc	Atropine 1 mg/ 10cc IV Push	IV SOLUTIONS						NURSE'S NOTES (Ph, PO₂, PCO₂, Color, Mental Status Temp, Pupils, procedures, ETC)
												Lidocaine ___gm ___cc	Dopamine ___mg ___cc	Isuprel ___mg ___cc				

CARDIO – PULMONARY RESUSCITATION FLOW SHEET

Page _____ of _____

FIGURE 9.13

*I*NCIDENTS

An **incident** is any event that is not consistent with the routine operation of the hospital or the routine care of the patients. It may be an accident to a patient or to a visitor, a theft, or another unusual event involving patients, visitors, or members of the hospital staff. The following are some examples of incidents:

- A patient or visitor is injured inside the hospital or an outlying hospital property such as sidewalks, parking lots, or entrances.
- There is a theft involving a patient, visitor, or hospital employee.
- A patient loses or misplaces property such as a hearing aid or false teeth.
- A nurse makes a medication error.

Whenever an incident occurs, a written report must be made. This is very important to the safety program of the hospital and so that the hospital can be prepared for possible lawsuits.

Incident or **quality occurrence reports** must be complete and accurate. They will be prepared under the direction of the nurse in charge. Nursing administration and the patient's physician are notified; a copy of the report is sent to the hospital's attorney (Fig. 9.14).

*L*EARNING ACTIVITIES

Complete the following.

1. Describe the mission of OSHA. _____
_____

2. List three programs OSHA requires hospitals to have.
(a) _____
(b) _____
(c) _____

3. List 10 general rules of hospital safety.
(a) _____
(b) _____
(c) _____
(d) _____
(e) _____
(f) _____
(g) _____
(h) _____
(i) _____
(j) _____

4. List three rules for lifting.
(a) _____
(b) _____
(c) _____

5. List three rules for changing direction.
(a) _____
(b) _____
(c) _____

I. OCCURRENCE:			(IF NO PLATE)		STATUS	
DATE	TIME	LOCATION	NAME		☐ INPT ☐ OUT PT	☐ VISITOR ☐ OTHER

AGE	SEX ☐ M ☐ F	Diagnosis or Procedure	Witness Yes ☐ No ☐ Name _____ Dept. _____

Condition Prior to Occurrence ☐ Alert ☐ Disoriented ☐ Asleep ☐ Anesthetized	Meds last 12 hrs (falls only)

II.

MEDICATION (all that apply)

☐ Wrong medication
☐ Wrong amount ☐ Wrong
☐ Wrong pt   date/time
☐ Wrong route
☐ Transcription error
☐ Allergic reaction
☐ Omission
☐ Incorrect narcotic count
☐ Other _____
Name of Med

Consent:
_____
☐ None written
☐ Mismatch
☐ Refused to sign
☐ Incomplete
☐ Other
_____

AMA

☐ AMA signed
☐ Not signed
☐ AWOL
☐ Other

INTRAVENOUS (Note all that apply)

☐ Wrong solution ☐ Wrong medication
☐ Wrong rate
☐ Wrong time
☐ Infiltration
☐ Transcription error
☐ PCA error
☐ Blood transfusion
☐ Hyperalimentation
☐ Other _____

Equipment

☐ Not available
☐ Disconnected
☐ Procedure not followed
☐ Nonsterile
☐ Malfunction
☐ Other _____
☐ Descript. of item _____

Pressure Sore (complete both sides)

☐ On admission
☐ Hospital acquired
☐ Picture taken

☐ Stage I
☐ Stage II
☐ Stage III
☐ Stage IV

FALL (Complete both sides)

☐ Ambulating
☐ In BR
☐ Out of bed
☐ To FRM B/R
☐ Other

☐ PT has fallen prev
☐ Restrained
☐ Side rails up
☐ Side rails down

Surgical — Please Comment

☐ Delay
☐ Consent mismatch
☐ Unplanned return
☐ Incorrect count
☐ Unplanned repair/removal
☐ Arrest
☐ Death
☐ Anesthesia related
☐ Other _____

Other

☐ Security   ☐ Self abuse
☐ Engineering   ☐ Lost/damaged article
☐ Combative pt.   ☐ Hazardous exposure
☐ Suicide attempt ☐ Burn
☐ Fire   ☐ Lab
☐ Respiratory   ☐ X ray
☐ Pharmacy   ☐ Food services
☐ Code blue, expired ☐ Housekeeping
☐ Code blue, survived ☐ Other (Comment)
☐ Complaint   _____

III   Severity of Outcome

☐ No Injury   ☐ Inconsequential   ☐ Consequential

IV   Comments & Action

Name of MD notified	Date	Time	Seen by MD?
			Yes ☐ No ☐

X-ray / Lab / Tests ordered?	Equipment
Yes ☐ No ☐ State _____	Sent for repair ☐ Removed from service ☐

V Follow up (Director to complete)

☐ Communicated with
_____
☐ Employee counseled
☐ Inservice
☐ Policy change / new
☐ Trend
☐ Other _____

Reported by — Date — Dept	Persons Involved Dept	Department Director Sign — Date

Ballpoint Pen Only

QUALITY OCCURRENCE REPORT

● **Not Part of Medical Record** ●
● **DO NOT Photocopy**
● **Complete all Sections and forward to QRS Immediately**

FIGURE 9.14

6. Define ergonomics. _____

_____

7. List the five most common causes of fire.
(a) _____
(b) _____
(c) _____
(d) _____
(e) _____

8. List five general fire safety rules.
(a) _____
(b) _____
(c) _____
(d) _____
(e) _____

9. Define RACE.
(a) _____
(b) _____
(c) _____
(d) _____

10. If you discover a fire, you must attend to the safety of the _____

_____.

11. List four responsibilities of the health unit coordinator in a medical emergency.
(a) _____
(b) _____
(c) _____
(d) _____

12. What is a defibrillator? _____

_____

13. What is a crash cart? _____

_____

14. What does the nurse mean if he says the patient has coded? _____

_____

Match the International Code in Column A with its description in Column B.

Column A	Column B
(a) Code Red	_____ There is a cardiac or respiratory arrest
(b) Code Blue	_____ Triage
(c) Code Yellow	_____ There is a fire in the hospital
(d) Code Green	_____ There is an uncontrolled individual or threatening situation

15. Why must the health unit coordinator practice good body mechanics? What kinds of situations could occur on the job that might require heavier than usual lifting?

   _____
   _____
   _____
   _____
   _____

16. Describe the kinds of HUC tasks that could potentially result in injury if not done properly.

   _____
   _____
   _____
   _____
   _____
   _____

17. List as many possible hazards on the job as you can think of. What can you do to work more safely?

   _____
   _____
   _____
   _____
   _____
   _____

18. A patient is being admitted to your unit, and the nurses need another person to help move the patient off the gurney and onto the bed. What should you do?

   _____

19. You are walking by a patient's room and hear cries for help. When you enter the room you see that the patient's pillow is on fire. What should you do?

   _____
   _____
   _____
   _____
   _____

20. The patient in room 412 has coded. The code team is in the room working to save the patient. Why should you stay at the nurses' station with the intercom to the room turned on? _____

   _____

21. The patient's family comes rushing down the hall toward room 412 because they have heard the page "code blue—Room 412." What should you do? How do you think they feel at this moment? As the HUC how do you think you will feel?

_____

_____

_____

_____

_____

_____

CHAPTER 10

Introduction to Management at the Nurses' Station

Meticulous   Extremely careful and precise about details

Multitask   To prioritize and do many things simultaneously

Nurses' station   Area of the nursing unit where the health unit coordinator sits that contains the telephone, computer, other administrative equipment and supplies, and the patients' records

Prioritize   To put first things first; to decide which is the most important to do at a given time

Time sheet   The nursing unit staff's work schedule

OBJECTIVES

When you have completed this chapter, you will be able to:

- Define the terms listed in the vocabulary.
- List three areas of health unit coordinator management.
- Discuss your responsibilities for medical and nursing supplies and equipment.
- Give examples of multitasking.
- Discuss your responsibilities for management of the nurses' station.
- List and explain the purpose of four clerical supplies or types of equipment used frequently at the nurses' station.
- List and define reference materials found at the nurses' station.
- Discuss the unit records and reports.
- State some of the ways you can better manage your time and health unit coordinator activities.

Now that you have learned about the hospital environment and your general duties, you are ready to become familiar with the management techniques that will help you organize and expedite your work.

In some areas of the country there is more than one position level for health unit coordinators, for example, the beginning level or Unit Coordinator I, the next level or Unit Coordinator II, and Unit Managers. Unit Coordinator II's assume more responsibility and may act as assistant unit managers. However, the health unit coordinator, unless he or she has been promoted, does not supervise and manage other staff members. The health unit coordinator does manage other facets of the job through the management of his or her own time and activities, the management of nursing and medical supplies and equipment, and the coordination of certain nursing unit activities at the **nurses' station.**

THE NURSES' STATION

Although most of your work is done at the nurses' station, it is not your private office. Doctors, nurses, aides, persons from other departments, and often student nurses come in and out freely to use the charts, computer, Kardex, and other forms and medical supplies. It will largely be your responsibility to keep the station neat and orderly and you should know what medical equipment and supplies you can expect to find there (Fig. 10.1).

FIGURE 10.1

OTHER WORK AREAS ON A NURSING UNIT

- **Treatment/examination room.** Patient physical examinations and treatments such as Pap smears, sigmoidoscopies and colonoscopies, and certain biopsies are performed here.
- **Medication room.** Usually adjacent to the nurses' station—contains locked drugs such as narcotics, certain medications, refrigerator, and usually a stock of intravenous solutions and supplies.
- **Utility rooms.**
  "Clean"—Contains nursing supplies from central supply.
  "Contaminated or Dirty"—Contaminated equipment and supplies are taken here for cleaning or for return to central supply.
- **Kitchen.** Patient snacks and sometimes meals are prepared here. Contains refrigerator, cupboards, sink, and usually a microwave oven.

- **Storage rooms.** Wheelchairs, gurneys, walkers, and other patient assistance equipment are stored here.
- **Dictation room.** Contains dictation equipment for physician and other professionals' use. Dictation is then transcribed by the medical transcriber in Health Information Services (Medical Records).
- **Waiting Room.** For visitors.
- **Nurses' lounge or office.** Area for conferences, change-of-shift report, and relaxation.

*N*URSING AND MEDICAL EQUIPMENT

Equipment used for physical examination of the patient is kept in the nurses' station. This may include:

- Stethoscopes
- Blood pressure machines (sphygmomanometers)
- Flashlights
- Percussion hammer
- Ophthalmoscope (for examining eyes)
- Otoscope (for examining ears)

If it is your responsibility to manage this equipment, always check it at the beginning of the shift. Replace any light bulbs that are not working and keep extra bulbs on hand. When the doctors and nurses have finished with the equipment be sure it is put in its proper place (Fig. 10.2).

FIGURE 10.2

NURSING UNIT SUPPLIES

To properly manage supplies for the nursing unit, you must know what you have on hand and what you need. It will be necessary to regularly inventory the supplies for which you are responsible and keep a "want list" so that other nursing personnel can let you know when they are getting short of supplies.

You should order only what you need and reorder regularly. Overstocking is called hoarding and is discouraged.

Keep a list of desirable quantities of each supply and order properly so that you keep that amount on hand. For example:

- Physician's Orders forms—3 packages of 100 each.
- Telephone record pads—10.
- Black pens—25.

Certain clerical equipment and supplies not previously discussed in Chapter 8 will be of particular interest to you since the health unit coordinator uses them so frequently:

- **Imprinter (or addressograph machine)**—a small machine that, when used with the patient's imprinter card (addressograph plate), prints the patient's name, unit number, room number, doctor's name, and other pertinent information on all the chart forms and requisitions that pertain to the patient's care.
- **Imprinter or addressograph card holder**—a holder placed by the imprinter machine for each patient's card on the nursing unit. These cards, which originate in the admitting department, are usually filed by room number and must be returned to their proper space in the card holder. Improperly placed cards can result in the stamping of a form or requisition for the wrong patient with resultant serious consequences.
- **Baskets**—for incoming and outgoing requisitions and test results. These should be neat and clearly labeled.
- **Files**—these will contain a supply of blank chart forms, blank requisitions, and other forms used frequently in your hospital. "Old charts" (charts from a patient's previous admissions and sent from Medical Records) may also be kept in a file during the patient's current hospitalization.
- **Computer**—for sending and receiving a variety of information.

REFERENCE MATERIALS

A small library of reference materials is kept on the nursing unit (Fig. 10.3). These include all manuals containing recorded material that might be of use to the medical and nursing staff. The following is a typical list:

- A **diet manual** lists and describes every type of diet the hospital kitchen provides (e.g., diabetic diet, ulcer diet).
- A **laboratory manual** describes in detail the various tests performed by the laboratory. It commonly lists the department regulations—when the laboratory is open, what constitutes an emergency laboratory test, and so forth. It may also include a list of "normal" values for each test.
- A **health unit coordinator manual** gives step-by-step descriptions of health unit coordinator procedures.
- A **nursing procedure manual** gives step-by-step descriptions of nursing procedures.

- A **hospital policy manual** gives administrative policies concerning such things as visiting hours, wage and salary scales, and smoking regulations.
- The *Physicians' Desk Reference* (PDR) contains descriptions of medications in common usage.
- A **hospital formulary** lists and describes all medications stocked and used in the hospital.
- **General medical and nursing reference texts** often constitute a small reference library.
- An **x-ray procedure manual** gives pertinent data about the patient preparation required for each x-ray ordered.

FIGURE 10.3

Vital Signs Books or Sheets Some hospitals require that after the nurse takes the vital signs, he or she record them in a special book to be graphed later by the health unit coordinator (see Chapter 13). You may fill in the skeleton form of this sheet by entering the patients' names, rooms, and bed numbers so that the nurse need only record the vital signs (Fig. 10.4).

Name	Room No.	8 a.m. TPR&BP	12 Noon TPR&BP	4 p.m. TPR&BP	8 p.m. TPR&BP
Jones, Wm.	449	97^6-78-20 120/80			
Clark, Geo.	450	99^2-80-20 110/70			

FIGURE 10.4

Schedules Working hours, vacations, tours, and days off for unit personnel are posted on the bulletin board. Most hospitals call this a **time sheet**.

It is your responsibility, as a health unit coordinator, to know where the patients' charts are at all times. To some degree it is also your responsibility to know where the patients are. You must be able to locate nursing personnel on your unit, and you are frequently asked to find a doctor who is on the unit.

One method for keeping track of patients and their charts is a **patient activity log.** At the beginning of each shift, you would list each patient's room number and name; next to this note any pertinent data relating to that patient's activity (Fig. 10.5). When a patient or chart has returned, draw a line through the notation.

Patient Activity Log		
Room		Date
100	Brown, John	8 A to surg c̄ chart
101A	Jones, Claire	
101B	Berol, Turquoise	10:15 to PT
102	Sevens, Dana	11:05 chart c̄ Dr. in dictation room
103	Park, Perry	
104	Austin, Ryan	8:30 to X-ray; rtd 10:05
105	Brazier, Nell	11:45 to OT
106	Siler, Linda	
107A		
107B	Dollar, Chris	7:35 to surg c̄ chart

FIGURE 10.5

Staff Activity Log When you are asked to locate unit personnel, you will first refer to the assignment sheet to find the general location of their patient assignment. This sheet also frequently includes staff break and lunch times. If a staff member leaves the unit for a special purpose, jot it down. Keeping notes on the location of staff members can be a great help on a busy day, when your memory may fail you (Fig. 10.6).

STAFF ACTIVITY LOG

7:25 Mr. Dean floated to 4 W for day
12:15pm Miss Brown to staff meeting - due back 1:30
12:30pm Mrs. Grey to help in O.B. for 1 hr.
1:15pm Dr. White to ER, back in about ½ hr.

FIGURE 10.6

A **census record** is an accurate count of all patients who have been admitted, transferred, or discharged, or who have died. It is prepared by the nursing unit to inform the hospital admitting department of the exact number of patients on each unit and therefore in the hospital. A **daily** or **summary report** is a report given by nursing to the nursing administration to inform them of critical patients and incidents.

The **change-of-shift report** is given by the nurses going off duty to those coming on as well as by the health unit coordinator to the oncoming health unit coordinator. The purpose is to relay what has occurred during the previous shift and what needs are to be given priority by the staff coming on duty.

MANAGING YOUR TIME AND ACTIVITIES

The following are some rules of efficiency to help you as a health unit coordinator manage time and tasks more efficiently:

- Always put things back when you are through with them.
- Try never to run out of supplies.
- Complete one task before you move on to another. This may not always be possible but it is a good rule and something for which to strive.
- Learn to **prioritize.** Your ability to decide what to do first is important to your success as a health unit coordinator.

Stat (do immediately) orders and emergencies take precedence over other priorities. Assisting a doctor or nurse should come before your routine health unit coordinator tasks. Patient and visitor requests should take priority over other health unit coordinator activities. Answering the telephone usually takes priority over other tasks.

Hospitals want health unit coordinators who can **multitask,** that is, to be able to do many things at the same time by constantly prioritizing.

Make good use of your time. If there is a period of the day when you are not busy, use this time to do some of your routine tasks. For example, you will learn that the chart of each new patient contains at least eight (and probably many more) different forms that must be arranged in a specific order. When you are not busy, you can arrange sets of these forms in the proper order. You will find this to be a great help to you on busy days when many admissions are expected.

- Make notes to yourself and lists of calls to make and things to do. When you have completed the task, draw a line through it on the list.
- Make out a daily work schedule.
- Look for ways to make your work more efficient. Avoid duplication of effort. Try to combine running errands with a coffee break or a lunch period. Don't waste energy by going to get a new supply of chart forms for your file only to discover an hour later that you also needed a supply of dietary requisitions. Do not, however, confuse efficiency with shortcuts. Meticulous attention to detail is part of your job.

TRAINING OTHERS

From time to time you will be asked to help train newly employed or student health unit coordinators. As you manage this part of your job responsibility you truly can use your human relations and communications skills discussed in the first chapters of this book. In your role as teacher you become many things—role model, evaluator, and, if you try, a friend. When this time comes, think back to one of the main functions of a hospital—to provide education for health care workers. Look at this experience as a challenge. Show others that you know your job well enough to impart that knowledge to others. If you don't know what is expected of you, seek guidance from the education department, your head nurse, and the student health unit coordinator's instructor. Use empathy and remember when you, too, were a student.

*L*EARNING ACTIVITIES

Complete the following.

1. List three areas of health unit coordinator management.
   (a) _____
   (b) _____
   (c) _____

2. Define the following.
   (a) Sphygmomanometer _____
   (b) Ophthalmoscope _____
   (c) Otoscope _____
   (d) Imprinter or addressograph machine _____

3. State the purpose of each of the following reference materials.
   (a) Laboratory manual _____
   _____
   (b) Nursing procedure manual _____
   (c) Hospital policy manual _____
   (d) *Physicians' Desk Reference* _____
   _____
   (e) Hospital formulary _____

4. State the purpose of the following.
   (a) Change-of-shift report _____
   (b) Census record _____
   (c) Daily or summary report _____
   _____
   (d) Vital signs book or sheet _____
   (e) Time sheet _____
   (f) Patient activity log _____
   _____

5. List six rules of efficiency.
   (a) _____
   (b) _____
   (c) _____
   (d) _____
   (e) _____
   (f) _____

6. Putting first things first is called _____.

7. To do many things at the same time is to _____.

8. Have you ever worked with someone who was very good at his or her job? What did he or she do that made an impression on you? List as many things as you can think of.

_____
_____
_____
_____
_____
_____
_____

9. Have you ever worked with someone who had poor work habits? What did he or she do that you didn't like?

_____
_____
_____
_____
_____
_____

10. It is a busy day at the nurses' station. You have a stack of charts with new orders. A doctor is trying to get your attention. A nurse is waiting to talk to you. The telephone is ringing. A patient's family member has just walked up to the desk, and a volunteer is waiting to ask you a question.

How will you prioritize and handle this situation?

_____
_____
_____
_____
_____
_____

What criteria did you use to make your decisions?

_____
_____
_____
_____
_____
_____

CHAPTER 11

The Patient's Chart

Cardinal symptoms	Temperature, pulse, and respirations
Chart back	Loose-leaf, vinyl notebook or metal cover that holds the patient's chart; also called the chart holder
Charting	The recording of information on the patient's chart
Chart rack	Device to hold all the charts on a nursing unit, which are arranged by room number
Concur	Agree
Patient's chart	Records that document a patient's care during hospitalization that are organized and kept together in a chart holder
Sequence	The order of something
Standard chart form	Forms that become a part of every patient's chart
Stuffing the chart	Adding new forms to the chart
Supplemental chart forms	Forms that are added to the chart as required by the circumstances of the patient's care during hospitalization
Thinned (chart)	A chart that has had some portions removed and filed on the unit because it has become so thick
Unit number	Number assigned to a patient on admission

When you have completed this chapter, you will be able to:

- Define the terms listed in the vocabulary.
- Explain the reasons for the patent's chart.
- Define terms used in this chapter that relate to the chart.
- List and explain the rules of charting.
- Describe the health unit coordinator's responsibilities in maintaining the chart and list the routine chart checks.
- List and discuss the standard chart forms.
- Assemble a patient's chart.
- List and describe the common supplemental chart forms.

The hospital keeps a vast collection of records for both medical and legal reasons. Probably the most important among these are those that make up the individual **patient's chart.**

The Joint Commission on Accreditation of Health Care Organizations (JCAHO) has established a number of reasons why all patients should have charts.

𝒫URPOSES OF CHARTS

1. To serve as a basis for the planning of patient care

2. To provide a practical means of communication between physicians and other members of the health team

3. To furnish documentation of the course of a patient's illness and care

4. To be used for legal purposes in a court of law

5. To provide data for use in research (Fig. 11.1)

FIGURE 11.1

𝓜AINTAINING PATIENT CHARTS

Each patient who enters the hospital has records kept on all phases of his or her medical progress. During the patient's hospital stay, all or most of these individual records are brought together, in proper order, and bound into loose-leaf metal or vinyl covers called **chart backs** or **chart holders.** New sheets may be added as necessary. Or, if the patient's stay has been a long one, the chart may be **thinned** or "split" by removing certain chart forms and filing them on the unit. Your instructor will explain which forms you may take out of the chart and which you may not. One chart holder is available in every nursing unit for each hospital bed. When not in use by doctors or nurses, all chart holders are kept in special devices called **chart racks.** The charts have special places in the rack, usually in the same order that the patient's rooms are located in the nursing unit. This arrangement makes them easy to find when needed. Each chart should be replaced in the rack after use.

After the patient is discharged, a health unit coordinator routes all record sheets relating to the patient to Health Information Services, where they are filed together, under a special **unit number** that was assigned to the patient on admission. All forms that were removed when the chart was thinned or split must be returned to the chart in proper sequence. If a patient is readmitted to the hospital at a later date, this "old" chart can be used as reference to the patient's previous medical history. For each admission, a new chart is always started and kept in the unit so that information can be continuously recorded. After the patient's discharge, this chart can be added to any previous records the hospital may have on the patient (Fig. 11.2).

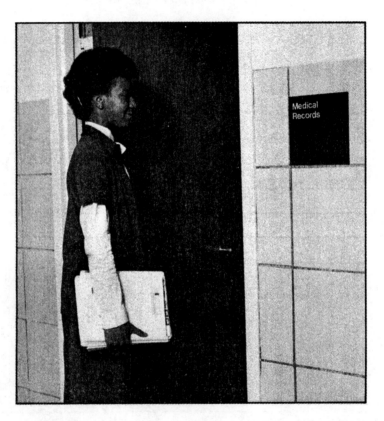

FIGURE 11.2 Storage of medical records in health information services or medical records.

*T*HE CHART FORM

The individual record forms that are assembled to make up the patient's chart have two things in common. The name of the hospital where it is used is printed on it, and a space is provided on each for the patient's name. Most hospitals use some variation of the chart forms described in this chapter, although the exact form varies from one hospital to another. Some hospitals print the forms according to their own needs and specifications and to satisfy documentation requirements of the JCAHO.

The space that identifies the chart form with the patient is recorded by means of a mechanical device (an imprinter), which was discussed in Chapter 6. One chart form varies in format from another according to the information to be recorded on it. Your instructor will help you identify the forms among those discussed in this chapter that are used in your hospital.

EXECUTION OF CHART FORMS

Health unit coordinators do not write on most chart forms. It is your responsibility to stamp these forms with the patient's imprinter card and place them in the proper sequence on the patient's chart. There are, however, several standard chart forms on which you may write or actually file diagnostic reports. Fig. 11.3 shows one hospital's method of chart organization.

Orders
  - Discharge Form
Hyperalimentation
Progress Notes
H & P/Consults
Vital Signs/Graphics
  - Patient Care Flowsheet
  - Restraint Flowsheet
  - Patient Transfer Sheet
Plan of Care/Patient Education
  - Plan of Care and Referral Summary
  - Multidisciplinary Plan of Care
  - Clinical Pathways
  - Patient Education Sheet
Medications/IVs/Diabetes Record
OP Reports/Consents
  - Op Report/Consents
  - Perioperative, Anesthesia, and PACU Records
  - Special Procedures Record
  - Sedation/ Analgesia Procedural Record
Admission Assessment
  - Patient Admission Form
  - Emergency Department Phyician Record/Flowsheet/Nurses Notes
Lab/Pathology
Radiology
  - X-rays, MRI, CT, Nuclear Medicine
Respiratory
  - Respiratory Care Flowsheets
  - Pulmonary Function Test (PFT)
Cardiology
  - EKG Reports, Echo Reports
EKG Monitor Strips
Neuro/Vascular
  - Neuro Studies
  - GI Lab
  - Ultrasound
PT/OT/Speech/Cardiac Rehab.
  - Initial Evaluation
  - PT/OT/Speech Treatment Record
  - Cardiac Rehab. Exercise Record
  - Progressive Ambulation Record
Miscellaneous
Advance Directives
Face Sheets/ Condition of Admission (COA)

FIGURE 11.3 Sample chart form organization.

STANDARD CHART FORMS

There are at least nine chart forms that usually become part of every patient's chart upon admission. These are referred to as **standard chart forms.** It is important that you learn to identify and describe each of these forms. Other chart forms, called **supplemental chart forms,** are used only when required. Many hospitals color-code their chart forms to make them easy to identify and have dividers in the charts printed with the names of the forms. Your hospital may have different names for the chart forms other than those used here. Some hospitals or special units within a hospital may include other forms that they consider "standard" for their hospital or special unit. Following are descriptions of the nine standard chart forms (Fig. 11.4).

STANDARD CHART FORMS

3. Graphic Chart

2. Nursing Record

4. History and Physical Examination

5. Medication Record

1. Conditions of Admission

6. Physician's Order Form

7. Progress Notes

8. Clinical Care Notes

9. Laboratory Results

FIGURE 11.4

Face Sheet and Conditions of Admission

The **face sheet** and **conditions of admission** are completed by the admitting department. The conditions of admission is signed by the patient or his or her guardian when the patient is admitted. This signature allows the hospital to treat the patient and indicates the patient accepts financial responsibility for the bill. Information on the face sheet form includes the patient's name, date and time of admission, age, date of birth, sex, religion, address, telephone number, occupation, social security number, financially responsible party, type of insurance, next of kin, name of person to notify in an emergency, and admitting diagnosis. Other information may be included as well. The patient is assigned a hospital number, which is recorded on the form, and typically the form is sent along

MEMORIAL HOSPITAL

DATE DISCHARGED - BY HOUR

| PATIENT NO. | ADMIT DATE MO DAY YR | TIME ADM. A/P | ROOM | PAT TYPE | HOSP SERV | ADMITTING PHYSICIAN | | DOCTOR NO. | FIN CL | IP |
| | | | A | | | | M.D. | | | |

| PATIENT NAME | LAST | FIRST | INITIAL | D | DATE OF BIRTH | AGE | BIRTHPLACE | SEX M STAT S/M | RELG |

| PATIENT ADDRESS | | CITY — STATE - ZIP | TELEPHONE NO. | DATE OF PREVIOUS ADMISSION |

| OCCUPATION - PATIENT | EMPLOYER | ADDRESS | CITY - STATE - ZIP | PHONE NO. |

| SOCIAL SECURITY NO. | MEDICARE NO. | ALPHA | FIN RESP. PARTY PHONE NO. AREA | ADMIT ELEC. EMER. 001 002 | FROM ER 003 | UR DAYS |

| INSURANCE CO. | SUBSCRIBER NAME | GROUP NO. | CERT. NO. | EFFECTIVE DATE |

| FINANCIALLY RESPONSIBLE PARTY (First Name, Middle Initial Last Name) | (Street, Address & City, State & Zip) | RELAT. CODE |

| SOCIAL SECURITY NO. | OCCUPATION | EMPLOYER | ADDRESS - CITY | PHONE NO. |

| INSURANCE CO. | SUBSCRIBER NAME | GROUP NO. | CERT. NO. | EFFECTIVE DATE |

| CR CA | NEXT OF KIN | PHONE NO. | NOTIFY IN EMERGENCY | PHONE NO. |

ADMITTING DIAGNOSIS

ADM. CLERK

FINAL DIAGNOSIS .... CODE

Physician's
Discharge
Summary

OPERATIONS

SEQUELAE OR INFECTIONS

| DISCHARGED WITH APPROVAL | RELEASED AGAINST ADVICE | TRANSFERRED TO | | EXPIRED | |
| | | OTHER HOSPITAL | EXTENDED CARE FACILITY | OVER 48 HRS. ☐ UNDER 48 HRS. ☐ | AUTOPSY NONE ☐ HOSP ☐ COR ☐ | SERVICE: REVIEWED BY COMMITTEE |

CONSULTANT

SURGEON

ANESTHESIOLOGIST   ATTENDING PHYSICIAN

201

CHART COPY

FIGURE 11.5 Face sheet.

with the patient's addressograph plate to the nursing unit. The face sheet and conditions of admission are usually placed as the first pages of the chart. When the patient is discharged, transferred, or expires (dies), the bottom portion of the face sheet is completed by the physician. This portion is called the **physician's discharge summary.** This information includes the final diagnosis, any operations, and complications including infections. This information is usually completed after the chart has been sent to health information services/medical records (Fig.11-5).

Nursing Record

Special forms are provided for nurses to record their observations of the patient's condition and the care they give. The nurses' notes are their written communication with the physician. Hospitals have strict regulations regarding the frequency and the manner in which these notes are made. A comprehensive admission nursing assessment begins the nursing record, and there is usually a separate form for this purpose. The nursing diagnosis, ongoing assessment, intervention, daily care, and discharge planning are all components of the **nursing record.** Figure 11.6 shows examples of the nursing record.

Graphic Chart

The **graphic chart** is so called because it is primarily a graph; the patient's temperature, pulse, respiration (TPR), and frequently blood pressure are recorded on the graphic chart as soon as possible after they are taken. Space is usually provided for recording this data for a period of one week. Many hospitals use the graphic chart to record other information about the patient's daily condition and progress as well. Information such as the patient's appetite, total fluid intake and output, weight, height, and daily bowel movements may also be recorded on this sheet.

    Temperature, pulse, and respiration rates of patients are taken at specified times during the day in most hospitals, and on certain patients more frequently as ordered. You may be responsible for entering this information on the graphic chart. Red ink may be used to record the temperature (although the trend is to use all black ink, because red ink doesn't copy as well) and blue or black ink to record the pulse and respiration rates. To graph you will make a dot representing the value of each *cardinal symptom* (the cardinal symptoms are the temperature, pulse, and respiration) and the blood pressure, if required, in the column of the graph that indicates the day and hour it was taken. Connect this dot to the previous dot with a straight line similar to the one shown in Fig. 11.7. It is very important to be accurate when performing this task. The cardinal symptoms in some diseases have a characteristic pattern of rising and falling, and the graph is an aid in seeing the pattern at a glance.

Bedside Computer Charting

Many hospitals have computers in each patient's room so that nursing care can be documented as it is given. These records are usually printed every 24 hours and then filed in the patient's chart. Hospitals that use bedside computer charting do not use the nursing records mentioned above because the information is printed directly from the computer (Fig. 11.8).

History and Physical Examination Record

Every patient admitted to a hospital has a medical history taken and undergoes some sort of physical examination. Observations by the doctor are recorded in full on the

NURSING RECORD

ASSESSMENT / PROGRESS NOTES (RN)

DATE ___/___/___

PRIORITY	NURSING DIAGNOSIS		PRIORITY	NURSING DIAGNOSIS
☐	Impaired Gas Exchange		☐	Potential for Infection
☐	Ineffective Coping - Anxiety		☐	Potential for Physical Injury
☐	Alteration in Comfort		☐	Impaired Communication
☐	Alteration in Nutrition		☐	Knowledge Deficit
☐	Impaired Skin Integrity		☐	Altered Mental Status
☐	Activity Intolerance / Immobility		☐	Alteration in Elimination
☐	Other:		☐	Other:

Time: Care Plan: ☐ Reviewed ☐ Revised   Reviewed w/ ☐Pt. ☐SO   RN Signature
Time: Care Plan: ☐ Reviewed ☐ Revised   Reviewed w/ ☐Pt. ☐SO   RN Signature
Time: Care Plan: ☐ Reviewed ☐ Revised   Reviewed w/ ☐Pt. ☐SO   RN Signature

TIME   FOCUS   D = DATA   A = ACTION   R = RESPONSE

MEDICAL / SURGICAL DAILY NURSING RECORD

189 3/96

ADDRESSOGRAPH

DAILY CARE RECORD - RN, LVN, CNA Shaded Areas   02 04 06 0

VITAL SIGNS
- Temperature: (R)ectal   (Ax)illary   (Tympanic)
- Pulse (A)pical
- Respirations
- Blood Pressure
- Orthostatic Blood Pressure

SAFETY
- Measurement: Type:
- Side Rails ↑, Bed ↓, Wheels Locked
- Call Bell In Reach
- Bands On: ID/ALLERGY (Circle)
- Protective Device - Type:
- Neuro-Vascular assessment q 2 h
- Food-Fluid needs assessed q 2 h
- Elimination needs assessed q 2 h
- Released, ROM, reapplied q 2 h
- Device removed
- Device reapplied
- Isolation - Category:
- Protocol Maintained

RESPIRATORY
- Cough/Deep Breathing
- Suction Frequency
- Pulse Oximetry   (% sat)
- Incentive Spirometry
- Oxygen ___ LPM per ___ Device

HYGIENE
- Bath: Type
- AM, PM, HS Care
- Linen Change
- Perineal/Catheter Care
- Denture/Oral Hygiene

ACTIVITY/EXERCISE
- Ambulate
- Chair
- Bedrest
- BSC/BRP
- Dangle
- Position Change
- ROM — Passive (P)   Active (A)

TREATMENTS
- Dressing Change(s)   1. Site ___   2. Site ___
- Drainage *
- Bowel Hygiene *
- Antiembolic Treatment: Seq TEDS ___ Stockings ___
  - Type: 1. ___ 2. ___ 3. ___
  - Location: 1. ___ 2. ___ 3. ___

IV MGT.
- IV Site Checked — Clear, Without Complications
- IV Patent & Infusing Well
- Dressing Dry & Intact
- IV(S) Discontinued—Without Difficulty-Catheter Intact
- ✓=Assessed/Completed   *=See Nsg Note   Blank=Does Not Apply   *=___ RN

02 04 06 08 10 12 14 16 19 20 22 24

PART I.   ADMISSION BASELINE – (RN, LVN, NA)

DATE ___   TIME ___   DIAGNOSIS ___   ROOM ___

IDBAND ___   VERIF ___

TRANSPORT MODE: ☐ AMBT FROM ☐ ER ☐ HOME ☐ SNF   VITAL SIGNS: TEMP ___
☐ W/C ☐ STR. ☐ AMB ☐ MD OFFICE ☐ OTHER HOSP.   HT. ___   WT: STATED ___   PULSE ___

EQUIPMENT WITH PT.: ☐ NONE ☐ DENTURES/PARTIALS ☐ U ☐ L ☐ CANE ☐ WALKER
☐ CONTACT LENSES ☐ GLASSES ☐ HEARING AID ☐ W/C ☐ OTHER:

ADVANCE DIRECTIVE: ☐ YES ☐ NO   IF NO, INFORMATION GIVEN?
COPY TO CHART: ☐ YES ☐ NO

PART II.   FUNCTIONAL HEALTH PATTERNS ASSESSMENT

INFORMATION DOCUMENTED BY: ☐ PATIENT ☐ SIGNIFICANT OTHER ☐ RN ☐ LVN

HEALTH PERCEPTION/HEALTH MANAGEMENT
☐ 1. REASON FOR HOSPITALIZATION (stated by patient/informant):
☐ 2. PERTINENT MEDICAL/SURGICAL HISTORY:
☐ 3. HOW DOES PATIENT DESCRIBE GENERAL HEALTH?
☐ 4. WHAT KIND OF THINGS DOES PATIENT DO TO KEEP HEALTHY?
☐ 5. USE OF   TOBACCO: ☐ NO ☐ YES HOW MUCH? ___ HOW LONG? ___
                ALCOHOL: ☐ NO ☐ YES HOW MUCH? ___ HOW LONG? ___
                REC. DRUGS: ☐ NO ☐ YES DESCRIBE: ___

CURRENT MEDS   DOSE   FREQ   LAST DOSE   CURRENT MEDS   DOS
NON RX (LAX./ANALG.)

☐ 6. HAS PATIENT BEEN ABLE TO FOLLOW PRESCRIBED MEDS/TREATMENTS: ☐ YES ☐
☐ 7. DISPOSITION OF MEDICATIONS: ☐ DID NOT BRING ☐ SENT HOME WITH FAMILY ☐
☐ NO KNOWN ALLERGIES   ☐ DID ☐ YES ☐ ALLERGY BAND ON
                        ALLERGY   TYPE OF

ALLERGIES
MEDS
FOODS
OTHER

ACTIVITY/EXERCISE
☐ 1. MOBILITY STATUS: ☐ AMBULATORY ☐ AMBULATORY WITH ASSIST ☐ TRANSFER WI
☐ 2. ASSISTIVE DEVICES: ☐ NONE ☐ CRUTCHES ☐ CANE ☐ WALKER ☐ W/C ☐
☐ 3. LIMITATIONS: ☐ NONE ☐ WEAKNESS ☐ FATIGUE ☐ RECENT (6 MO. <) FALL?
☐ 4. ACTIVITIES OF DAILY LIVING: ☐ INDEPENDENT IN ALL ADL
  FEEDING ___ TOILETING ___ GROOMING ___ DRESSING ___ BATHING ___
☐ 5. EXERCISE REGULARLY? ☐ NO ☐ YES, DESCRIBE

SLEEP/REST
☐ 1. SLEEP: ☐ NO PROBLEM ☐ DIFFICULTY FALLING ASLEEP ☐ DIFFICULTY STAYING
  ☐ DOES NOT FEEL RESTED AFTER SLEEP ☐ OTHER:
☐ 2. WHAT HELPS PATIENT SLEEP?
☐ 3. SLEEP ROUTINE: BEDTIME ___ NO. HOURS ___ ☐ NAPS ___ NO. PILLOWS ___

ADMISSION ASSESSMENT

185 (12/60)

FIGURE 11.6

247

GRAPHIC CHART

FIGURE 11.7

FIGURE 11.8

history and physical examination record. The report may be handwritten, but most commonly the physician dictates the report, which is then typed (transcribed) by a medical transcriptionist. If this is the case, the report must be filed in the chart in the proper place when it arrives from the medical transcription department, which is often a part of health information services. Many hospitals use more than one type of history and physical record. Occasionally, a very long form may be used for research or educational purposes. An abbreviated form may be used for patients admitted for 48 hours or less or for certain outpatient procedures (Fig. 11.9).

Medication Record

The **medication administration record** or **MAR** is a chart form used for recording all medications given to the patient. Each time the nurse gives a medication, the nurse records that the prescribed medication was given at the appropriate time. A separate form may be used for intravenous (IV) medications.

If your hospital uses a record similar to the one described, you will have certain clerical duties to perform. When the medication administration record in progress has been filled, you must stamp a new form with the patient's name and unit number and place it in the chart. You may also be asked to transfer the information, including the names of drugs currently being administered to the patient to the new chart form (Fig. 11.10). Your instructor will explain the precise methods used in your hospital.

Physician's Order Form

The **physician's order form** has primary importance and will be placed at the front of the chart in most hospitals. The doctor uses this standard chart form to write all orders for the patient. The form is dated and signed each time the physician writes an order. All changes and cancellations of orders are written here as well. If a nurse takes a telephone or verbal order from the physician, it is recorded here. The doctor will sign those orders on the next visit. There is often a space on the physician's order form asking if another brand of drug identical in form and content may be dispensed by the pharmacy. If the doctor concurs, the space is checked.

Once written, doctor's orders are then transcribed to other hospital records. These orders guide the care that is given to the patient. The physician's order form serves as a blueprint of the care the patient is to receive.

Some of the clerical duties you will soon learn will require you to "take off" or transcribe the doctor's orders. You will then requisition the various tests, medications, procedures, treatments, services, supplies, and equipment either by computer or by filling out order forms (Fig. 11.11).

Progress Notes

Progress notes contain the recorded observations, impressions, and recommendations of all physicians who examine and treat the patient during the patient's hospitalization. Entries are not always made after each visit by the physician, however, if the patient's condition is unchanged since the previous visit. The JCAHO requires that progress notes must be written as often as needed to thoroughly document the patient's care. Most hospitals require that a doctor's note appear on every patient's chart at designated intervals. Generally, doctors will write at least one note a day while the patient is hospitalized and more often if the patient is very sick. Learn the regulations as to admission notes, postoperative notes, other progress notes, and discharge notes in effect in your hospital (Fig. 11.12).

(A)

Chief Complaint; Present Illness
Past History; Family History
Systemic Review
Physical Examination
ALL POSITIVE AND IMPORTANT NEGATIVE FINDINGS

MEMORIAL HOSPITAL   **PHYSICAL EXAMINATION & HISTORY**

(B)

Patient Name: _____

Chief Complaint:

History of Present Illness:

Past History:

     Illness & Injuries

     Operations

     Medications

     Habits

     Bleeding

     Allergies

Family History:

Review of Systems:

Physical Examination:

     General Appearance

     Head-Eye, Ear Nose and Throat

     Heart and Lungs

     Abdomen

     Genitourinary

     Extremities

     Neurologic

     Other

Pertinent Lab/Diagnostic Results:

Physician Signature _____ Date_____

MEMORIAL HOSPITAL

SHORT HISTORY AND PHYSICAL
(To be used for patients in hospital less than 48 hours)

FIGURE 11.9 (A) Physical examination and history; (B) Short history and physical.

ALLERGIC TO:
NO KNOWN ALLERGIES

CONSENT DATES: LITHIUM
ANTICHOLINERGICS
ANTIPSYCHOTICS
ANTIDEPRESSANTS

ROOM NO.

DIAGNOSIS

START RE ORDER	RN	DRUG DOSE FREQ.					DATE DC	SCHEDULE RATE	DATE	
		PO	IM	IVPB	IVP	SQ.	R			A.M. / SITE / P.M. / SITE
		PO	IM	IVPB	IVP	SQ.	R			A.M. / SITE / P.M. / SITE
		PO	IM	IVPB	IVP	SQ.	R			A.M. / SITE / P.M. / SITE
		PO	IM	IVPB	IVP	SQ.	R			A.M. / SITE / P.M. / SITE
		PO	IM	IVPB	IVP	SQ.	R			A.M. / SITE / P.M. / SITE
		PO	IM	IVPB	IVP	SQ.	R			A.M. / SITE / P.M. / SITE
		PO	IM	IVPB	IVP	SQ.	R			A.M. / SITE / P.M. / SITE
		PO	IM	IVPB	IVP	SQ.	R			A.M. / SITE / P.M. / SITE
		PO	IM	IVPB	IVP	SQ.	R			A.M. / SITE / P.M. / SITE
		PO	IM	IVPB	IVP	SQ.	R			7A / 7P

SLASH THROUGH TIME WHEN MEDICATION GIVEN.

CIRCLE MED NOT GIVEN & NOTE REASON:

NPO-FOR SURG/X-RAY   REF-REFUSED
N/V-NAUSEA   HELD-NOTE REASON

REFER TO MEDICATION SCHEDULE GUIDE TO DETERMINE APPROPRIATE
ADMINISTRATION TIMES.

RECOPIED   RN:

K   INJECTION SITE: (R or L)
E   D-Deltoid   G-Gluteal
Y   A-Abdominal   T-Thigh
    IC-Iliac Crest

Page ____ of ____

MEDICATION RECORD

ROUTINE   PRN/NOW

FIGURE 11.10 Medication administration record (MAR).

251

MEMORIAL HOSPITAL
PHYSICIAN ORDERS

Room No.

ANOTHER BRAND OF DRUG IDENTICAL IN FORM AND CONTENT MAY BE DISPENSED UNLESS CHECKED. ☐

Date	Time	R.N.	Date	Time	M.D.

1

Room No.

ANOTHER BRAND OF DRUG IDENTICAL IN FORM AND CONTENT MAY BE DISPENSED UNLESS CHECKED. ☐

Date	Time	R.N.	Date	Time	M.D.

2

Room No.

PHYSICIANS: WRITE ORDERS IN NEW SECTION EACH TIME. ORDERS MUST BE SIGNED.

ANOTHER BRAND OF DRUG IDENTICAL IN FORM AND CONTENT MAY BE DISPENSED UNLESS CHECKED. ☐

Date	Time	R.N.	Date	Time	M.D.

SC0108
(REV. 5/93)

CHART

3

252

NOTE PROGRESS OF CASE, COMPLICATIONS, CONSULTATIONS, CHANGE IN DIAGNOSIS,
CONDITION ON DISCHARGE, INSTRUCTIONS TO PATIENT.

DATE/TIME

**MEMORIAL HOSPITAL
PROGRESS NOTES**

FIGURE 11.12 Progress notes.

Clinical Care Notes

The **clinical care notes** chart form is usually used by health care professionals other than doctors or nurses. It may be used by respiratory therapy, physical therapy, occupational therapy, nutrition services, and the like to describe the care and progress given to the patient by personnel from these departments. A supplemental form designed for a specific department may be used instead if available (Fig. 11.13).

Laboratory Report or Clinical Pathology Record

All hospitals require certain laboratory tests to be performed on every patient admitted. The most common method of reporting the results is for the laboratory to send a computerized printout to the nursing unit. The results are then filed in the patient's chart.

Some hospitals have a system in which test results come back from the laboratory on special slips that are then attached to a type of **laboratory report form** (Fig. 11.14). Hospitals have an established method for alerting the physician

NOTE PROGRESS OF CASE, COMPLICATIONS, CONSULTATIONS, CHANGE IN DIAGNOSIS,
CONDITION ON DISCHARGE, INSTRUCTIONS TO PATIENT.

DATE

MEMORIAL HOSPITAL
Clinical Care Notes

FIGURE 11.13 Clinical care notes.

about abnormal test results. This is usually done by the laboratory. You will learn to follow the routine of your hospital before you are asked to post test results into the chart.

SUPPLEMENTAL CHART FORMS

Supplemental chart forms may or may not be included in the individual patient's chart. Their use will depend on the tests, treatments, and procedures required to treat the patient's specific condition. The details of using supplemental chart forms vary among different hospitals. Learn to use the forms in your hospital (Fig. 11.15).

Radiology and Other Diagnostic Test Results

Whenever a test is ordered, a report must be sent back to the nursing unit in dictating the results of the test. All results of x-rays, CT scans, MRIs, nuclear medicine studies,

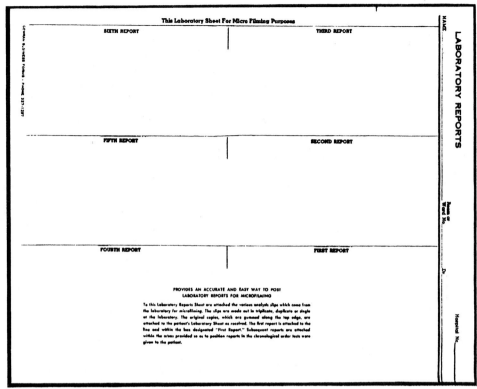

FIGURE 11.14 Laboratory report form.

SUPPLEMENTAL CHART FORMS

FIGURE 11.15

electrocardiograms, echocardiograms, ultrasounds, electroencephalograms, or any other diagnostic test must be filed in the patient's chart.

Surgical Records

Patients admitted to the hospital for surgery will have many specialized records in their charts before they are discharged. Prior to surgery, a **consent to surgery** must be signed by the patient, giving the surgeon and his or her assistants permission to perform the operation, and a **consent for anesthesia** explaining the risks of anesthesia and giving consent for the procedure. Other preoperative forms such as a **preoperative checklist** and **preanesthesia patient questionnaire** may be included at this time. At least two more records are added in the operating room—one to record the anesthesia given and the general progress of both the operation and the patient during surgery, and another record to describe the operative procedures performed. When tissue is removed for laboratory examination, a third record, **surgical pathology,** is added to the chart. In the recovery room, a record is kept of the patient's condition while awakening from the anesthetic. This is often called the **postanesthesia care unit (PACU) record.** A **transfusion record** may be necessary for a patient who has received blood before or during the operation.

Special Therapy Records

Sometimes a patient receives special treatments from personnel in other hospital departments. When this occurs, special records are kept of these treatments. Examples of these records follow:

- **Respiratory therapy records**—used when a patient has a condition requiring some type of inhalation therapy or pulmonary therapy (Figs. 11.16 (a) and (b)).
- **Physical therapy records**—used when the patient is undergoing rehabilitative treatment because of injury or disease (Fig. 11.17).
- **Radiation therapy records**—used for patients who are receiving doses of radiation, generally for the purpose of killing cancerous cells.
- **Nutrition therapy records**—used to record a patient's nutritional status, treatment, and dietary progress.
- **Social service records**—kept on a patient being seen by personnel from the Social Services Department, who work to help patients adjust to personal or emotional problems brought on by illness.

Consultation Form

This form is used when a physician wants advice from another doctor. Often a physician will be consulted who specializes in the type of condition or symptoms the patient presents. The consulting doctor records his or her impressions on the form, which is then included in the patient's chart. Before a consultation is done, the patient's doctor must write an order requesting it on the patient's chart.

Vital Signs Record

This chart form may be used when a patient's condition requires that his TPR and blood pressure be taken frequently (Fig. 11.18).

RESPIRATORY THERAPY DEPARTMENT

Care Plan Date:_____   Ed Log Date:_____   Eval Due Date:_____

The following is a repeating treatment record form (five identical blocks). Each block contains the following fields:

Date	HHN IS CPT/PD AERO	MODE MP MASK Blowby TRACH	Objective Complete ☐ / 72° Eval ☐	MEDICATION cc / cc / cc	Pulse 1.___ 2.___ Resp. Rate	Duration / Volumes	Position HF___ SF___ LF___	PEF 1. / PEF 2.	☐ Cough ☐ Suction / ☐ Productive ☐ Non-Prod.	SPUTUM Vol.___ Vis.___ Color___	Adverse Reaction ☐ NO ☐ YES
Time											
Missed TX___	Initial s/u ☐	Circuit Δ ☐	Care Plan ☐ / Ed Log ☐	___ cc ___ Nacl	1.___ 2.___	CPT: RUL RML RLL / LUL LLL		Breath Sounds: ā___ p̄___			

COMMENTS: SIGNATURE:

(This block repeats five times down the page.)

MEMORIAL HOSPITAL
RESPIRATORY THERAPY TREATMENT RECORD

FIGURE 11.16a Respiratory therapy records.

Respiratory Therapy Continuous Flow Sheet

Date	Time	Physician's Orders

Date	Time	Cool/Htd Aerosol	Mask	NC	F102	Pulse Oximeter Sa O_2	COMMENTS

MEMORIAL HOSPITAL

FIGURE 11.16b Respiratory therapy records.

DIAGNOSIS	
M.D. ORDERS	

REFERRING M.D.	CHIEF COMPLAINT

HISTORY

_____

_____

_____

_____

TEST RESULTS/MED	COGNITION

PREVIOUS FUNCTION LEVEL

SOCIAL HISTORY

PRESENT FUNCTIONAL LEVEL

_____ BED MOBILITY	_____ SIT TO STAND	_____ BED TO CHAIR/COMMODE	_____ DISTANCE
_____ SUPINE TO SIT	_____ STATIC STANDING BALANCE	_____ AMBULATION LEVEL SURFACE	_____ ASSISTIVE DEVICE
_____ STATIC SITTING BALANCE	_____ DYNAMIC STANDING BALANCE	_____ STAIRS	OTHER _____

_____ DYNAMIC SITTING BALANCE

STRENGTH (0 - 5)

KEY:

N = NORMAL	* = LIMITED BY PAIN
G = GOOD	MIN = MINIMAL ASSIST
F = FAIR	MOD = MODERATE ASSIST
P = POOR	MAX = MAXIMAL ASSIST
I = INDEPENDENT	U = UNABLE
S = SUPERVISED	NT = NOT TESTED
C = CONTACT GUARD	

ROM: WITHIN NORMAL LIMITS	LIMITATIONS	ABNORMAL MOTOR FINDINGS (INCLUDING TONE, COORDINATION, ETC.)
LUE		
RUE		
LLE		
RLE		
TRUNK		
OTHER		

**MEMORIAL HOSPITAL
PHYSICAL THERAPY
INITIAL EVALUATION PAGE 1 of 2**

FIGURE 11.17 Physical therapy records.

MEMORIAL HOSPITAL **VERSUS CHECKLIST**						
DATE	TIME	ARM B.P.	PULSE	RESP.	TEMPERATURE	LEVEL OF CONSCIOUSNESS

FIGURE 11.18 Vital signs record.

Intake and Output Record

This form is used to measure all fluids taken into the body and all fluids leaving the body (Fig. 11.19).

Special Medication Records

Special records are kept when a patient is being given a particular type of medication. Some examples include the following:

- **Diabetic record**—used when a patient is receiving insulin and is being carefully monitored. The diabetic record contains much information about the diabetic patient in addition to the medication he or she requires, primarily insulin (Fig. 11.20).
- **Anticoagulant record**—used when a patient is receiving medication such as heparin or Coumadin to keep the blood from clotting too rapidly and is being carefully monitored (Fig. 11.21).
- **Patient-controlled analgesia (PCA) record**—used when a patient is receiving self-administered pain medication intravenously (Fig. 11.22).
- **Epidural/spinal analgesia record**—used when a patient is receiving medication for pain relief into the spaces of the spinal cord (Fig. 11.23).

There are many supplemental chart forms. The preceding examples will help you recognize some of the more common types used in your hospital.

FLUID / ELECT. / NUTRITION

Date: _____

IV SOLUTION / RATE			PUMP	TUBE FEEDING SOLUTION
A.			☐	
B.			☐	
C.			☐	
D.			☐	
I.V. Site			☐	

TUBE FDG.
PUMP BAG CHANGE TIME
☐ ☐
☐ ☐

N/G TUBE TYPE: _____ DATE LAST B.M.: _____
PLACEMENT VERIFIED: _____ SUCTION: N Y LIS LCS

TIME	PO	KEY TUBE FEEDING	Credit/Absorbed	INTAKE IV Solutions – Absorbed				TOTAL INTAKE	OUTPUT URINE	NG	IRRIG	B.M.	O.B.	TOTAL OUTPUT	
0700															
0800															
0900															
1000															
1100															
1200															
1300															
1400															
8-HR TOTAL															
1500															
1600															
1700															
1800															
1900															
2000															
2100															
2200															
8-HR TOTAL															
2300															
2400															
0100															
0200															
0300															
0400															
0500															
0600															
8-HR TOTAL															
24-HR TOTAL															

7A SIGNATURE / 3P SIGNATURE / 11P SIGNATURE
24° Amount: FLUID RESTRICTION? Y N

DAILY MEASUREMENT

ADMISSION WEIGHT

TODAY'S WEIGHT ST. CH. BED

DIET TYPE
Breakfast ___% Lunch ___% Dinner ___% Snacks

**MEMORIAL HOSPITAL
INTAKE-OUTPUT**

FIGURE 11.19 Intake and output record.

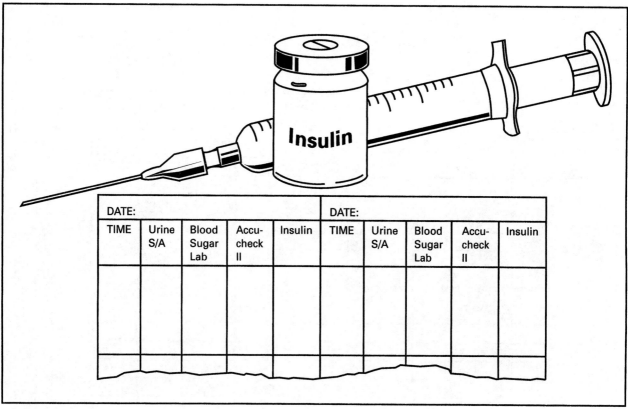

FIGURE 11.20 Diabetic record.

ANTICOAGULANT RECORD				
DATE	PROTHROMBIN X	COUMADIN	HEPARIN	PTT

FIGURE 11.21

CHARTING RESPONSIBILITIES

CONFIDENTIALITY AND THE PATIENT'S CHART

In your work with patients' charts, you will have access to information of a very personal nature. Always remember that this information, as well as all data related to the patient's medical condition, *must* be kept confidential. You are not permitted to reveal this information to the patients or to their visitors, nor should you discuss it with your fellow workers or friends. You may discuss a patient's chart only with hospital personnel who are directly involved with the care of that patient. Keep the charts closed when not in use and put out of the view of patients and visitors who may come to the desk.

PCA

Date: _____

Drug: _____   Concentration: _____

Time	# DOSES Given	# DOSES Attempted	Clinician Activated Bolus (mg)	Total GIVEN (mg)	LOC	Respiratory Rate / Quality	Level of Pain	Side Effects
						Assessment		
7-8								
8-9								
9-10								
10-11								
11-12								
12-13								
13-14								
14-15								
Total								
15-16								
16-17								
17-18								
18-19								
i9-20								
20-21								
21-22								
22-23								
Total								
23-24								
24-01								
01-02								
02-03								
03-04								
04-05								
05-06								
06-07								
Total								
24 Hr Total								

TIME	AMT. IN SYRINGE	SIGNATURES IN	OUT
7A			
3P			
11P			

SYRINGE/CHANGE:

DOSAGE/CHANGES   TIME:

Drug:

Incremental Dose (mg)

Basal Rate (   )

One Hour Limit

ASSESSMENT
Before and after the first dose, then
Every hour X 4 hours, then
Every 2 hours X 4, then
Every 4 hours until PCA discontinued
or as ordered
PRN as indicated
    Level of consciousness
    Respiratory rate & quality
    Level of pain
    Side effects
    IV Site check every shift

LEVEL OF CONSCIOUSNESS CODE
1. awake
2. drowsy, dozing intermittently
3. only awakens when aroused
4. difficult to awaken / lethargic
5. non-responsive

RESPIRATORY QUALITY CODE
S - Shallow   A - Absent
O - Obstructive   NL - Normal

LEVEL OF PAIN
1-10
Scale

SIDE EFFECTS CODE
1. Nausea
2. Vomiting
3. Pruritius
4. Respiratory depression
5. Urinary Retention
6. Other

**MEMORIAL HOSPITAL
PCA FLOW SHEET**

FIGURE 11.22 Patient-controlled analgesia record.

EPIDURAL/SPINAL
Analgesia

Date:_____

Drug:_____ Concentration:_____

Time	Continuous RATE (ml/hr)	Clinician Activated Bolus (ml)	Total GIVEN (ml)	LOC	Respiratory Rate / Quality	Level of Pain	Side Effects
7-8							
8-9							
9-10							
10-11							
11-12							
12-13							
13-14							
14-15							
Total							
15-16							
16-17							
17-18							
18-19							
19-20							
20-21							
21-22							
22-23							
Total							
23-24							
24-01							
01-02							
02-03							
03-04							
04-05							
05-06							
06-07							
Total							
24 Hr Total							

TIME	AMT. IN BAG ML	SIGNATURES IN	OUT
7A			
3P			
11P			
BAG CHANGE:			

DOSAGE/CHANGES
Continuous Dose (ml/hr)
Titrate from   to   ml/hr
Bolus Dose (ml)
Accelerated Infusion Dose

ASSESSMENT
Level of consciousness qh
Respiratory rate & quality qh
Level of pain as indicated
Side effects as indicated
Site check every shift

LEVEL OF CONSCIOUSNESS CODE
1. awake
2. drowsy, dozing intermittently
3. only awakens when aroused
4. difficult to awaken / lethargic
5. non-responsive

RESPIRATORY QUALITY CODE
S - Shallow   A - Absent
O - Obstructive   NL - Normal

LEVEL OF PAIN
1-10 Scale

SIDE EFFECTS CODE
1. Nausea
2. Vomiting
3. Pruritius
4. Urinary Retention
5. Other_____

ADDITIONAL COMMENTS: _____

MEMORIAL HOSPITAL
EPIDURAL FLOW SHEET

FIGURE 11.23 Epidural/spinal analgesia record.

Charts are the legal property of the hospital. It is the health coordinator's responsibility to protect all charts and the information they contain from loss, damage, alteration, or use by unauthorized persons.

Information in the chart cannot be released to another physician without written consent of the admitting doctor. Charts can be inspected at any time by court order and can be removed from a hospital only if requested by court order.

Members of the nursing and medical staff will often need to inspect or record in the charts. As a health unit coordinator, in fairly constant attendance at the desk, you will be expected to keep track of the charts that are used by others. Always remember to do the following:

- Replace all charts in the rack after use.
- Take care to replace each chart in its designated position in the chart rack.
- Keep a written record of all charts removed from the nurses' station by medical personnel.
- Before reporting off-duty each day, check to see that all charts are at the nurses' station, in the rack, or in use.

$\mathcal{R}$ OUTINE CHART CHECKS

Now that you are familiar with the chart forms used in your hospital you are ready to learn what facts to look for in all patients' charts at specified intervals throughout the day.

- All forms included in the chart must be checked to be sure that the patient's name and unit number are entered correctly.
- Each chart must be checked for the proper **sequence** of pages.
- Each chart must be reviewed for forms that are completed; new forms must be stamped properly and added to the chart as necessary. Adding new forms is called **stuffing the chart.**
- All charts belonging to new admissions must be checked routinely for inclusion of laboratory reports and completed medical history and physical examinations. If any reports have been omitted, appropriate personnel should be requested to supply the missing information.
- All preoperative charts must be checked on the morning of surgery to make certain all prescribed laboratory tests have been completed and the results posted in the chart. They should also be checked for inclusion of blank surgical records.
- Charts must be reviewed periodically to see that progress notes have been recorded at required intervals. If any of these have been omitted, physicians responsible must be notified.
- Doctors' order sheets from all charts must be reviewed frequently for orders that need transcription and for orders calling for requisitions.

$\mathcal{R}$ ULES OF CHARTING

Four basic rules should guide all the **charting** you do, not only on patients' charts but on other hospital forms as well.

1. **BE ACCURATE.** Information on charts must be recorded accurately. Data recorded incorrectly can lead physicians to wrong conclusions about their patients. Treatments ordered on the basis of incorrect conclusions can significantly retard or otherwise affect the patients' medical progress. You must not be responsible for errors of this sort.

2. **WRITE LEGIBLY.** Your handwriting must be neat and legible. If a doctor or nurse is unable to read what has been recorded, both your time and theirs has been wasted.

3. **DO NOT ERASE.** The patient's chart is considered a legal document. It can be admitted as evidence in a court of law in the case of a suit against the hospital or physician. Any chart with erasures will not be admitted as legal evidence. Despite all precaution, recording errors will occasionally be made. One accepted way to make corrections is to draw a single line through the error, write in the correction, initial and date. Some hospitals will want the word error written as well (Fig. 11.24).

4. **WRITE ALL ENTRIES IN INK.** To further strengthen the status of chart records in court as legal documents, hospital regulations require that all recording be done in ink.

FIGURE 11.24 Correcting errors.

LEARNING ACTIVITIES

Complete the following.

1. Define
   (a) Chart holder or chart back _____
   (b) Chart rack _____
   (c) Chart _____
   (d) Unit number _____
   (e) "Old chart" _____
   (f) Splitting or thinning _____
   (g) Stuffing the chart _____

2. List three purposes of the chart.
   (a) _____
   (b) _____
   (c) _____

3. In keeping track of the charts always remember to do the following:
   (a) _____
   (b) _____

(c) _____
(d) _____

4. Before use, each chart form must be _____ .

5. Define and give an example of each of the following categories of supplemental chart forms.
  (a) Special therapy records _____
    Example _____
  (b) Surgical records _____
    Example _____
  (c) Special medication records _____
    Example _____

6. List five of the routine chart checks.
  (a) _____
  (b) _____
  (c) _____
  (d) _____
  (e) _____

Match the standard chart form in Column A with its definitions in Column B.

Column A

(a) Doctor's order sheet
(b) Progress notes
(c) Nurses' notes
(d) Graphic chart
(e) Summary sheet
(f) Clinical pathology report
(g) Medication record
(h) Surgical records
(i) Special therapy records
(j) Diagnostic examination

Column B

____ X-ray reports
____ Nurses' communication with doctor
____ Face sheet
____ Laboratory test results
____ Inhalation therapy reports
____ Regular medications
____ Blueprint of care
____ Operative consent
____ TPR
____ Recorded observations of physician

7. List five things to know about keeping the information in the chart confidential.
  (a) _____
  (b) _____
  (c) _____
  (d) _____
  (e) _____

8. List the nine standard chart forms discussed in this chapter and state the purpose of each.

    Chart Form   **Purpose**

(a) _____   _____
(b) _____   _____
(c) _____   _____
(d) _____   _____

	Chart Form	**Purpose**
(e)	_____	_____
(f)	_____	_____
(g)	_____	_____
(h)	_____	_____
(i)	_____	_____

9. Complete the following:
   (a) If a patient is on Coumadin or heparin, which form will be added to the chart? _____

   (b) If a patient is receiving insulin, which form will be added to the chart? _____

   (c) Which standard chart form is completed in the admitting department and is signed by the patient or his or her guardian? _____

   (d) When the patient is receiving self-administered pain medication intravenously, which record is added to the chart? _____

10. What must a physician do if he or she wants advice from another doctor not on the case about a patient's condition? _____

    _____

11. What could be the consequences of not stamping each of the patient's chart forms with the proper imprinter plate? _____

    _____

    _____

    _____

    _____

12. Why is it important for the health unit coordinator to know the proper order of the chart? _____

    _____

    _____

13. A patient has been admitted to the unit without admitting orders, and the nurse is about to call the physician to get those orders. On what form will the nurse write these new orders? _____

14. Although you, as the health unit coordinator, try very hard to keep track of the charts, one or two of the nurses tend to leave charts lying all over the desk, and one of the nurse's aides frequently puts the charts in the wrong place in the chart rack. What can you do about this, and how will you handle the situation? _____

    _____

    _____

    _____

    _____

    _____

    _____

15. Why is it so important that charts be legible, accurate, in ink without erasures, and signed? _____

_____

_____

_____

16. In performing the routine chart checks you come across two sets of orders from the same doctor written on the previous shift that have not been transcribed. The charts were not flagged and were put back in the chart rack. How could this have happened? How serious do you think it is? Is there anything you can do to keep it from happening again? _____

_____

_____

_____

_____

_____

17. What should you do if you can't find a chart? Think of the places you should look. _____

_____

_____

_____

_____

CHAPTER 12

The Health Unit Coordinator and Computers

VOCABULARY

Cathode ray tube (CRT)   Viewing screen

Central processing unit   Working unit of the computer, the "brain"

Command   User's instruction to tell the computer to process information

Cursor   Flashing indicator that denotes where information input will begin

Debug   Remove problems in a computer program that keep it from working

Enter key   Key that gives the computer the command to process information

Ergonomics   The science of fitting a job to workers' physical and psychological needs in terms of their bodily position and ability to see in relation to the equipment they are using. This is done to make the work safer and more comfortable for the worker.

Hard copy   Printed page of computer information

Input   To enter information into computer

Keyboard   Computer typewriter

Light pen   Input device that looks like a pencil but is capable of sensing information typed on screen

Machine language   The computer's language made up of binary digits. Does not require translation to work

Mainframe   The largest of all computers; capable of performing multiple tasks at rapid speeds

Menu   List of computer functions available

Microcomputer   The smallest of computers; also called the personal computer

Minicomputer   A medium-sized computer that is capable of stand-alone functions or auxiliary to a mainframe

Monitor   Viewing screen or CRT

Mouse   A device used for data input that serves as a pointer and moves the cursor around the screen so that different items may be selected

On-line   Done while the computer is connected to a system

Output   What comes out of the computer as processed information

Password   Secret code that allows access to a computer system

Program   Instructions given to computer that cause it to perform functions

Terminal   Computer station that is capable of sending and receiving information to the mainframe via telephone lines, cables, or dedicated digital lines

When you have completed this chapter, you will be able to:

- Define the terms listed in the vocabulary.
- List and describe types of computers.
- List the basic components of all computer systems.
- Identify the single technology that has contributed to the growth of computerization.
- Identify input devices.
- Identify output devices.
- Name the working unit of the computer system.
- Describe what computers do.
- Name the functions of computers in hospital patient care areas.
- Identify the most important computer key.
- Describe possible ethical concerns of using computers in hospitals.
- List rules of computer confidentiality.

*I*NTRODUCTION

Computers have been used in some hospital departments for many years. For example, central supply has used them to keep track of inventories, and the accounting department has used them to itemize statements sent to patients or to prepare paychecks for employees. It was only a matter of time before the computer appeared in the patient care areas, and today computers are widely used there. There is no doubt that health unit coordinators entering the job market today will encounter a computer in their job environment.

The health unit coordinator is a primary operator of the computer system in the patient care area. Computers are designed to help you do your job more efficiently, consistently, and easily. Computers soon lose their mystique as you learn what they can do, what they cannot do, and how you can operate them.

*C*OMPUTERS IN GENERAL

Since the 1950s, computer technology has seen growth at an unbelievable rate. The early computers were made of vacuum tubes and required large, environmentally controlled rooms. Even then they often overheated and became inoperable for many hours. Repairing them was time consuming. Large systems were very expensive, and only the largest organizations were able to afford them. The heart of today's computers are large-scale circuits integrated (LSIC) or microprocessor chips that are often as small as ⅛-inch square. Each LSIC allows thousands of microscopic electronic circuits to be mounted together to do what tons of equipment did in the early years. This technology has allowed computers to become smaller, more powerful, and less expensive.

Today, computers come in three basic sizes: small, medium, and large. The small computers, known as **microcomputers** or personal computers, have become very popular with individuals who use them in organizing their work at home or in a small business. Schools have introduced the microcomputer into the curriculum from elementary grades through high school. Such computers are self-contained and can do all the things a larger computer can do but on a limited scale. They are easy to use, just like typing on a typewriter. Programs have been written for the microcomputer that can be used by anyone, even without knowledge of programming or how the computer works. Microcomputers can even connect with larger computer systems over telephone lines with a device called a *modem* or even through wireless technology (Fig. 12.1).

The medium-sized computer is called a **minicomputer.** The minicomputer is a desktop or stand-alone computer that is capable of processing data like a large computer but does not need a special environmentally controlled room or heavy electrical wiring. Minicomputers were first used for specific or predefined functions such as a front-end machine in data-entry editing but today have become complete database systems or main systems. Minicomputers use high-level languages and are not dependent on the larger system.

The largest of all the computer systems is called a **mainframe system.** It is capable of processing large amounts of information at unbelievable speeds. Mainframe computer systems can access information at unbelievable speeds. Mainframe computer systems can access information from auxiliary storage devices as well as send information to other computers or terminals located in remote sites. Most large organizations have their own mainframe computer; some smaller businesses purchase computer time from the large organizations.

In the hospital, you will most likely work on a minicomputer system that may or may not be connected to a mainframe system or on a remote terminal connected to a microcomputer or a mainframe system. Regardless of the system, operating it is basically the same.

FIGURE 12.1

ℬASIC COMPUTER SYSTEM

Whether you operate a small microcomputer or interact with a large mainframe computer you are working on a computer system with three basic components. All computers must have a means to *input* information, a means to *process* information, and a means to *output* information (Fig. 12.2).

FIGURE 12.2

ℐNPUT

There are several ways to enter information into the computer. The most common one used by the health unit coordinator is the **keyboard.** The keyboard looks like a typewriter with a few extra keys. One key plays a very important function—the **Enter** key. When you are finished putting your information into the computer, you must signal the computer "I'm done, now it's your turn." You do this with the ENTER key. Some computer companies color this key red because of its importance. It is not absolutely necessary to have typing skills to operate the computer keyboard; however, being familiar with the keyboard will help you develop computer keyboard skill (Fig. 12.3).

FIGURE 12.3

A second common input device is the **light pen.** The light pen looks like a pencil, but it is designed to sense the writing on the computer screen. The operator selects a choice, then moves the light pen across the choice and across the Enter statement. The information is entered into the computer's processing unit.

A **mouse** is an input device used for pointing that moves the cursor around the screen so that a selection can be made from items listed on the screen. The **cursor** (flashing light or lighted mark of some sort) is a symbol that indicates where the user is on the screen. It takes some practice to become competent at using a mouse. The clicking of mouse buttons and movements of the mouse elicit various commands and require some eye–hand coordination.

Other input devices of computer systems include floppy disks, magnetic disks or tapes, or compact discs. These become storage devices of the hospital computer system and are "behind the scene" of the health unit coordinator using the computer. Stored information must be retrieved from the computer and replaced with current information. This is usually not done at the keyboard of a hospital system.

𝒫ROCESS

A computer processes information that is input to it and returns that processed information to the person putting it in or to someone else in another department. This **central processing unit (CPU)** is the working unit of the computer and consists of many electronic components and microchips. The computer performs its processing function in computer or machine language based on digital logic. It is given instructions to do a specific task in a program. The person using the computer does not have to understand the computer's language nor the program in detail but must understand the commands the computer needs to initiate its functions. The processing unit can process only the information it receives; if it receives wrong information, it processes wrong information. Thus it is very important for the health unit coordinator to input only correct information. So far computers have not been designed to "think" as we do, they just process information in a logical, rapid, and consistently accurate manner.

𝒪UTPUT

What goes in must come out. Such is also true for computers. Just as there are several ways to enter information into the computer, there are several ways to get it out. The most common ways are **visually on the monitor** or **video screen** and **printed copy via a printer.** The health unit coordinator will work with both these methods. A monitor or video screen is also called a **cathode ray tube,** or **CRT.** It looks much like a television. As you input information it can be seen on the screen of the monitor. When it is processed, it returns to you and can be seen on the screen. Information that is stored can also be called to the screen. If you need a printed copy of the results of the processing, a printer is used to type information on paper. Information printed on paper is called **hard copy** and can be subsequently filed with the patient's record. Information can also be output to floppy disks or magnetic disks or tapes. Stored information can also be output to your screen or printer

There is no mystery to a computer. Information to be used must first be input, it is then processed via electronic components in digital logic, and it is returned as output. The health unit coordinator is involved in inputting information and receiving the output for the patient's record.

WHAT COMPUTERS DO IN HOSPITALS

By now you are aware that hospitals process information (i.e., records, charges, charts, supplies, and files). Today virtually all accounting and purchasing functions are done with computers. Some hospitals even have computer diagnostic services that allow individuals to have their complete physical examination analyzed by a computer and be told the results at the end of the examination. Depending on the hospital and its needs, the hospital may either own its own computer system or purchase computer services. It may design its own program to meet its needs or purchase a computer system from a supplier of programs. Computers are widely used in patient care areas as well as in accounting and purchasing. The health unit coordinator has become a processor of information via the computer. Using a computer helps health unit coordinators with their job responsibilities, cuts down the required writing and potential errors, and increases the speed with which orders can be carried out.

COMMON SYSTEMS IN PATIENT CARE AREAS

It is not possible to describe each computer system that may be found in the hospital, since many companies have designed systems. Familiar names are IBM, EDS, SMS, TDS, and Med-Pro. Computer systems can be designed solely for one hospital, or they can be designed with general applications to a variety of hospitals. Much research goes into selecting a computer system. Putting a hospital on-line can often take months or years. Problems often develop that have to be worked out. Solving these problems is called **debugging.** Those individuals who work with the system often develop new skills in identifying computer problem areas and can be very helpful to the computer department. The department in the hospital responsible for computers is often called **information systems.** It is staffed with specialists in computer science, who often plan and implement the computer training of hospital personnel.

What functions can a computer perform in the patient care area? Computers are being used to:

- Order medications
- Order or change diets
- Order unit supplies
- Process charges for nursing care equipment

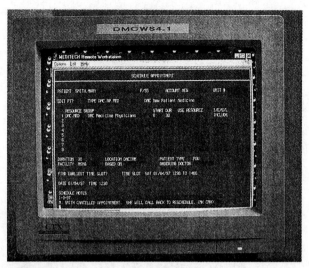

FIGURE 12.4 Computerized charting.

- Order lab work
- Record lab results for patient records
- Document nursing care at the beside (Fig. 12.4)
- Schedule x-rays, special tests, or surgery
- Process discharges

Computers can obtain a census listing names of patients, room numbers, bed assignments, and conditions. They can transfer patients to another unit and even send appropriate departments a message of the change (e.g., pharmacy, the business office, and dietary). They can print out a complete record of all the patient's orders since admission. Computer systems can even print routine preparation or procedure orders that can be used to instruct patients or notify a department with a sound when a stat request has been ordered or a stat report is available. If this list sounds like what you do, you are correct. Remember, we said computers process information (Fig. 12.5).

*T*HE HEALTH UNIT COORDINATOR AND THE COMPUTER

You will be using a computer for many of the tasks you will be performing. There are some general skills you can learn now that will be useful regardless of the computer system you must use. If you have a computer in your school, you should practice these skills.

1. Signing on
2. Moving the cursor
3. Entering data
4. Verifying orders
5. Inquiring about orders
6. Correcting mistakes

FIGURE 12.5

7. Deleting orders

8. Notifying other departments

9. Planning for contingencies

Signing On

Although a computer is easy to operate, access is limited to special persons. When you have been cleared, you will be given a security ID and/or a password. It will identify you as an eligible user of the computer. You should never give this information to anyone.

Most systems require a sequence of operations to sign on. You will learn the required sequence for your hospital's system. When requested, enter your security ID and/or password. When you have completed your sign-on (if it is correct), you will see a **menu** displayed, showing all the possible requests you can make of your computer. Typically, submenus are displayed as well.

Moving the Cursor

Somewhere on the screen you will see a flashing indicator called a **cursor,** which identifies the starting point of your request. The cursor can be moved all over the screen. When an order is sent to the computer, the cursor will automatically reset itself to the point where you will begin to enter the order. You should practice moving the cursor around the screen.

Entering Data

The most important key on the computer keyboard is the Enter key. Once you have selected the function you wish the computer to perform, you must press the Enter key. This signals the computer processor to process your order. If you use a light pen, you must pass the pen over the ENTER command. *The computer awaits your command; you are in control!* If you make a spelling or a selection error, you can easily correct it by moving the cursor prior to entering your order. You should always check what you have typed to be sure it is correct. Once you press Enter, the computer tries to process your order. If it does not recognize the request, it will tell you so; if it recognizes the request it will process it, even if it is wrong. For example, you request a barium enema procedure for a patient. In typing your order you spell *barium* as *bareum.* The computer will not recognize the spelling and will tell you so. If you request a barium enema when a barium swallow is really wanted, the computer will schedule the barium enema. *Remember, it is possible to correct errors even after they are entered.*

Inquiring about Orders

Requesting "order inquiry" will allow you to see all orders or orders placed on a certain day (like today). You can trace orders to see where they were lost. You can even learn the identification of the person who entered the order as well as if another department placed an order. This function also allows you to perform a similar inquiry order to allow you to locate patients by their name should a visitor be looking for someone in the hospital.

Correcting Mistakes

All computer systems have ways to correct mistakes. There is one procedure to use prior to entering the order, such as cursor movement and backspace, and another after the order has been entered, such as deleting orders. You will want to become familiar with both of these ways. Some computers use order verification, a second Enter step, to allow a review of the order to be sure it is correct.

Verifying Orders

After an order has been placed, the request will appear on the screen. If the information is correct, you should press the Enter key. If it is not correct, correct it at this time. When you have entered all orders, you can request an inquiry of the orders as another check.

Deleting Orders

If, after you have entered an order, you find it is not correct, you can request that the computer delete the order. This command is also used when an order is canceled, such as when a new medication is ordered and the old one is no longer needed.

Notifying Other Departments

Many times an order request affects another department such as dietary, laboratory, radiology, accounting, or admitting. Hospital computers are designed to forward messages to departments that need this information. For example, when an x-ray is ordered that requires the patient to be NPO, the dietary request to hold the next meal is made at the same time. The charge for the procedure is then sent to accounting. All this can be done through the computer without additional paperwork or phone calls.

Contingency Planning

Whenever humans depend on machines, contingency plans need to be made in case the machine is out of order. When a computer is not functioning, it is *down*. Downtime can be scheduled to allow a new program to be entered into the computer's memory or to make changes. Downtime can also be unexpected—due to power failure or component failure. Hospitals have alternative plans in case failure occurs. Despite modern technology, you still need to know manual methods of entering orders. You will probably prefer the computer once you have mastered the technique of using it.

*E*THICS AND CONFIDENTIALITY

By now you should realize how important ethics and confidentiality are in your work. When using a computer, you must not let your identification code or password get in the hands of the wrong person. The consequences could be disastrous to patients. If you were tempted to alter patient information, serious consequences would result. Although there are many safeguards built into the computer system, they can be bypassed by an unethical person with a knowledge of computers. Ethics and confidentiality are essential when computers are used. The patient's privacy must be maintained.

Rules of Confidentiality

1. The type and amount of information gathered and recorded about a patient by a caregiver, employee, and the like shall be limited to that information required for legitimate purposes.

2. All individuals engaged in the collection, handling, or dissemination of information shall be specifically informed of their responsibility to protect confidential data and of the penalties for violation of this trust. Proven violation of confidentiality of private information may be cause for disciplinary action or termination of employment. Breach of confidentiality is considered to be a very serious employment offense.

3. Access to material that contains confidential information shall be limited to situations in which legitimate need and purpose can be demonstrated.

4. Access to areas where confidential information may be discussed, such as patient treatment areas, shall be limited to only those individuals whose presence is required for a legitimate purpose.

5. Confidential information shall be protected from access by unauthorized individuals in both manual and automated systems.

6. Computerized information and access codes shall be authorized by directors based on the "need to know" concept.

7. All caregivers who receive a computer access code shall be required to read and sign a confidentiality statement at the completion of the system training period (Fig. 12.6).

8. Special confidentiality/security procedures for sensitive records, e.g., payroll records, will be documented in the individual department policy and procedure manual.

MEMORIAL HOSPITAL
Computer User's Access Codes (Log-ins)
Confidentiality Statement

Obtaining access to the Hospital's computerized information system requires a clear understanding of your responsibilities regarding access and adequate training on the system. The following statements will provide an understanding of the significance of the User Access Code you receive following your training. Please, read them **carefully**.

1. My User Access Code (password) is confidential. It identifies me in a *unique* manner. I am responsible for all data entered into Merlin under my code.

2. I will not disclose my User Access Code to anyone, nor will I attempt to learn another person's access code.

3. I will not use another person's access code to enter, update, or retrieve data on Merlin.

4. If I have reason to believe the confidentiality of my code has been compromised, I will notify Information Systems Services immediately so that my code can be deleted and a new code issued to me.

5. I understand that all patient data viewed, printed, or entered is confidential patient data and part of the medical-legal record. I will not access data on patients for whom I have no responsibilities and for whom I have no "need to know."

6. I understand that any misuse of my confidential User Access Code is a violation of Hospital policy, and will subject me to disciplinary action up to and including termination of employment.

Your signature below acknowledges agreement with and understanding of these statements.

Signature _____ Name Printed _____

Department _____ Date _____

Trainer's Initials/ I.S. Issuer _____ Date _____

DISTRIBUTION: ORIGINAL - HUMAN RESOURCES, Employee File   PHOTOCOPY - DEPT. DIRECTOR

- -

Employee# _____ **Access Code** _____
            (if known)   (PRINT password CLEARLY)

Please Note: If you have not received a certificate of class completion and/or access is not available within 4 days, please notify your director.

FIGURE 12.6

Summary

Not all hospitals have installed computers in the patient care areas where the health unit coordinator will be working, but most have done so or are moving in this direction. You may be one of the pioneers in your hospital as computer technology helps you do your job more efficiently and consistently. Computers are only machines. They were designed by humans and help humans. Humans are in control of the computer.

Sample Computer Use for Laboratory Oder

Screen	Input
Step #1—PASSWORD	
return	
ENTER FUNCTION	ORDER ENTRY (F2) (will select from menu of many functions, each with own letter).
return	
PATIENT NUMBER (#), e.g., #123456	FROM ADDRESSOGRAPH PLATE
return	Will echo name
DEPARTMENT	
PRESS "HELP" TO CHOOSE FROM CRC-CV-CAR-CT-CS-EPI-LAB-MIC-NEU-NUC-NCS-OT-PT-RAD-RT-SS-US-ST-PF-MRI.	
Enter one group of initials	
Example: LAB	
COLL BY LAB?	If yes, press return
DATE TO COLL	If today, press return
TIME TO COLL (RETURN)	If tomorrow, press T + 1
	IT WILL SHOW THE APPROPRIATE DATE
PRIORITY (HELP)	ROUTINE—STAT, ASAP, PREOP, AM DRAW
	(If press R, will show routine)
TEST	■ In this system at this point HUC must go to book of codes to select valid item number and will enter that number. *For example:* #1020 = CBC
ORDER DR. NAME	If the same as chart, push Return. Will echo name
COMMENTS	Type in anything special
ENTER	Press return
ORDER ENTRY #	■ Screen shows number which is to be copied on Physician's Order Sheet next to order and on Kardex.
PUSH EXIT TO GET OUT	

SAMPLE COMPUTER ABBREVIATIONS

Abbreviations	Departments
CRC	Cardiac Rehabilitation
CV	Cardiovascular
CAR	Cardiology
CT	CAT Scan
CS	Central Supply
EPI	Epidemiology
LAB	Laboratory
MIC	Microbiology
NEU	Neurology
NUC	Nuclear Medicine
NCS	Nutrition Care Services
OT	Occupational Therapy
PT	Physical Therapy
RAD	Radiology
RT	Respiratory Therapy
SS	Social Services
US	Ultrasound
ST	Speech Therapy
PF	Pulmonary Therapy
MRI	Magnetic Resonance Imaging

SAMPLE COMPUTER FUNCTION

Codes	Function
F1	NAME INQUIRY SELECT
F2	ORDER ENTRY
F3	CANCEL REQUEST
F4	ORDER INQUIRY
F5	PATIENT FILE REVISION
F6	INPATIENT DISCHARGE
F7	TRANSFER/SWAP SELECT
F8	POST BED STATUS
F9	MAINTENANCE SELECT
F10	SEND/RECEIVE MESSAGE SELECT
F11	FACE SHEET INQUIRY
<NBM>	NEWBORN MINI-ADMIT
<ORS>	ORDER SET INQUIRY
S1	NAME INQUIRY—HELD OUTPATIENT
S2	VERIFY HELD PATIENT
S7	CORRECT DISCHARGE
S8	CENSUS SELECT
S9	PRINT CENSUS UTILITIES (Diets, Nursing Worksheets, etc.)
S10	VACANT BED LIST
S11	PRINTER UTILITIES
S12	REQUEST CHART PULL
<PC3>	PRINT CENSUS UTILITIES

LEARNING ACTIVITIES

Complete the following.

1. List and describe three categories of computers.
   (a) _____
   (b) _____
   (c) _____

2. List the three basic components of all computer systems.
(a) _____
(b) _____
(c) _____

3. List two input devices.
(a) _____
(b) _____

4. List two output devices.
(a) _____
(b) _____

5. Describe what computers do. _____
_____

6. List eight functions computers perform in hospital patient care areas.
(a) _____
(b) _____
(c) _____
(d) _____
(e) _____
(f) _____
(g) _____
(h) _____

7. Name the most important function key on the computer keyboard. _____
_____

8. What is the significance of the cursor? _____

9. List four rules of computer confidentiality.
(a) _____
(b) _____
(c) _____
(d) _____

Match the word in Column A with its definition in Column B.

Column A

(a) Cursor
(b) Debug
(c) Light pen
(d) CRT
(e) Program
(f) Command
(g) Menu
(h) Password

Column B

_____ An input device
_____ Secret code
_____ Listing of available functions
_____ Flashing indicator
_____ Viewing screen
_____ Instructions
_____ Request
_____ Problem solving

Complete the following:

10. Although you are very computer literate, a new nurse who has come back to nursing after staying home to raise her children is not. She frequently asks you to help her with computer issues. She is nice and so are you; however, you are also very busy. How can you handle the situation?

_____

_____

_____

11. A recovering patient likes to come to the desk and visit. He also likes to look at the computer screen as you order. What can you do to protect the patient's privacy in this situation?

_____

_____

_____

_____

12. Your hospital has decided to put in a new computer system, and many of the staff are concerned and complaining because they know how much extra effort it is going to be to get used to a new system. How do you think you would feel about this? In what ways could you be a positive influence on your fellow staff members?

_____

_____

_____

_____

_____

13. In a worst-case scenario what might happen if the wrong person got access to the private information contained in the hospital's computer system?

_____

_____

_____

_____

_____

Introduction to Order Transcription

Computer-generated Kardex	Form printed by the computer for each patient that contains consolidated information from the doctor's order sheet regarding diagnostic and therapeutic orders
Flagging	The use of a red or other colored tag on the chart by the physician to indicate that new orders have been written
Kardex	A patient care record card used for consolidating information regarding the patient's diagnostic and therapeutic orders
Kardex holder	A vinyl or metal-backed rectangular device with a series of graduated inserts that holds the patient care record card by room number for each patient on the nursing unit
Kardexing	The act of transcribing orders from the chart and placing them on the Kardex
NCR	No carbon required
One-time or limited order	An order that is to be done only once or is limited to the number of times specified by the doctor's order
Sign off	The placement of the nurse's signature, date, and time on the doctor's order sheet to indicate that the nurse has carefully checked the transcribed orders and verified that they have been done correctly
Standing prn order	Orders that remain as written until changed but that are carried out on an as-needed basis
Standing routine orders	Orders that once written remain unchanged until changed by the physician and are carried out on a regular basis
Stat orders	Orders that are to be carried out immediately
Take off orders	Transcribe physician's orders
Telephone order	An order received by telephone from the physician that is written on the chart by the nurse and later signed by the physician
Transcription of orders	The process of transferring orders written by the physician to other forms and into the computer, and the ordering of supplies, equipment, and services so that the orders may be carried out
Verbal order	An order given orally by the physician in person that is written on the chart by the nurse and later signed by the physician

OBJECTIVES

When you have completed this chapter, you will be able to:

- Define the terms listed in the vocabulary.
- State two reasons for doctors' orders and the three methods by which they may be obtained.
- List and discuss the tools of transcription.

- List and explain the seven steps of order transcription.
- State the purpose of symbols in order transcription.
- List and define the seven general classifications of doctors' orders.
- List and discuss the four categories of doctors' orders.
- Discuss ways to avoid errors in order transcription.

GENERAL INFORMATION

All medical and many nursing services performed in a hospital for the patient require written orders from the patient's doctor. There are two main reasons for this:

1. Only the doctor knows what medical treatment will best meet the needs of the patient.
2. Legal safeguards are necessary to protect the patient from incorrect medical treatment.

METHODS OF OBTAINING ORDERS

Often the doctor will give the nurse orders over the telephone. The nurse will write these on the physician's order sheet, write T.O. (**telephone order**) Dr. _____, and sign his or her name. The physician must sign these orders when he or she comes to the hospital. Occasionally, you will see doctors' orders written by the nurse and followed with VO (**verbal order**) Dr. _____ and the nurse's signature. This means that the doctor told the nurse to do something (often in an emergency) and will sign the order later.

Sometimes doctors will have their routine orders printed to reduce the need for handwriting, make individual corrections as necessary, and sign these when they visit; but most frequently, doctors will write their own orders in handwriting and sign them at that time.

ORDER TRANSCRIPTION

For both medical and legal reasons, then, medical care orders for the patient originate and are given with the doctor's direction and consent.

Once an order has been written by the doctor, the responsibility for seeing that the order is carried out rests with the nurse. As a health unit coordinator, you will share this responsibility with the nurse by performing the clerical task called **transcription of orders.** For purposes of carrying out a doctor's orders, equipment or services often must be ordered from other departments. The orders themselves must be transferred to other records that will be available to all nursing staff members who will care for the patient. In transcribing or **taking off** doctor's orders, you are simply ordering by computer or rewriting them on requisitions, patient chart forms, and special records.

The most important hospital records are those concerning doctors' orders for the treatment of patients. Errors in these records, and resulting errors in treatment, may have immediate as well as long-term effects on the condition of a patient. Consider, for example, what may happen to a patient who is given the wrong dosage of a medicine because the written order was copied incorrectly on a medication administration record. Consider a newly admitted patient with bleeding ulcers who, by clerical error, has a regular diet ordered for him and begins to hemorrhage violently after eating the meal. As you learn the principles and methods of transcribing orders **always remember that any error can have disastrous effects.** If you do not understand an order or are unable to read the doctor's writing, the nurse is present to answer your questions.

- Always **ASK** when in doubt.
- Always be **ALERT** when transcribing doctor's orders.
- Always be **ACCURATE.**

$\mathcal{T}$OOLS OF TRANSCRIPTION

$\mathcal{D}$OCTOR'S ORDER SHEET

The tools of transcription are the doctor's order sheet and the Kardex. The doctor's orders are written on the doctor's order sheet and then transferred to the Kardex via computer or by hand by the health unit coordinator. The doctor's order sheet and the Kardex serve as the order communication tools of the nursing unit. Review the discussion of the doctor's order sheet in Chapter 11, then study Fig. 13.1 until you have a general understanding of what the term *doctor's order* means. Note that the doctor does not indicate how or where you should transcribe the order, nor identify the type of order for you. When you finish learning transcription of orders, you will know these facts solely by what is written.

DATE	ORDER	SIGNATURE
6-1-xx	*Hot soaks to elbow q4h*	
	Aspirin 600 mg. p.o. q4h for Temp > 103°F.	
	Out of bed ad lib.	
	Allow shower in A.M.	
	Electrolytes in A.M.	
	IVP	
	Transfer to semiprivate in P.M.	
	Remove restraints. Replace if necessary.	

FIGURE 13.1

$\mathcal{K}$ARDEX (PATIENT CARE RECORD CARD)

You already know that the Kardex is used for consolidating information about the patient and the diagnostic and therapeutic orders written by the physician. Nursing personnel use this form to learn their specific duties regarding a patient without having to refer constantly to the chart or order sheet. You have probably used it too, to answer some of the many questions about patients directed to you during the day. As a health unit coordinator, you will be engaged in much of the actual recording of information on the Kardex. You will need to understand fully the information it contains and how this information is recorded.

Kardex systems vary widely from one hospital to another. Many use **computer-generated Kardexes,** discussed on page 289. The example used in this chapter consolidates nearly all the information that is ordinarily included. Your hospital will use a Kardex best suited to its needs and will have other methods of consolidating any information not included on its card.

The **Kardex holder** is usually a vinyl or metal-backed rectangular device with a series of graduated inserts (Fig. 13.2).

FIGURE 13.2

The Kardex, one for each patient, is placed in the inserts with the identifying information (patient's name, room number, etc.) visible at the bottom of the card. Each card can be flipped upward to expose the additional information on a particular patient. The cards are filed by room number.

- Permanent recording on the Kardex, such as the patient's name and doctor's name, is usually done in ink.
- Different colors of ink may be used to record certain data, such as a patient's allergies, so that such information will be easy to see.
- Some of the recording is done in pencil so it can be erased and replaced with new orders when the original orders are canceled.
- Sometimes small "throwaway" cards are used with the more permanent Kardex for recording orders to be carried out only once. These cards are kept primarily to provide information to the nursing staff through one 24-hour period and are discarded on a daily basis or when full.
- If a Kardex becomes mutilated after long use or many erasures, the orders currently in effect may be recopied on a new card and the old card destroyed or marked "copied" and kept behind the new card.
- The Kardex is removed when the patient is discharged, and a blank card, to be used for the next patient to occupy the bed, is then inserted.
- The Kardex is often used to construct staff patient care assignments, to give change-of-shift reports, and to check on specific orders for a patient.

Sample Construction of Kardex

On Side 1, as indicated in Fig. 13.3, a place is provided to list all diagnostic tests and special procedures on the patient. These may include laboratory tests, x-rays, electrocardiograms, endoscopies, and isotopic examinations. Surgical procedures might be recorded in red ink for emphasis. With this record, the doctor is able to tell at a glance what tests have been ordered and performed; and the nursing staff is able to order necessary preparations of patients for medical and surgical procedures and to see that all ordered procedures have been performed. Side 2 is an acuity assessment used to plan staffing. Side 3 shows medications, IVs, and treatments, as carried out by nursing personnel. At the very bottom of this page, visible on each card when the file is closed, is the summary information for identification of the patient. Sample Kardexes are provided at the end of Chapter 17 for order transcription practice.

FIGURE 13.3

The Computer-Generated Kardex

Many hospitals are using computers in the patient care areas and many no longer use the Kardex just described. Instead, the computer prints out a Kardex for each patient on demand. This means that instead of handwriting all the orders into the various spaces on the Kardex each time an order is transcribed, all the work is done for you at the time the orders are entered into the computer. The printout is the most up-to-date information available on the patient and is used by nursing in the same way that the older Kardex was used. The individual Kardexes may be kept in a notebook or on a clipboard at the nurse's station, but the Kardex holder will no longer be used. Figure 13.4

```
                              KARDEX              Pg. 1 of 3

   41001   EXAMPLE, IMA      1234567890 66 F  ADM-042197 053097 16:49 4MS
   DX ADM  BRONCHITIS        ADM   000022  GOODDOCTOR, GEO. AL1 pcn
   DX CUR  pneumonia         ATT   000022  GOODDOCTOR, GEO. AL2 asa
      DX1  ARDS              CON1  000023  ALSOGOOD, ALVIN  AL3 codeine
      DX2                    CON2  000024                  AL4
      DX3                    CON3  000026                  AL5
      DX4                    CON4  000027                  AL6
     SUR1  lobectomy 1995    CON5  000000                   HT 64
     SUR2                    CON6  000000                   WT 150
     SUR3                    CON7  000000
     SUR4                    INVS  LNE
    HIST1                    DIAB
    HIST2                                            IV
    HIST3                    IS TY                   OXYGEN
    HIST4                    COMM                       MRN-00219218


----- SKIN ASSESSMENT ----------------!----- ALLERGY/HT/WT -----------------
___ Assess skin q shift.             !  ___ Allergies/Ht/Wt entered in Merlin
                                     !      (If ht/wt/allergies do not show in
___ Begin Pressure Ulcer Protocol.   !      upper right hand corner of this
                                     !      Kardex, then they still need to be
                                     !      entered.)
----- LABORATORY ---------------------!----- NUTRITION SERVICES -------------
   483 053097 ROUTINE URINE, CREATI-  !   186 042197 CAFFEINE,BLAND,RESIDUE
       NINE RANDOM COLLECT BY NURSE   !       OR FIBER CONT BLAND LOW RESIDUE
   717 053097 ROUTINE TYPE & SCREEN   !   296 042197 ORAL NUTRITION /
       COLLECT BY LAB                 !       SUPPLEMENTS - SUSTACAL PLUS
   718 053097 ROUTINE TYPE AND        !       FLUID RESTRICTION
       CROSSMATCH PACKED RBCS         !   385 042197 STANDARD TUBE FEEDING
   719 053097 STAT CSF PANEL (INCL.   !       FORMULA T.F.PRO CONTINUOUS 40CC
       CELL CT., GLUC, T.P.)          !       HR
   720 053097 STAT CSF IMMUNOSUPPRES- !   387 042197 STANDARD PROTOCOL: REG.
       SED PANEL                      !       DIETITIAN TUBE FEEDING CONSULT
   737 053097 STAT INDIA INK PREP (CSF)!  1057 051497 STANDARD TUBE FEEDING
   738 053097 STAT CRYPTOCOCCUS       !       FORMULA T.F.PRO CONTINUOUS 40CC
       ANTIGEN (CSF)                  !       HR
   739 053097 STAT CULTURE/GM. STAIN  !  1058 051497 STANDARD PROTOCOL: REG.
       (CSF)                          !       DIETITIAN TUBE FEEDING CONSULT
   740 053097 STAT CULTURE, FUNGUS    !       TESTING SORT SORTING TEST
       (CSF)                          !   313 052897 STANDARD TUBE FEEDING
   741 053097 ROUTINE CULTURE, BLOOD -!       FORMULA T.F.PRO CONTINUOUS 60CC,
       IMMUNOSUP (HIV) COLLECT BY NURSE!      HR
   742 053097 ROUTINE CULTURE,        !   315 052897 STANDARD PROTOCOL: REG.
       RESPIRATORY (BRONCH-IMMUNOS)   !       DIETITIAN TUBE FEEDING CONSULT
       COLLECT BY NURSE               !   484 053097 PROTEIN CONTROLLED DIET-
   743 053097 COLLECTION OF AUTOLOGOUS !      RENAL,HEPATIC 35 GM PRO 2.5 GM
       BLOOD                          !       K+ FLUID RESTRICTION 700 CC
                                     !
```

FIGURE 13.4 Example of computer-generated Kardex.

```
                          KARDEX              Pg. 2 of 3

  41001  EXAMPLE, IMA           1234567890 66 F ADM-042197 053097 16:49 4MS
```

----- CARDIOPULMONARY -----------------!----- BEHAVIORAL MEDICINE ------------
  192 042197 ROUTINE OXYGEN ORDER 4L   !
  204 042197 ROUTINE COLOR FLOW   !
  205 042197 STAT COMPLETE ECHO   !
  206 042197 STAT HOLTER MONITOR   !
  485 053097 VENTILATOR ORDER 100% 14   !----- NURSING ORDERS -----------------
      SIMV   ! 231 042197 14H ACCUCHECKS BY NURSING
  486 053097 VENTILATOR CHANGES ORDER   ! 275 042197 Q6HR ACCUCHECKS BY
      90%   !   NURSING
  487 053097 Q6H IPPB TERBUTALINE   ! 276 042197 BATH NURSING ORDER
  488 053097 ROUTINE CAROTID DUPLEX   !   PARTIAL BATH
      ULTRASOUND CARDIZEM   ! 277 042197 DIET NURSING ORDER
  713 053097 ROUTINE ELECTROCARDIO-   !   CALORIE COUNT
      GRAM DIGOXIN   ! 278 042197 DRESSINGS NURSING ORDER
  714 053097 ROUTINE TREADMILL BETA   !   SUBCLAVIAN/SWAN DRESSING CHANGE
      BLOCKERS   ! 279 042197 GASTRO NURSING ORDER
                                        !   COLOSTOMY CARE
                                        ! 289 042197 Q6H ACCUCHECKS BY
                                        !   NURSING
                                        ! 292 042197 Q8GR STANDARD PROTOCOL:
----- DISCHARGE/SOCIAL SERVICES -------!   CHECK GASTRIC RESI 500CC OR
                                        !   MORE, HOLD TUBE FEEDING X 1
                                        !   HOUR AND RECHECK RESIDUAL.
----- RADIOLOGY/NUC MED ---------------!   NOTIFY M.D. IF TUBE FEEDING
  482 053097 STAT ENTIRE SPINE LTD   !   HELD MORE THAN 2 CONSECUTIVE
      PAIN   !   HOURS.
                                        ! 293 042197 STANDARD PROTOCOL:
                                        !   RECORD WEIGHT Q 3 DAYS FIRST
                                        !   WEEK, THEN Q WEEK
                                        ! 386 042197 HYDRATION/TUBE FEEDING
----- PHYSICAL THERAPY ---------------!   ORDER: IRRIGATE TUBE WITH 50 CC
  201 042197 PHYSICAL THERAPY   !   OF H2O AT LEAST Q 8 HRS
      EVALUATION REQUEST   ! 388 042197 STANDARD PROTOCOL: TUBE
  225 042197 GAIT TRAINING   !   CONFIRMATION: CHECK FEEDING
  226 042197 PHYSICAL THERAPY   !   TUBE PLACEMENT PRIOR TO
      EVALUATION REQUEST   !   BEGINNING TUBE FEEDING
  227 042197 THERAPEUTIC EXERCISE   ! 389 042197 STANDARD PROTOCOL:
  228 042197 TRANSFER TRAINING   !   TOLERANCE EVAL: ADVANCE TUBE
  715 053097 GAIT TRAINING S/P TOTAL   !   FEEDING AS ORDERED IF RESIDUAL
      HIP   !   NO GREATER THAN 100 CC OR ABOVE
                                        !   SPECIFIED LEVEL, NO ABDOMINAL
                                        !   DISTENTION, NO GREATER THAN 5
----- REHAB SERVICES -----------------!   LIQUID STOOLS PER 24 HOURS.
                                        ! 390 042197 STANDARD PROTOCOL: ELEV.
                                        !   HEAD OF BED > 30 DEGREES DURING
                                        !   FEEDING & 30 MIN. AFTER DELIVERY
                                        ! 391 042197 TUBE ORDER: INITIATE
                                        !   FEEDING THROUGH CURRENT
                                        !   NASOENTERIC TUBE
                                        ! 1063 052897 Q6HRS STANDARD PROTOCOL:

FIGURE 13.4 (*Continued*)

KARDEX   Pg. 3 of 3

41001   EXAMPLE, IMA   1234567890 66 F   ADM-042197 053097 16:49 4MS

```
        CHECK GASTRIC RESI 400CC OR     !  291 042197 PO MED: DIGOXIN
        MORE, HOLD TUBE FEEDING X 1     !  744 053097 SQ Q6HR REGULAR HUMAN
        HOUR AND RECHECK RESIDUAL.      !      INSULIN 4UNITS ACCUCHECKS Q 6 HRS
        NOTIFY M.D. IF TUBE FEEDING     !  746 053097 SQ Q4HRS SLIDING SCALE
        HELD MORE THAN 2 CONSECUTIVE    !      REGULAR INSULIN IF <150=0 U; IF
        HOURS.                          !      151-200 = 2 U; IF 201-250 = 4U;
  1064 052897 STANDARD PROTOCOL:        !      IF >251, CALL IF >251, CALL MD.
        RECORD WEIGHT Q 3 DAYS FIRST    !  747 053097 75 ML/HR IV ORDER D5W
        WEEK, THEN Q WEEK               !      20MEQ KCL
   314 052897 HYDRATION/TUBE FEEDING    !
        ORDER: IRRIGATE TUBE WITH 50 CC !
        OF H2O AT LEAST Q 8 HRS         !
   316 052897 STANDARD PROTOCOL: TUBE   !
        CONFIRMATION: CHECK FEEDING     !----- MESSAGES RE THIS PATIENT -------
        TUBE PLACEMENT PRIOR TO         !  716 053097 TO ADMITTING - ADMITTING
        BEGINNING TUBE FEEDING          !      INFO FORM ADMITTING CLERK MAY
   317 052897 STANDARD PROTOCOL:        !      COME & SEE PATIENT NOW FAMILY
        TOLERANCE EVAL: ADVANCE TUBE    !      IS HERE TO INTERPRET
        FEEDING AS ORDERED IF RESIDUAL  !
        NO GREATER THAN 100 CC OR ABOVE !
        SPECIFIED LEVEL, NO ABDOMINAL   !----- HOME HEALTH SERVICES -----------
        DISTENTION, NO GREATER THAN 5   !
        LIQUID STOOLS PER 24 HOURS.     !
   318 052897 STANDARD PROTOCOL: ELEV.  !
        HEAD OF BED > 30 DEGREES DURING !
        FEEDING & 30 MIN. AFTER DELIVERY!
   319 052897 TUBE ORDER: INITIATE      !
        FEEDING THROUGH CURRENT         !
        NASOENTERIC TUBE                !
   481 052897 ANY MISCELLANEOUS         !
        NURSING ORDER ANY FURTHER       !
        INFORMATION ANY REMARKS ANY     !
        MORE REMARKS                    !
   745 053097 Q6HR ACCUCHECKS BY        !
        NURSING                         !
                                        !
                                        !
                                        !
----- CENTRAL SUPPLY -----------------!
   270 042197 AIR MATTRESS DAILY        !
                                        !
                                        !
----- MEDICATIONS --------------------!
   232 042197 SQ Q4H SLIDING SCALE      !
        REGULAR INSULIN                 !
   280 042197 SQ Q4H REGULAR HUMAN      !
        INSULIN 3U                      !
   290 042197 75 ML/HR IV ORDER D5NS    !
        10MEQKCL                        !
```

FIGURE 13.4 (*Continued*)

shows a three-page computer-generated Kardex for a patient on the medical floor. All the information that would have been on the handwritten Kardex is available; it simply looks different.

Step 4 in the transcription procedure described in the next section will not be used if a computer-generated Kardex is used.

TRANSCRIPTION PROCEDURE

STEPS OF TRANSCRIPTION PROCEDURE

Seven steps are necessary for the transcription of each order. Learn these steps, and use them as a checklist when performing this task.

1. Recognize

You must first recognize and note that an order needs transcription. Every hospital has a method by which doctors indicate to the nursing and clerical staff that new orders have been written. The patient's chart, or the order sheet alone, may be marked or placed in a designated container such as an "in-basket." A red or other color tag contained in the chart holder may be pulled up; this is called **flagging** the chart. A new order or set of orders will show the current date and will be signed by the doctor. No other writing, initials, or marks will be present to alert you that new orders exist. Sometimes doctors will forget to flag their orders or otherwise bring new orders to your attention. The chart may even be put back in the chart rack with new orders without your knowledge. It is for this reason that you must, during your shift, regularly check the charts for new orders.

2. Rip

Many hospitals use a doctor's order sheet that has several copies (**NCR,** no carbon required copies). The disposition of the copies varies widely with the hospital. Whereas once the copies were used along with handwritten requisitions to notify other departments of orders, now this is largely done by computer. However, these copies are frequently sent to the pharmacy because it is desirable to have the pharmacist actually see the physician's orders to avoid misinterpretation. Know the system in your hospital and tear off the back copies of the doctor's order sheet as soon as you recognize that an order exists. Always be sure that all doctors' orders are stamped with the correct patient's addressograph plate before tearing off the copies.

3. Prioritize

Now you must read the doctor's orders and do those orders first that have the highest priority. When you see words like **stat, now, immediately,** and this AM, you should call the nurse's attention to it at once, that is, **without delay.** Sometimes the order will simply make a statement such as DC IV (discontinue intravenous) or electrolytes (a blood test). If you have several charts and all have orders, you must prioritize the orders on each chart. The order to DC IV and electrolytes should be given priority over less urgent orders but not as high a priority as stats.

4. Kardex

Next, you must transfer the order to the special records and forms. From these the nursing staff will carry out the order or make sure that it has been done if that remains the process in your hospital. As stated earlier, you will omit this step if your hospital uses the computer-generated Kardex. Most orders are copied directly from the doctor's order sheet to the patient care record card. This process is called **Kardexing.**

5. Requisition

Then, you must requisition all equipment and services necessary to carry out the order. You will select and complete the requisitions you need to order the various laboratory tests, x-rays, treatments, diet changes, and so on that the doctor may have ordered for the patient. If you are ordering by computer, it is still termed requisitioning. You just don't have to fill out all those forms! (Fig. 13.5).

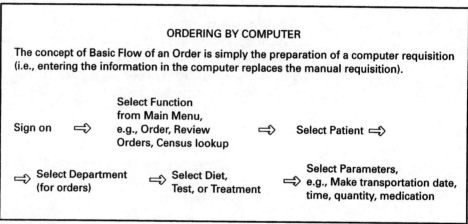

FIGURE 13.5

6. Symbols

At this point, the order itself is in the process of being carried out. Before the transcription procedure is complete, however, you must indicate in writing on the doctor's order sheet what you have done to set the order in motion. You may use symbols—which you will learn more about in the next section—for this purpose.

7. Nurse Checks

The final step in transcribing orders is designed to protect both you and the patient. Because your knowledge of medicine is often limited to the instructions you receive in this course, and because you are directly responsible to the registered nursing staff on your floor, **all orders you have transcribed must be checked by the nurse.** The nurse will check all requisitions, tickets, and special records, as well as the orders themselves for accuracy and completeness. This procedure saves the nurse's time and effort in transcribing the order and doubly assures the accuracy of the transcription by the efforts of two persons. In this way, too, the nurse is kept informed of the orders in effect for his or her patients.

   REMEMBER: Be sure the nurse sees any **stat** or other high priority orders without delay. Do not wait until he or she checks your transcription (Fig. 13.6).

Steps of Order Transcription

1. Recognize
2. Rip
3. Prioritize
4. Kardex

5. Requisition or Computer Order
6. Write Symbols
7. Have Nurse Check

FIGURE 13.6

*T*RANSCRIPTION SYMBOLS

You can use letters and symbols to indicate to the nurse the work you have completed. Figure 13.7 shows one set of symbols and letters; those used in your hospital might be entirely different. The important lesson to be mastered is that you thoroughly learn and use those indicators applied in your hospital to show that the work has been accomplished (Fig. 13.7).

O𝑛S	to indicate that	An order has been input into the computer or that a slip or requisition for equipment or services has been filled out.
K	to indicate that	An order has been transcribed to the Kardex.
T	to indicate that	A ticket has been filled out.
AP	to indicate that	An appointment has been made. The date of the appointment should accompany this symbol on the doctor's order sheet.
P or *called*	to indicate that	The appropriate department or persons have been notified of an order by telephone.
V	to indicate that	All activities necessary to complete transcription, and not indicated by any of the symbols included above, have been carried out.

FIGURE 13.7

To simplify the nurse's checking task, you may be asked to write these symbols in red ink, because most orders are written in blue or black ink. It may sometimes be necessary to include other information besides the symbols alone, as in connection with appointments. After the nurse checks your order transcription, she or he will sign, state the time, and date the orders.

Figure 13.8 shows how the doctor's orders would look after they had been transcribed, using the proper symbols.

SIGNATURES

When the doctor writes an order, the doctor signs it in the space provided. As previously stated, if the nurse takes a telephone or verbal order, the nurse signs it and the doctor signs it later.

After the registered nurse has carefully checked your transcription, the nurse will **sign off** the orders as shown in Fig. 13.8.

DATE	ORDER	
6-1-xx	✗ Hot soaks to elbow q4h ✗ Aspirin 600 mg po q4h for temp > 103°F ✗ Out of bed ad lib ✗ Allow shower in AM ✗0 Electrolytes in AM ✗0 IVP Ap 6-3 ✗0 Transfer to semiprivate in PM. Called ✗ Remove restraints. Replace if necessary.	
Date Time R.N. 6-1-xx-2100 L. Bowman, R.N.	Date Time M.D. 6-1-xx-2100 J. Stevens	Date Time H.U.C. 6-1-xx-2200 D. Jones, C.H.U.C.

FIGURE 13.8

It is recommended that the health unit coordinator also sign off as the person who transcribed the order. Use the first letter of your first name, your last name, your title, and HUC for health unit coordinator or CHUC if you are a certified health unit coordinator. Example:

> Date   Time
> 6-1-xx   2200   D. Jones, CHUC

Be very careful when writing anything on the physician's order sheet that you do not write over the doctor's orders. It is very important, from a legal standpoint, that the orders be completely visible.

GENERAL CLASSIFICATION OF ORDERS

Doctors' orders can be classified according to the subject of the order. You will probably encounter all of the following seven general types of orders.

Medication Orders

All medication orders on a patient are written in a similar form and are a major class of orders in themselves. The orders will be discussed in Chapter 14, Understanding Medication Orders.

Treatment/Monitoring Orders

Treatment orders include a wide variety of procedures to be performed for a patient. Such diverse activities as oxygen administration and ice pack applications are all treatments. Monitoring orders include orders for vital signs and circulation check. Nursing treatment and monitoring orders will be discussed in Chapter 15. Radiation, respiratory, and physical therapy orders are covered in Chapter 16.

Diagnostic Procedure Orders

All laboratory tests, x-rays, isotopic procedures, electrocardiograms, and other diagnostic procedures fall into this category. The orders are discussed in Chapter 16.

Diet Orders

These include orders that refer to any nourishment to be given to the patient by any method. Special fluid restrictions, tube feedings, as well as meal orders, are all part of this category of orders. Diet orders are covered in Chapter 16.

Intravenous Orders

These include the various types of intravenous fluids given to the patient. These are discussed in Chapter 15.

Activity Orders

These refer to orders governing the level or type of activity the patient is to be allowed. A subcategory of activity orders are position orders. These are also found in Chapter 15.

Miscellaneous Orders

This group is a catchall term for all orders not already included. Miscellaneous orders are alike in that they generally indicate quite precisely a special task to be performed or limitation to be accepted and understood. As examples: The doctor may request, by order, that a patient's family be informed of impending surgery or that x-rays be sent with the patient to the operating room. The doctor may place a patient on the critical list or in isolation, or sign an order for his discharge. The doctor may order special permissions, such as "may go on pass," restrictions such as orders for side rails on the patient's bed, or protection orders such as restraints. These are discussed in Chapter 15.

*F*OUR MAIN CATEGORIES OF DOCTORS' ORDERS

In addition to looking at doctor's orders according to the classifications just listed, you must also be aware of their duration or how long they are to continue. Based on those criteria, there are four main categories of doctors' orders:

1. **Standing routine orders.** Once these orders are written, they remain unchanged until changed by the physician. Standing routine orders are done on a regular basis. Examples of standing routine orders are:
   - VS qid (vital signs four times a day)
   - PT ROM bid. (physical therapy with range of motion twice a day)

- OOB in WC. 30 min tid (out of bed in wheelchair 30 minutes three times a day)
- BS q AM (blood sugar every morning)

2. **Standing PRN orders.** These orders stand as written until changed but the order is carried out on an as-needed basis. For example, SSE qod prn (soap suds enema every other day as needed); may wash hair prn.

3. **One-time or limited orders.** This type of order is to be done only once or is limited to the number of times it is to be performed as specified in the order. For example:
- Remove NG (nasogastric) tube this morning
- ECG today (electrocardiogram today)
- Hct X 3 days (hematocrit to be drawn for 3 days only)

4. **Stat orders.** These orders are to be carried out immediately. For example, DC IV stat (discontinue the intravenous immediately), tracheal suction now; FC/SD stat (Foley catheter (retention catheter), to straight drainage immediately).

In order for you to intelligently transcribe doctors' orders you must learn many medical abbreviations. A glossary of abbreviations is included in Chapter 4, Medical Terminology, for easy reference.

*A*VOIDING MISTAKES IN ORDER TRANSCRIPTION

Order transcription is one of the primary duties of the health unit coordinator. It requires skill and an ongoing sense of responsibility. You must make every effort to ensure that doctors' orders are transcribed accurately, completely, and in a timely manner. The following are suggestions for avoiding errors in order transcription:

- Try to scan new orders before a doctor leaves the floor. This is particularly important if the doctor's handwriting is known to be difficult to read.
- If the doctor has left the floor, try to contact the doctor before he or she leaves the hospital if you cannot read or do not understand an order
- Most physician's order forms are divided in thirds, with the back NCR copies perforated so they can be torn off and routed to the appropriate places. The top copy is not perforated and remains the permanent chart record. Because of this design, if orders extend part way into the next third of the page, draw diagonal lines to block off the remaining portion so the doctors won't accidentally write in that block the next time instead of the one below (Fig. 13.9).
- Most physician's order forms are designed so that the orders begin at the top of the page, and the doctor writes down the page. When orders begin at the top of a page, always look on the preceding page for more orders.
- Because doctors do not always flag or otherwise indicate that they have written new orders, regularly check the charts for new orders or orders that were missed by a previous shift. (See Chapter 11, Routine Chart Checks.)
- Prioritize. Expedite the orders that must be done first.
- Never guess. Always ask when in doubt.

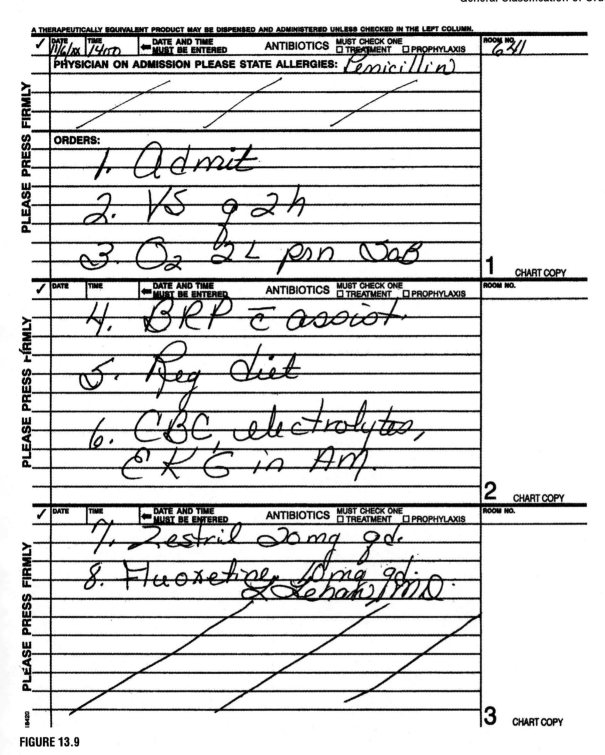

FIGURE 13.9

L̲EARNING ACTIVITIES

Complete the following.

1. List the primary reasons for doctors' orders.
   (a) _____
   (b) _____

2. List the three methods of obtaining doctors' orders.
   (a) _____
   (b) _____
   (c) _____

3. No matter what the method of obtaining orders, they must always be _____ by the doctor.

4. List the tools of order transcription.
   (a) _____
   (b) _____

5. List the seven steps of order transcription.
   (a) _____
   (b) _____
   (c) _____
   (d) _____
   (e) _____
   (f) _____
   (g) _____

6. List the seven general classifications of doctors' orders.
   (a) _____
   (b) _____
   (c) _____
   (d) _____
   (e) _____
   (f) _____
   (g) _____

7. List the four main categories of doctors' orders.
   (a) _____
   (b) _____
   (c) _____
   (d) _____

8. What does *flagging* a chart mean, and what is its purpose?
   _____
   _____

9. If the nurse asks you to *take off* orders, what does the nurse want you to do?
   _____
   _____

10. What is the purpose of *ripping* the NCR copies from the back of the doctor's order sheet?
    _____
    _____

11. What is meant by the term *signing off* doctors' orders?

   _____

   _____

12. Doctor Veryfine writes new orders on several of his patients' charts, sets the charts in a pile on your desk, and turns to leave. What should you do immediately and why?

   _____

   _____

   _____

13. You now have a stack of charts, each with numerous orders. Describe how you will proceed. What criteria will you use to decide what to do first? Be as detailed as possible in your answer. _____

   _____

   _____

   _____

   _____

   _____

   _____

   _____

14. Can you always assume that doctors will flag charts after writing new orders?

   _____

15. What could happen if charts are put back in the chart rack with new orders that are missed?

   _____

   _____

   _____

CHAPTER 14

Understanding Medication Orders

Admixture A mixture created by adding a medication to an IV solution

Anti-infective A category of antimicrobial drugs that acts on susceptible bacteria, rickettsiae, and spirochetes by inhibiting their growth and replication

Automatic stop A period of time after which a drug order must be reordered by the physician, or it may not be continued

Controlled substances Drugs that by law are put into schedules I–V based on their potential for abuse

Hospital Formulary A list of all drugs approved for use by the hospital

IV push Medications given into a vein in a short period of time rather than into the bag of intravenous solution and given over a long period of time

MAR Medication Administration Record

PDR Physician's Desk Reference; a reference book published yearly by Medical Economics that provides detailed information on prescription drugs and diagnostic products

Peak level A drug's highest level in the blood

Pharmacology The study of drugs

Schedule Categories of controlled substances from I to V, with I having the most potential for abuse and V the least

Sliding scale Term indicating that the amount of drug (insulin) is to be given based on the results of a blood test for glucose

Thrombolytic therapy Medication given to break down blood clots

Trough level Lowest concentration of a drug in the blood

Unit dose system A common method used in hospitals for dispensing medication in which the pharmacy stocks drawers on the nursing unit's medication carts with the exact amount of medication to be given with each prescribed dose

OBJECTIVES

When you have completed this chapter, you will be able to:

- Define the terms listed in the vocabulary.
- Define the terms *antimicrobial, pharmacodynamic,* and *chemotherapeutic drugs.*
- Define new terms related to pharmacology in this chapter.
- Recognize common drug names and state their purpose.
- Define common drug categories.
- Discuss your responsibilities in relation to anticoagulants and antidiabetic drugs and the laboratory tests to monitor these drugs.
- Discuss intravenous medication orders.

- Demonstrate knowledge of the abbreviations used in this chapter.
- Demonstrate the ability to transcribe medication orders.

Pharmacology is the study of drugs. A **drug** is a substance that, when taken into the body, can change the way the body functions. There are three primary uses for drugs:

Therapeutic—a drug given to treat symptoms or the cause of the disease or to replace substances in the body that are depleted, such as vitamins, minerals, or hormones

Diagnostic—a drug used in diagnostic testing such as during x-ray or laboratory testing

Preventive—A drug such as a vaccine given to immunize and therefore protect a patient against a certain disease

Drugs come from many sources such as plants, animals, and minerals. Drugs that are produced in laboratories of pharmaceutical companies are called **synthetic drugs.** Another method of creating new drugs is through the process of genetic engineering.

Many factors affect the action of drugs. These include how rapidly the drug is absorbed into the body, how quickly it is transported by the bloodstream, how quickly it is broken down in preparation for elimination, and how quickly the body is able to eliminate it.

The type of drug, its route of administration, and the patient's condition all affect how well the drug works and is eliminated from the body. Many disease processes such as kidney, liver, respiratory, gastrointestinal, and cardiovascular disease may alter the effectiveness of a drug. A patient's age and size also are factors in drug administration. Older patients and children usually require smaller amounts of drugs.

A **local action** of a drug occurs when it is applied directly to a certain area. A **systemic action** is one that occurs when the drug is carried in the bloodstream and affects tissues and organs away from the site of entry. **Selective action** occurs when the drug affects only certain tissues and organs. **Synergistic action** occurs when one drug increases the effects of another. **Antagonistic action** occurs when one drug counteracts the effects of another. A **drug interaction** occurs when a drug, food, or alcohol reacts with another drug. Undesirable drug interactions can be very serious and are avoided whenever possible.

A **side effect** is an action of a drug other than what was intended. A patient taking a cardiac medication may complain of dry mouth. An **adverse reaction** is an undesirable and harmful side affect. Vomiting or fainting after taking a drug would be an adverse reaction to the drug. All staff must be alert to patients' complaints about symptoms that may be related to their medication.

Before you can learn to transcribe orders for medication, you must learn more about the medications themselves and how they are ordered. Understanding a new set of medical terms will be necessary. In this chapter you will learn about the general types of medication used in hospitals. Then you will study specific drug names and preparations, drug dosages, and routes and times of administration.

You will also learn about the types of medication orders and how to transcribe these orders.

Remember that errors in medication transcription may have disastrous effects for the patient. Pay close attention to the material presented in this chapter.

Remember, too, that there is much to learn about medications and that new or different medications will frequently come to your attention. Be inquisitive and listen and learn about medications whenever you can.

TABLE 14.1	***A*** NTIMICROBIAL DRUGS THAT AFFECT DISEASE-CAUSING ORGANISMS
Category	**Description**
Antiseptics	Chemicals that kill or inhibit the growth of micororganisms and are used on living tissue
Disinfectants	Chemicals that kill or inhibit the growth of microorganisms and are applied to inanimate objects
Antibiotics	Drugs produced by bacteria that prevent the growth of, or destroy, other bacteria
Antifungals	Drugs that inhibit or stop the growth of fungus
Anti-infectives	Drugs that act on susceptible bacteria, rickettsiae, and spirochetes by inhibiting their growth and replication
Antivirals	Drugs that inhibit or stop the growth of viruses
Antituberculars	Drugs that inhibit or stop the growth of the bacteria that cause tuberculosis, the tubercle bacilli
Sulfonamides	Chemical substances that weaken susceptible bacteria; commonly called "sulfa drugs"

C LASSIFICATIONS OF MEDICATIONS

Medication is one of the most effective methods of treating many diseases. Drugs may be categorized in different ways.

1. They may destroy or render harmless microorganisms in the body that cause disease. Drugs acting in this manner are called **antimicrobial drugs.** The most common groups of antimicrobial drugs are listed in Table 14.1.

2. They may either stimulate or depress normal body functions in such a way that the nature or course of a disease is altered. These drugs are called **pharmacodynamic drugs.**

3. They may treat neoplastic disease and have a selective effect on the invading cells or organisms. These are called **chemotherapeutic drugs.**

Drugs are ordinarily grouped according to the disease or symptom they treat or the body function they affect. You will often hear drugs referred to by category and should be familiar with the most common groups of medications. However, some drugs, because they affect different body parts and functions, can be used to treat a number of different diseases. Table 14.2 describes the major drug categories. This is not a complete list of categories, nor does it include all the possible uses for each drug.

TABLE 14.2	***P*** HARMACODYNAMIC DRUGS AND THE BODY SYSTEMS THEY AFFECT
Category	**Description**
Nervous System	
Analgesics	This type of medication is given primarily for relief of pain without loss of consciousness.
Narcotic analgesics	Habit-forming analgesics that when withdrawn from the addicted patient produce certain uncontrollable physical symptoms.
Nonnarcotic analgesics	This group differs from narcotics in that they are not habit forming. In addition to relieving pain, some of the drugs in this group such as aspirin and tylenol also reduce fever (antipyretics).
Nonsteroidal anti-inflammatories (NSAIDs)	Drugs such as ibuprofen that inhibit prostaglandin synthesis and reduce inflammation and fever.

TABLE 14.2	CONTINUED
Category	**Description**
Nervous System	
Anesthetics	Drugs that produce loss of sensation and an inability to perceive pain.
General	General anesthetics produce loss of sensation and muscle relaxation accompanied by loss of consciousness. They are administered by inhalation of a gas, by intravenous injection, or by a combination of the two.
Local	Local anesthetics produce loss of sensation in a limited area of the body by "deadening" the nerves in that area and are usually administered by injection. *Topical* anesthetics are applied to the skin, usually to mucous membranes.
Antianxieties	Reduce anxiety or tension; however, this group of drugs differs from the hypnotics in that they do not usually produce sleep. Also called tranquilizers.
Anticonvulsants	Drugs that suppress convulsions or seizures.
Antidepressants	Drugs that elevate the mood and relieve depression. They are divided into three categories: tricyclics, MAOIs, and miscellaneous antidepressants.
Antipsychotics	Drugs that treat psychosis.
Hypnotics and sedatives	Compounds that exert a general depressant effect on the central nervous system and are defined based on the dose and degree of effect.
Barbiturates	Drugs that decrease the transmission of impulses to the cerebrum. They are frequently used to control seizures. They include amobarbital, aprobarbital, butabarbital, mephobarbital, pentobarbital, phenobarbital, and secobarbital. The body may develop a strong dependence on barbiturates.
Nonbarbiturate hypnotics	These drugs are used as sleeping medications when the doctor chooses not to order barbiturates.
Stimulants	Drugs such as amphetamine that produce increased functional activity. They are used to treat attention deficit disorder, narcolepsy, and obesity.
Endocrine System	
Antidiabetics	
Insulin	Hormones that aid in the metabolism of sugars; used in the treatment of diabetes—Type I: insulin-dependent diabetes mellitus (IDDM) and Type II: non-insulin-dependent diabetes mellitus (NIDDM).
Oral antidiabetics	Chemicals taken by mouth to lower blood sugar in certain types of diabetes, such as NIDDM, and as an adjunct to insulin therapy.
Corticosteroids	Hormones produced by the adrenal glands; often used to treat inflammatory conditions.
Other hormones	Examples are estrogen and thyroid replacement used when the individual gland is not producing enough of its hormone.
Respiratory System	
Antihistamines	Drugs that help relieve allergic symptoms by counteracting the effect of histamine in the body. They also relieve allergic symptoms of the skin such as hives and other reactions of the body due to allergy.
Antitussives	Drugs given to relieve coughing by affecting the cough center (medulla) in the brain.
Bronchodilators	Drugs that widen the bronchial tubes, especially in the treatment of asthma.
Expectorants	Drugs that increase or liquify secretions in the bronchi and aid the expulsion of mucus.
Gastrointestinal System	
Antacids	Drugs that lower the acidity of the gastric secretions. Commonly used to treat the symptoms of indigestion.
Anticholinergics	Drugs that decrease gastric secretions and motility.
Antidiarrheals	Drugs used in the treatment of diarrhea.
Antiemetics	Drugs that stop vomiting and relieve nausea.
Antiflatulents	Drugs that decrease amount of gas in the gastrointestinal tract.

TABLE 14.2 CONTINUED	
Category	**Description**
Gastrointestinal System (continued)	
Antispasmodics	Drugs used to relieve spasm of the digestive tract.
Cathartics	Drugs that aid in causing bowel movements.
Emetics	Drugs that produce vomiting such as ipecac syrup.
Histamine H$_2$ antagonists	Drugs that treat gastric and duodenal ulcers and gastric reflux disease.
Circulatory System	
Alpha-adrenergic blockers	Drugs that dilate peripheral blood vessels.
Antianginals	Drugs that dilate coronary arteries to increase the coronary blood flow. They are divided into three categories: nitrates, calcium channel blockers, and beta-adrenergic blockers.
Anticoagulants	Drugs that inhibit the clotting of blood. In disease, they are used most frequently on patients with abnormal clotting within blood vessels.
Antidysrythmics	Drugs such as calcium channel blockers and beta blockers that help correct abnormal heart rhythms.
Antihyperlipidemics	Drugs that lower cholesterol levels in the blood.
Antihypertensives	Drugs that lower the blood pressure.
Cardiotonics	Drugs that affect the heart, usually improving the quality of the heart's action.
Diuretics	Drugs that increase the flow of urine. They are used primarily to reduce blood pressure by reducing fluid retention.
Hematinics	Drugs such as iron supplements used to treat some anemias.
Thrombolytics	Drugs that aid in breaking down blood clots. They are used to treat deep-vein and arterial thrombosis, various types of embolism, and certain evolving myocardial infarctions.
Vasoconstrictors	Drugs that cause the blood vessels to constrict or narrow. They are often used in emergencies to counteract shock by raising the blood pressure.
Vasodilators	Drugs that cause the blood vessels to dilate or widen. They may be used to treat hypertension and other diseases of circulatory impairment, where the blood vessels have narrowed such as intermittent claudication and various types of ischemia.
Musculoskeletal System	
Antiarthritics	Drugs that treat symptoms of arthritis and other related diseases.
Antigouts	Drugs that treat gout, a bone and joint disease often involving the great toe.
Muscle relaxants	Drugs that reduce painful spasms of the skeletal muscles.

Antimicrobial Drugs

Many types of microorganisms, by definition too small to be seen without a microscope, can cause disease. In addition to viruses and bacteria, there are others such as fungi, protozoa, rickettsiae, and spirochetes. Many of them can be destroyed by drugs (Fig. 14.1). Anti-infectives are divided into a number of groups including penicillins, cephalosporins, tetracyclines, and aminoglycosides.

One category of antimicrobials is the **antivirals.** Antiviral drugs act on viral DNA synthesis that is needed for its replication.

Pharmacodynamic Drugs

Diseases may be caused by the malfunction of an organ or body part. Such malfunctions can usually be traced to either an excess or a decrease in the normal activity of the organ concerned. For this reason, pharmacodynamic drugs serve either to depress specific body functions or to stimulate them. Table 14.2 lists common pharmacodynamic drug categories and some of the body systems they affect. Table 14.3 lists categories of chemotherapeutic drugs.

MAY DESTROY OR INHIBIT
GROWTH OF MICROORGANISMS

FIGURE 14.1 Antimicrobials.

TABLE 14.3	*C*HEMOTHERAPEUTIC DRUGS
Category	**Description**
Antineoplastics	Drugs that are used to kill cancerous cells.
Antiparasitics	Drugs that are used to treat diseases caused by such animal parasites as helminths (worms), amoeba, and protozoa.

*C*OMMONLY ORDERED DRUGS

There are many drugs that doctors frequently order. Add any medications commonly used in your health care institution to the appropriate categories. Examples of these drugs are listed by category below, although in medicine, many drugs are used for more than one purpose and so don't always fit neatly into one category. Generic names (which are not capitalized) follow in parentheses. If a drug is a combination of drugs, only one name (brand or generic) is given. Keep in mind that this is not a complete list of all the drugs a doctor may order and that you will need to become most familiar with the drugs approved to be used in your hospital. (*Note:* An asterisk indicates those categories of drugs that are usually **automatic stop** and must be reordered by the doctor within a hospital-specified time period to be continued.) The following categories with commonly ordered drugs are listed:

Analgesics	Antidiarrheals
Anesthetics	Antidysrhythmics
Antacids	Antiemetics
Antianginals, Vasodillaters	Antiflatulents
Antianxieties	Antigouts
Antiarthritics	Antihistamines
Anticoagulants	Antihyperlipidemics
Anticonvulsants	Antihypertensives
Antidepressants	Anti-infectives
Antidiabetics	Antineoplastics

Antipsychotics   Emetics
Antisecretory Agents   Hematinics
Antispasmodics   Hormones
Antituberculars   Muscle Relaxants
Antitussives   Nasal Decongestants
Antivirals   Neuromuscular Blockers
Bronchodilators   Potassium Replacements
Cardiotonics   Sedatives/Hypnotics
Carthartics, Laxatives, and Stool Softeners   Thrombolytics
Corticosteroids   Vasopressors
Diuretics   Vitamins

TABLE 14.4 *COMMONLY ORDERED DRUGS*

Analgesics

NONNARCOTIC

Advil, Naprosyn, Motrin (ibuprofen)
Aspirin (acetylsalicylic acid)
Bufferin
Darvon (propoxyphene)
Fiorinal
Norgesic
Oruvail (ketoprofen)
Percogesic
Talwin (pentazocine)
Tylenol (acetaminophen)

NARCOTIC*

Codeine
Codeine in combination with other drugs such as:
   Tylenol c̄ codeine (*Note:* Numbers are assigned to analgesics containing codeine to designate the
   amount of codeine found in the medication.)
      Tylenol #2 = acetaminophen c̄ codeine 15 mg
      Tylenol #3 = acetaminophen c̄ codeine 30 mg
      Tylenol #4 = acetaminophen c̄ codeine 60 mg
   Empirin c̄ codeine—*Example:* Emp. #3 po q4h prn headache *means* Empirin with 30 mg of
   codeine by mouth every four hours as needed for headache
Demerol (meperidine)
Dilaudid (hydromorphone)
Dolophine (methadone)
Duragesic (fentanyl)
MSIR, MS Contin, Roxanol, MS (morphine)
Pantopan (opium tincture)
Percocet
Percodan
Vicodin

Anesthetics

Local
   Ambesol (benzocaine)
   Novocain (procaine)
   Xylocaine (lidocaine)—with or without epinephrine
General
   Diprivan (propofol) for sedation of mechanically ventilated patients

Antacids

Amphojel (aluminum hydroxide)
Gelusil
Maalox
Mylanta
Riopan (magaldrate)

(continued)

TABLE 14.4 CONTINUED

Antianginals/Vasodilators

Apresoline (hydralazine)
Cardene (nicardipine)
Cardizem (diltiazem)
Imdur (isosorbide mononitrate)
Isordil (isosorbide dinitrate)
Loniten (minoxidil)
Nitrobid, Nitrostat (nitroglycerin)
Nitropress (nitroprusside)
Persantine (dipyridamole)
Priscoline (tolazoline)
Procardia (nifedipine)
Vascor (bepridil)

Antianxieties

Atarax, Vistaril (hydroxyzine)
Ativan (lorazepam)
Buspar (buspirone)
Compazine (prochlorperizine)
Equanil (mebrobamate)
Inderal (propranolol)
Klonopin (clonazepam)
Librium (chlordiazepoxide)
Serax (oxazepam)
Sinequan (doxepin)
Stelazine (trifluoperazine)
Thorazine (chlorpromazine)
Valium (diazepam)
Xanax (alprazolam)

Antiarthritics

Ascriptin
Feldene (piroxicam)
Motrin (ibuprofen)
Naprosyn (naproxen)
Tolectin (tolmetin)

Anticoagulants*

Coumadin (warfarin)
Fragmin (dalteparin)
Heparin Sodium, Liquaemin Sodium (heparin)
Lovenox (enoxaparin)
Normiflo (ardeparin)
Orgaran (danaparoid)
Refludan (lepirudin)

Anticonvulsants

Cerebyx (fosphenytoin)
Dilantin (phenytoin)
Luminal (phenobarbital)
Mysoline (primidone)

Antidepressants

Aventyl (nortriptyline)
Elavil (amitriptyline)
Marplan (isocarboxazid)
Nardil (phenelzine)
Parnate (tranylcypromine)
Paxil (paroxetine)
Prozac (fluoxetine)
Sinequan (doxepin)
Tofranil (imipramine)
Triavil
Zoloft (sertraline)

Antidiabetics

ORAL HYPOGLYCEMICS

Actos (pioglitazone)
Avandia (rosiglitazone)
Glucophage (metformin)
Glucotrol (glipizide)
Micronase (glyburide)
Precose (acarbose)

(continued)

TABLE 14.4	CONTINUED

INJECTABLE HYPOGLYCEMICS

Humalin L: insulin, Lente
Humalin N: insulin, NPH
Humalin 70/30: insulin, NPH and regular
Humalin U; Ultralente: insulin, ultralente
Humalog: insulin, analog injection (lispro)
NovolinR: insulin, regular

Antidiarrheals

Imodium (loperamide)
Kaolin/pectin
Lomotil (diphenoxylate and atropine)
Paregoric (opium)
Pepto-Bismol (bismuth subsalicylate)

Antidysrhythmics

Adenocard (adenosine)
Atropisol (atropine)
Bretylol (bretylium)
Calan (verapamil)
Cordarone (amiodarone)
Cardioquin (quinidine)
Inderal (propranolol)
Isuprel (isoproterenol)
Norpace (disopyramide)
Pronestyl (procainamide)
Xylocaine (lidocaine)

Antiemetics/Antinauseants

Antivert (meclizine)
Compazine (prochlorperazine)
Dramamine (dimenhydrinate)
Phenergan (promethazine)
Thorazine (chlorpromazine)
Tigan (trimethobenzamide)
Torecan (thiethylperazine)
Vistaril (hydroxyzine)

Antiflatulents

Mylicon, Flatulex (simethicone)

Antigout

Anturane (sulfinpyrazone)
Benemid (probenecid)
Indocin (indomethacin)
Zyloprim (allopurinol)

Antihistamines

Actifed
Allegra (fexofenadine)
Benadryl (diphenhydramine)
Chlor-Trimeton (chlorpheniramine)
Claritin (loratadine)
Dimetane (brompheniramine)
Ornade
Triaminic

Antihyperlipidemics

Colestid (colestipol)
Lipitor (atorvastatin)
Mevacor (lovastatin)
Pravachol (pravastatin)
Questran (cholestyramine)
Zocor (simvastatin)

(continued)

TABLE 14.4 **CONTINUED**

ANTIHYPERTENSIVES

Aldomet (methyldopa)
Apresoline (hydralazine)
Atacand (candesartan)
Brevibloc (esmolol)
Calan, Isoptin (verapamil)
Capoten (captopril)
Cardura (doxazosin)
Catapres (clonidine)
Corgard (nadolol)
Diovan (valsartan)
Ismelin (guanethidine)
Lexxel (enalapril/felodipine)
Lopressor (metoprolol)
Minipress (prazosin)
Norvasc (amlodipine)
Plendil (felodipine)
Resserpine
Tenormin (atenolol)
Trandate (labetatol)
Vasotec (enalapril)
Zestril (lisinopril)

Anti-infectives*

Achromycin, Panmycin, Tetracyn (tetracycline)
Amikin (amikacin)
Amoxil (amoxicillin)
Bicillin (penicillin G benzathine)
Cipro (ciprofloxacin)
Cleocin (clindamycin)
Duricef (cefadroxil)
Floxin (ofloxacin)
Gantrisin (sulfisoxazole)
Garamycin (gentamicin)
Ilosone (erythromycin)
Kantrex (kanamycin)
Keflex (cephalexin)
Keflin (cephalothin)
Kefzol, Ancef (cefazolin)
Mefoxin (cefoxitin)
Monurol (fosfomycin)
Mycifradin Sulfate (neomycin)
Nebcin (tobramycin)
Principen, Omnipen, Polycillin (ampicillin)
Prostaphilin (oxacillin)
Rocephin (ceftriaxone)
Septra (trimethoprim: sulfamethoxazole)
Staphcillin (methicillin)
Streptomycin
Vantin (cefpodoxime)
Vibramycin (doxycycline)
Vira-A (vidarabine)
Wycillin (procaine penicillin G)
Zinacef (cefuroxime)

Antineoplastics

Adrucil, 5-FU (fluorouracil)
Cytoxan (cyclophosphamide)
Folex PFS (methotrexate)
Nitrogen mustard, Mustargen (mechlorethamine)
Platinol AQ (cisplatin)
Tamofen Nolvadex (tamoxifen)

Antipsychotics

Compazine (prochlorperazine
Haldol (haloperidol)
Lithane (lithium)
Mellaril (thioridazine)
Navane (thiothixene)
Prolixin (fluphenazine)

(*continued*)

TABLE 14.4 **CONTINUED**

Antipsychotics (continued)

Risperdal (risperidone)
Serentil (mesoridazine)
Sparine (promazine)
Stelazine (trifluoperizine)
Tegretal (carbamazepine)
Thorazine (chlorpromazine)
Trilafon (perphenazine)
Vesprin (triflupromazine)

Antisecretory Agents

Pepcid (famotidine)
Prevacid (lansoprazole)
Prilosec (omeprazole)
Tagamet (cimetidine)
Zantac (ranitidine)

Antispasmodics

Bentyl (dicyclomine)
Clindex
Donnatal
Pro-Banthine
Reglan (metoclopramide)

Antituberculars

INH (isoniazid)
Mycobutin (rifabutin)
pyrazinamide
Rifidin (rifampin)
Seromycin (cycloserine)
streptomycin

Antitussives

Benylin DM (dextromethorphan)
codeine
Hycodan (hydrocodone)
Mucosal (acetylcysteine)
Sudafed, Dorcol (pseudoephedrine)

Antivirals

Cytovene (ganciclovir DHPG)
dideoxycytidine HIVID (zalcitabine)
Epivir (lamivudine)
Famvir (famciclovir)
Flumadine (rimantadine)
Foscavir (foscarnet)
Invirase (saquinavir)
Retrovir (zidovudine)
Symadine (amantadine)
Valtrex (valacyclovir)
Videx (didanosine)
Zerit (stavudine)
Zovirax (acyclovir)

Bronchodilators

Adrenalin (epinephrine)
Atrovent (ipratropium)
Brethaire (terbutaline)
Choledyl (oxytriphylline)
ephedrine
Isuprel (isoproterenol)
Metaprel, Alupent (metaproterenol)
Phyllocontin (aminophylline)
Proventil, Ventolin (albuterol)
Theolair-SE (theophylline)

Cardiotonics

Crystodigin (digitoxin)
Dobutrex (dobutamine)
Inocor (amrinone)
Lanoxin (digoxin)
Primacor (milrinone)

(continued)

TABLE 14.4 CONTINUED

Cathartics, Laxatives, and Stool Softeners

cascara
Colace, Dialose, D-S-S, Modane (docusate sodium)
Dulcolax (bisacodyl)
Metamucil (psyllium)
Milk of Magnesia (magnesium hydroxide)
Peri-Colace
Petrogalar Plain (mineral oil)
Senokot (senna)

Corticosteroids

Celestone (betamethasone)
Cortef, Solu-Cortef (hydrocortisone)
Cortone Acetate (cortisone)
Decadron (dexa methasone)
Medrol, Depo-Medrol, Solu-Medrol (methylprednisone)
Orasone (prednisone)
Prelone (prednisolone)

Diuretics

Aldactazide (spironolactone/hydrochlorothiazide)
Aldactone (spironolactone)
Bumex (bumetanide)
Diamox (acetazolamide)
Diuril (chlorothiazide)
Dyazide (hydrochlorothiazide/triamterene)
Edecrin (ethacrynote)
Esidrix HydroDiuril (hydrochlorothiazide)
Hygroton (chlorthalidone)
Lasix (furosemide)
Midamor (amiloride)
Osmitrol (mannitol)

Emetics

ipecac syrup

Hematinics

Feosol (ferrous sulfate)
Imferon (iron dextron)
Ircon (ferrous fumarate)

Hormones

Delestrogen (estradiol)
DES (diethylstilbestrol)
Norplant (levonorgestrel)
Premarin (conjugated estrogens)
Provera, Depa-Provera (medroxyprogesterone)
Synthroid (levothyroxine T_4)
Thyroid Strong (thyroid)

Muscle Relaxants

Flexeril (cyclobenzaprine)
Paraflex, (chlorzoxazone)
Robaxin (methocarbamol)
Soma (carisoprodol)
Valium (diazepam)

Nasal Decongestants

Afrin Sudafed (pseudoephedrine)
Neo-Synephrine (phenylephrine)
Otrivin (xylometazoline)

Neuromuscular Blockers

Norcuron (vecuronium)
Pavulon (pancuronium)

(continued)

TABLE 14.4	**CONTINUED**

Potassium Replacements

K-Dur, K-lyte/cl, Slow k (potassium chloride)
Kaon (potassium gluconate)
SSKI (potassium iodide)

Sedatives/Hypnotics

Dalmane (flurazepam)
Halcion (triazolam)
Luminal (phenobarbital)
Nembutal (pentobarbital)
Nersed (midazolam)
Noctec (chloral hydrate)
Restoril (temazepam)
Seconal (secobarbital)
Versed (midazolam)

Thrombolytics

Abbokinase (urokinase)
Activase, TPA (alteplase)
Eminase (anistreplase)
Streptase (streptokinase)

Vasopressors

Adrenalin Chloride (epinephrine)
Intropin (dopamine)
Levophed (norepinephrine)
Neo-Synephrine (phenylephrine)

Vitamins

Centrum
Niacar (niacin)
Optilets
Solu-B c̄ C
Therabid
Theragran

*D*RUG MONITORING

Therapeutic Drug Monitoring

Therapeutic drug monitoring (TDM) is done to measure the levels of drugs in the blood to determine if an effective level has been reached (therapeutic level) or if the level is too high and is toxic (poisonous). Blood is drawn and analyzed by the laboratory. Timing is a factor with this test. The results of a test in which the blood is drawn at the drug's peak level (its highest concentration) is helpful in determining if the drug has reached a toxic level in the patient's body. The result of a blood test taken at the **trough level** or lowest concentration can help determine if a therapeutic level has been reached.

Drugs with narrow therapeutic margins, those for which the range between the therapeutic and toxic level is small such as ones from the categories of anti-infectives, anticonvulsants, antidysrhythmics, bronchodilators, and cardiotonics may require TDM.

Digoxin, digitoxin, quinidine, phenytoin, aminophylline, chloramphenicol, lidocaine, and lithium are a few examples of drugs that are often therapeutically monitored.

Anticoagulant drugs require careful monitoring also. They are given to reduce the potential for the formation of blood clots. If a patient receives too little of the medication, dangerous blood clots may form. If the patient receives too much, hemorrhage may occur. Therefore, patients on anticoagulants will frequently have daily blood tests to monitor the effects of the drug. Two common laboratory tests are **prothrombin time (PT)** and **partial thromboplastin time (PTT)** or **activated partial thromboplastin time (APPT).**

The doctor will decide to increase, continue, decrease, or discontinue the anticoagulant based on the results of the laboratory tests.

The health unit coordinator must understand the significance and extreme importance of these orders. Often an **anticoagulant record** is added to the chart to help monitor the results of each blood test and the amount of the anticoagulant given. This is a *supplemental chart form* (see p. 262). Results of the blood tests may be telephoned to the doctor before the next dose of anticoagulant is ordered.

Thrombolytic Therapy

Thrombolytics are given to break down blood clots by converting plasminogen to plasmin. Serious side effects can occur that include abnormal gastrointestinal, genitourinary, intracranial, and retroperitoneal bleeding. Therefore, blood studies are done before treatment is begun (PT, PTT, APTT, TT, Hct, and platelets), and the PT or TT is done every three to four hours during therapy. A **thrombolytic therapy record** is added to the chart when this procedure is begun.

Insulin

Insulin is given to reduce the amount of sugar in the blood. Careful monitoring of both the urine and blood of the diabetic is necessary to ensure that the patient is receiving the correct amount of insulin. The **diabetic record** (a supplemental chart form) is often added to the patient's chart to help monitor the results of blood and urine tests and record insulin dosages (see p. 262).

The doctor will select the type of insulin based on how quickly or slowly it acts and how long that action lasts. Some patients will receive more than one type of insulin. Here are two types:

- Regular insulin is quick-acting and of short duration.
- NPH insulin is slower to act but of longer duration.

Other types of antidiabetics or hypoglycemics are ordered for their intermediate action. Each diabetic condition is unique and requires a careful decision by the doctor.

Sliding Scale Insulin Orders

Sliding scale is a term indicating that the amount of insulin is to be given according to the results of a test to measure the amount of sugar in the urine or in the blood. These tests are done on the nursing unit by the nursing staff and not by the laboratory. No requisition or computer-generated order to the laboratory is necessary.

Urine Test. Using a chemically treated test strip, the nurse tests the patient's urine. A common order would require this test be done ac & hs (before meals and at bedtime).

Blood Test. Most commonly, however, the nurse performs a simple bedside blood test, using a device to prick the patient's finger and then analyze the results on a glucometer such as an Accucheck or Glucometer. Insulin is given to the patient based on the results of the blood test, using an **insulin sliding scale order** such as the following:

If Accu-chek

190–240 5 U regular insulin
241–290 10 U regular insulin

If >290, notify physician.

MEDICATION ORDER FORM

The nurse must have precise directions from the physician for each medication to be administered to a patient. For this reason, every medication order is written according to a specific form that includes all necessary directions. There are four primary categories in this form and often one additional category.

1. **Name of drug**—what is the name of the drug to be given?

2. **Dosage of drug**—how much of the drug should be given at one time?

3. **Route of administration**—by what means is the drug to be introduced into the patient's body?

4. **Frequency of administration**—how often is this drug to be given?

5. **Qualifying phrase**—the doctor may want to qualify the order. For example, the doctor may specify that the medication be given "with milk," or "for pain in feet."

A typical form of a medication order follows.

Aspirin	*600 mg*	*po*	*q4h prn*	*for headache*
1	2	3	4	5

NAMES OF DRUGS

You will soon become familiar with the names of the drugs most frequently ordered by the doctors in your hospital. At first many names will sound alike to you, and you will need to pay close attention to spelling variations. Each drug usually has at least three names and *may* have many more (Table 14.5).

- **Chemical name:** This is a precise description of the chemical constitution of a drug. It is rarely, if ever, used in writing a doctor's order.
- **Generic name:** This is usually proposed by the company that has developed the drug. Generic names are established by the U.S. Adopted Name Council. Once the generic name is agreed on, it is never changed. It cannot be used as a name for a new drug, and it can be used in all countries. The generic name

TABLE 14.5 **EXAMPLES OF DRUG NAMES FOR SINGLE PREPARATION**

	Drug	Manufacturer
Chemical name	4-dimethyl-amino-1,4,4a,5,5a,6,11, 12a-octahydro-3,6,10,12, 12a-pentahydroxy-6-methyl-1,11-dioxo- 2-naphthacene-carboxamide.	
Generic name	tetracycline	
Brand name	Achromycin®	Lederle
	Panmycin®	Pharmacia and Upjohn

is often derived from the chemical name but it is much simpler. It is never capitalized. Many hospitals require their pharmacies to label all medications with their generic names.

- **Trade or brand name:** This is the special name given to a drug by its manufacturers.

In addition to the name of the drug itself, the way in which it is pharmaceutically prepared is often indicated. Examples are: Zinc Oxide *Ointment; Enteric-Coated* Aspirin; Darvon® *Capsules;* and *Spirits* of Ammonia. Enteric-coated tablets are specially coated so they can pass through the stomach without dissolving until they reach the small intestine.

Pharmaceutical preparations are usually indicated by abbreviations. Table 14.6 lists the English names and their usual abbreviations. These abbreviations are important for at least two reasons:

1. You are much less likely to make errors, particularly when deciphering difficult handwriting, if you *know* the meanings of the abbreviations.

2. Many of the abbreviations are used not only with medication orders but as parts of other orders and frequently in conversation.

The health unit coordinator should note that drug names are often preceded or followed by other letters or numbers such as Argesic-SA (sustained action), Bicillin LA (long acting), EC Naprosyn, or Infumorph 200. Often the drug is also available without these additional designations. The health unit coordinator must take special care to transcribe the complete order as written.

*D*OSAGES OF DRUGS

Drug dosages are measured either by weight or by volume. There are two systems of weights and measures used in hospitals today; however, the apothecary system is being replaced by the metric system. Until that process is complete, both systems will be addressed.

1. **Apothecary system:** Because the United States originated as a colony of England, its system was widely used here until modern times.

2. **Metric system:** This system, like our money system, is based on multiples of 10 and is a simpler system by which to compute dosages.

TABLE 14.6   *N*AMES AND ABBREVIATIONS FOR PHARMACEUTICAL PREPARATIONS

Name	Abbreviation	Name	Abbreviation
Ampules	Amp	Oil	Ol
Capsules	Caps	Ointment	Ung
Compound	Comp	Pills	Pil
Elixir	Elix	Powder	Pulv
Emulsion	Emul	Solution	Sol
Enteric-coated	EC	Spansules	Spans
Extract	Ext	Spirits	Spt
Fluidextract	Fldext	Suppository	Supp
Liniment	Lin	Syrup	Syr
Liquid	Liq	Tablets	Tab
Lotion	Lot	Tincture	Tr, Tinct
Mixture	Mixt	Troches, lozenges	Troch

Unless your hospital has strict rules about the use of one system or the other, you will have to be familiar with both. You will not be required to convert dosages from one system to another. However, you must be able to recognize the abbreviations and copy them accurately from the doctor's order sheet (see Table 14.7).

TABLE 14.7 Measures in the Apothecary and Metric Systems

	Apothecary System		Metric System	
	Terms	Abbreviations	Terms	Abbreviations
Measures of weight	Grain	gr	Microgram	mcg
	Dram	ʒ	Milligram	mg
	Ounce	oz or ʒ	Gram	Gm or g
	Pound	lb	Kilogram	kg
Measures of volume	Minim	min or ṃ	Milliliter	
	Fluidram*	flʒ	(Cubic	
	Fluidounce*	fl oz or flʒ	centimeter)	ml (cc)
	Pint	pt	Liter	L
	Quart	qt		
	Gallon	gal		

*In practice, the "fluid" in these two terms is not commonly used.

Other variations in recording drug dosages exist between the two systems, as shown in Table 14.8.

TABLE 14.8 Variations in Drug Dosages

Apothecary System	Example	Metric System	Example
1. Quantities less than one are written as common fractions; a half is designated by the symbol ss.	gr 1/4 gr s̄s̄	1. Quantities less than one are written as decimal fractions, with a zero placed in front of the decimal point if no number precedes it.	0.25 mg 0.6 mg
2. Lowercase Roman numerals are used to indicate whole numbers.	ʒ iii ṃ v̄ gr ii s̄s̄	2. Arabic numerals are used to indicate whole numbers	3 mg 5 cc
3. Labels designating measurements are placed before the numerals.	As above	3. Labels designating measurements follow the numerals.	As above

Other abbreviations for measures of drug dosages you will occasionally encounter follow here.

Term	Abbreviation
Drop	gtt
Teaspoon	tsp or t
Tablespoon	tbsp or T
Unit	U
Milliequivalent	mEq

ROUTE OF ADMINISTRATION

The same drug can often be prepared in different ways and administered to patients by different routes (Fig. 14.2). For example, codeine comes in tablet form and can be given to a patient by mouth, but if the doctor wants a patient to have much faster pain relief he or she may order the codeine to be given by injection. Most routes of administration are abbreviated in the written order, as indicated in Table 14.9.

INTRAVENOUS MEDICATION ORDERS

Types of intravenous orders are discussed in detail in Chapter 15, Nursing Procedure Orders. In that chapter it is explained that doctors often order medications to be placed directly into the IV bag. The most common orders are for potassium chloride (KCl) or for vitamins, although other medications are also ordered.

ROUTES OF ADMINISTRATION

BY MOUTH, ORALLY (p.o.)

INTRAMUSCULAR (IM)

INTRAVENOUS (IV)

FIGURE 14.2

TABLE 14.9	ROUTES OF ADMINISTRATION
Route	**Abbreviation**
by mouth—orally	po
subcutaneous	sc, subcut
hypodermic	H
intramuscular	IM
intravenous	IV
intravenous push	IVP
in right eye	OD
in left eye	OS
in both eyes	OU
in right ear	AD
in left ear	AS
in both ears	AU
sublingual—under the tongue	subling

These types of orders mean that the medication, dissolved in the IV fluid, will drip into the patient's vein at the rate of flow of the existing IV.

> *1000 cc 5% DW c̄ 20 mEq KCl*
> *1000 cc 5% DW c̄ 1 amp MV1-12.*

Intravenous Push (IVP)

When the doctor orders medication by IVP, it is given directly into the vein by syringe and needle or into the IV tubing via a special part of the tubing designed for this purpose.

> *Lanoxin 0.5 mg IVP*
> *Demerol (meperidine) 25 mg IVP*

Some IVP medications may be injected into a minibag and allowed to drip into the patient's vein rather than by actual injection into the tubing (discussed further in Chapter 15).

IV Heparin Lock (Hep-Lock)

There are times when the doctor wishes a patient to receive IV medication on a regular basis, but the doctor does not want the patient to suffer the inconvenience of being attached to IV tubing, or the patient has no need for an IV, so a **heparin lock** is ordered. A needle with a small length of tubing is inserted into the vein. The end of the tubing has a resealable stopper. The ordered IV medication is instilled into this stopper, and the needle is kept open (unclogged by clotted blood) by flushing a small amount of heparin solution (an anticoagulant that prevents the blood from clotting) into the tubing each time after the medication is injected into the stopper. Heparin lock flush solution, USP, may be ordered for this purpose.

PCA Device

The PCA device allows a patient to administer his/her own pain medication (see p. 362, Chapter 15).

$\mathcal{T}$IMES OF ADMINISTRATION

The nurse must be given special directions concerning *when* a medication is to be given. Some drugs, such as sleeping medications, should be given only at night before bedtime. Others, given to affect digestion, are best administered before meals. Some must be given three or four times a day to produce the desired level of medication in the blood. Abbreviations are often used to denote how often a drug is to be given. Most hospitals have a precise schedule of hours equivalent to each of these expressions. For

TABLE 14.10 $\mathcal{T}$YPICAL TIMES OF ADMINISTRATION AND THEIR COMMON ABBREVIATIONS	
Times	**Abbreviations**
every other day	qod
every day	qd
twice a day	bid
three times a day	tid
four times a day	qid
every hour	qh
every ____ hours	q____h
at hour of sleep (once only)	hs
at hour of sleep (when necessary)	hs prn
before meals	ac
after meals	pc
at once, without delay	stat
when necessary or required	prn
may be repeated once if necessary	sos

example, qid may mean that a medication should be given at 10 A.M., 2 P.M., 6 P.M., and 10 P.M. In other hospitals, qid may indicate that the medication is to be given at 9 A.M., 1 P.M., 5 P.M., and 9 P.M. (see Table 14.10).

European or Military Time

Many hospitals prefer to use European or military time to eliminate the need for A.M. or P.M. The clock in Fig. 14.3 illustrates military time.

FIGURE 14.3

Each nursing station will have a schedule of medication times posted. An example of medication times using military time is shown in Table 14.11. Your hospital will provide a schedule of medication times, which will be posted at your desk at the nurses' station. Table 14.12 shows examples of working shifts in military and standard time. Table 14.13 shows examples of medication times.

TABLE 14.11 *H*OURS OF DAY

Military Time	Standard Time	Military Time	Standard Time
0030	12:30 A.M.	1230	12:30 P.M.
0100	1:00 A.M.	1300	1:00 P.M.
0130	1:30 A.M.	1330	1:30 P.M.
0200	2:00 A.M.	1400	2:00 P.M.
0300	3:00 A.M.	1500	3:00 P.M.
0400	4:00 A.M.	1600	4:00 P.M.
0500	5:00 A.M.	1700	5:00 P.M.
0600	6:00 A.M.	1800	6:00 P.M.
0700	7:00 A.M.	1900	7:00 P.M.
0800	8:00 A.M.	2000	8:00 P.M.
0900	9:00 A.M.	2100	9:00 P.M.
1000	10:00 A.M.	2200	10:00 P.M.
1100	11:00 A.M.	2300	11:00 P.M.
1200	12:00 P.M. (NOON)	2400	12:00 A.M. (MIDNIGHT)

TABLE 14.12 *S*HIFTS IN MILITARY AND STANDARD TIME

Military Time	Standard Time
0700–1530	7:00 A.M.–3:30 P.M.
1500–2330	3:00 P.M.–11:30 P.M.
2300–0730	11:00 P.M.–7:30 A.M.

TABLE 14.13 *E*XAMPLES OF MEDICATION TIMES

Order	Military Time	Order	Military Time
DAILY	0900	c̄ MEALS	0800–1200–1700
BID	0900–1700	ac	0800–1200–1700
TID	0900–1300–1700	pc	0900–1300–1800
QID	0900–1300–1700–2100		
Q2H	0100–0300–0500–0700–0900–1100 1300–1500–1700–1900–2100–2300	COUMADIN	1800
Q3H	2400–0300–0600–0900 1200–1500–1800–2100	HEPARIN BID	0900–2100
Q4H	0100–0500–0900–1300–1700–2100	Q6H	0300–0900–1500–2100
Q6H	0600–1200–1800–2400	Q8H	0100–0900–1700
Q8H	0600–1400–2200		
Q12H	0900–2100		

*Q*UALIFYING PHRASES

Most phrases in doctors' orders that qualify the administration of a drug will be written out in longhand. They need only be copied as written when you are transcribing the order. Sometimes, however, you will encounter the following abbreviations, and you should know what they mean.

Phrase	Abbreviations
of each	āā
with	c̄
without	s̄
freely, as desired	ad lib
do not repeat	non rep

THE PHYSICIAN'S DESK REFERENCE (PDR)

The **PDR,** published by Medical Economics each year, is a very helpful reference. You can use it for clarifying drug dosages, drug usage, and correct spelling of drugs for order transcription.

The PDR has different sections listed in the table of contents, and each section is printed on different colored paper. The sections you will use most often are:

- Alphabetical index by product name
- Section by generic name
- Product information section

On the page number listed following the drug name you will find product identification that will describe and explain the drug. It is recommended that you use the PDR as you study drugs to learn spelling, drug category, and purposes of each.

THE HOSPITAL DRUG FORMULARY

The **Hospital Formulary** lists all the drugs that are approved for use in your hospital. There is an ongoing review of the formulary by a committee such as a pharmacy and therapeutics committee. Drugs are added to or deleted from the formulary based on efficacy, existence of other (more effective) drugs, cost, demand or usage, bio-availability, and drug availability. If a doctor orders a drug that is not in the formulary, the pharmacist will contact the physician to see if a formulary item can be substituted without compromising patient care. The pharmacy department is responsible for keeping the formulary up to date and relaying formulary changes to physicians and nurses. Unless the physician indicates otherwise on the physician's order form, the pharmacist will substitute a generic drug as long as the generic product meets the standards required. There will be a copy of the hospital formulary at each nursing station.

TYPES OF MEDICATION ORDERS

There are three main types of medication orders, identified by the time and frequency of administration. Your responsibilities in transcribing each of these will vary, so you must be able to tell them apart. The three main types are:

- Standing—routine and prn
- Single-dose
- Stat

Standing Orders

This most common type of medication order designates that medication should be given to the patient on a regular schedule for a predetermined number of days or until further notice by the physician. In other words, the order stands as written until it is changed or canceled.

A special category of standing order is the **prn** order. As you have learned, prn is an abbreviation of Latin words meaning "whenever necessary." The prn order is transcribed like routine standing orders but differs in that there is no specific time schedule designated for administration. A sample of standing orders follows.

> *Aspirin gr x̄ po qid*
> *Procaine Penicillin 600,000 U IM q8h*
> *Codeine 30 mg po q4h prn for headache*

Single-Dose Orders

Occasionally, the doctor wants a patient to have just one dose of a medication for a specific purpose. Preoperative medications would be examples of this type of order. Often, before being sent to the operating room, the patient is given an injection containing a narcotic, a barbiturate, or perhaps another medication. Since this is to be given once only, it qualifies as a single-dose order.

The time of administration is the factor that generally identifies an order as a single-dose order. No time of administration may be indicated at all; or a specific time of day or date may be written; or an abbreviation such as hs or tonight (which indicates the drug is to be given once only) will identify single-dose orders.

Other medications, commonly ordered as a short series of injections of various dosages—for example, anticoagulants—may also be classified as single-dose orders according to the methods used to transcribe them in your hospital. Examples of single-dose orders follow.

> *Resperine 50 mg IM at 2 pm*
> *Heparin 40,000 U IM ac noon*
> *Nembutal 100 mg po hs*

Stat Orders

Stat is an abbreviation for the Latin word **statim,** meaning "immediately." In serious or emergency situations, a medication may be ordered stat. This requires that the nurse administer the medication as soon as possible. Typical stat orders follow.

> *Morphine sulfate gr 1/6 SC stat*
> *Nitroglycerine 0.9 mg po stat*
> *Compazine 50 mg IM stat*

BASIC TRANSCRIPTION PROCEDURE

Transcribing a standing order entails a number of specific tasks. The seven-step procedure described in Chapter 13 may help simplify your duties.

First, Recognize the Order

Remember: Standing orders can be identified by the time-of-administration schedules accompanying them. Any medication of a specific dosage ordered for an unstated period of time or for longer than 24 hours will generally qualify as a standing order. Refer again to the example of standing orders on p. 324.

Second, Rip

Tear off the NCR copy and route it to the pharmacy if this is your hospital's method for obtaining patient drugs. Another NCR copy may go to the nurse to notify him or her of the medication order. Hospitals have different ways of letting the pharmacy know about medication orders. In hospitals with integrated computer systems, entering of orders into the computer is the form of notification. Some hospitals fax the new orders to the pharmacy. Learn your hospital's rules regarding this procedure.

Third, Prioritize

Always select those orders of highest priority to transcribe first.

Fourth, Transfer the Order to Special Records (Kardex)

There may be as many as three special records on which a medication order should be noted—Kardex, medication records, and medication ticket.

Kardex. The order must be transcribed, exactly as written, to the appropriate section of the Kardex. It must be written legibly and accurately. The order is often recorded in pencil so it can be erased when canceled. Often, you are required to specify the time schedule of administration in terms of hours.

When computer-generated Kardexes are used, orders are entered into the computer and a printout is obtained. No handwriting is necessary.

Medication Record. All hospitals have some kind of medication record, which is one of the standard chart forms. When orders for a newly admitted patient are received, it is usually the nurse who transcribes the orders onto the medication administration record (MAR). In a computerized system, the pharmacy usually prints out an MAR for every hospitalized patient, and these are distributed at a designated time to each nursing unit (usually at night). The night nurse then compares the computerized sheet with the initial sheet that was completed on admission, updates the computerized sheet, places a copy in the chart, and returns a copy to pharmacy. This serves as a double check of all medication orders. The copy given back to pharmacy is also used for charging purposes (Fig. 14.4).

M.A.R. VERIFIED

BY: _____

MEDICATION ADMINISTRATION RECORD
M.A.R.

Name: EXAMPLE, IMA   Allergies ==> PENICILLINS   MEMORIAL HOSPITAL

Room: 000   Patient ID: 12345

Sex: F Age: 62 Hgt: 149cm Wgt: 49.09kg MR#:

Diagnosis: DEPRESSION

Physician: JOHN GOODDOCTOR   MD Phone: 000-0000

Comments: OWN CALCIUM

CONSENT DATES:
LITHIUM   ANTIPSYCHOTICS
ANTICHOLINERGICS   ANTIDEPRESSANTS

ADMINISTRATION PERIOD: 05/30/9 @ 2301 thru 05/31/5 @ 2300

Medication	Start	Stop	s1 2301 thru 0700	s2 0701 thru 1500	s3 1501 thru 2301
CALCIUM CARBONATE TAB 500MG TUMS PO 1 TAB x 500MG/EA BID LOT #: EXP DATE: **CHEWABLE TABLET**	2000 05/22 JML			0900	1700
ESTROGENS, CONJUGATE TAB 1.25MG PREMARIN PO 1 TAB x 1.25MG/EA DAILY	1800 05/21 RS			0900	
NEFAZODONE TAB 200MG SERZONE PO 2 TAB x 100MG/EA BID	1800 05/21 RS			0900	1700
PATIENT'S OWN MED 1 PT OWN MED PO UD OTC CALCIUM SUPPLEMENT	2000 05/21 RS				
RISPERIDONE TAB 1MG RISPERDAL PO 1 TAB x 1MG/EA HS	1800 05/21 RS				2100
TRIMETHOPRIM/SULFAME 800-160 TAB 1 SEPTRA DS PO 1 TAB BID Total Doses: 20 X 10 DAYS	2000 05/22 JML	1701 06/01		0900	1700

RESPONSE	MEDS NOT GIVEN	INJECTION SITES	SIGNATURE	INITIALS	SIGNATURE	INITIALS
A. ... in 30 Minutes B. Relief in 60 Minutes C. No Relief	B. BP Changes N. Med Not Avail. P. Patient Asleep Q. Off of Unit R. Refused S. NPO/Studies T. NPO/Surgery	INDICATE INJECTION SITE – R OR L 1. Deltoid 2. Abdominal = 1-10 Scale 3. Iliac Crest Pre & Post Analgesic 4. Thigh Pain Assessment 1 = Least Pain 10 = Most Pain				

Printed: 13:02 on 05/30/2xxx   Page 1 of

SCHEDULED

FIGURE 14.4

DATE	MEDICATION	5/30 MON.	5/31 TUES.	6/1 WED.	6/2 THUR.	6/3 FRI.	6/4 SAT.	6/5 SUN.
5-27-XX	Digitoxin 0.2 mg po qd	A.J.T. 10am	A.J.T. 10am	10am				
6-1-XX	Aspirin gr x̄ po qid			10-2 6-10				
6-1-XX	Procaine Penicillin 600,000U IM q8h			4P 12Mn	8 am 4 pm 12 Mn			

FIGURE 14.5

As new orders come in, the health unit coordinator inputs them into the computer, and they are printed out onto the Kardex. The nurse (or the health unit coordinator if specially trained) writes the new orders on the medication administration record, the pharmacy receives the new information via the computer or fax, and the cycle repeats.

If it is your responsibility to record medications on the medication record, you must be particularly careful to demonstrate your skill of accuracy. Be sure when writing a dosage that includes a decimal to always write a zero before the decimal point to exclude any possibilities that a fraction will be interpreted as a whole number (see Fig. 14.5—digitoxin **0.2 mg**).

Medicine Ticket In many hospitals using the **unit dose system,** which provides medications in single doses each time during the day that the medication is ordered, the medicine ticket is no longer used. However, medicine tickets are sometimes used in long-term care or psychiatric facilities. The nurse refers to this ticket as the medication is prepared, keeps each ticket with the appropriate medication, and makes a final check just before it is administered to the patient. Medicine tickets vary in form but will ordinarily include the date of order, patient's name, room and bed number, name of medication, dosage, route of administration, and any qualifying phrase (Fig. 14.6).

Standardized rules almost always apply to the filling out of medicine tickets:

- *All* information included in the order must be transferred to the ticket *accurately, legibly, and exactly as written.* Abbreviate where the doctor has done so; write out any words or phrases the doctor has written out. This rule should apply whenever orders are transcribed.
- If any information in the order, such as qualifying phrases, cannot be included on the front of the ticket for reasons of space, show *clearly in large, bold letters* that the ticket must be turned over for further inspection.
- Medicine tickets may be color-coded or size-coded to distinguish among different types of medications (e.g., hypnotics, narcotics) or different types of orders (e.g., standing, single dose). Your instructor will explain any variations of this type used in your hospital.

Fifth, Requisition Equipment and Services

To carry out a medication order, the nurse must have the medication on hand. Step two, tearing off the appropriate NCR copy from the doctor's order sheet and sending it to the pharmacy, is the common method of obtaining drugs. Some hospitals use a pharmacy requisition (Fig. 14.7). Many order by computer.

SPECIAL RECORDS
NEEDED FOR
TRANSCRIBING
MEDICATION ORDERS

DOCTOR'S
ORDERS
FOR
MEDICATIONS

PATIENT CARE RECORD CARD   MEDICATION RECORD

MEDICINE
TICKET

FIGURE 14.6

Memorial Hospital				
PHARMACY — DRUGS Requisition and Charge				

Date_____   Are drugs to be taken home?   ☐ Yes ☐ No

Room No._____   Signature (R.N.)_____

Name_____   Prescribed by _____

Hosp. No._____   Rx No. _____

Doctor_____

Order filled and charged by

QUANTITY	ITEM	STRENGTH OR DOSAGE	DIRECTIONS FOR USE	ORAL OR HYPO	CHARGE	
				TOTAL CHARGE		

FIGURE 14.7

Sixth, Write Correct Transcription* Symbols *on the Doctor's Order Sheet (Fig. 14.8)

Date	Order	Signature
6-1-xx	Ҟ Aspirin grx̄ po qid	
	Ҟ Procaine Penicillin 600,000 U IM q8h	
	Ҟ Codeine 30 mg po q4h prn for headache	*AJ Stahl*

FIGURE 14.8

Seventh, Have Transcribed Orders Checked

This final step is as important as the others. The orders you have transcribed cannot be put into effect until your work has been checked by the nurse. With the help of the nurses with whom you work, you will be able to establish a method of accomplishing this task that is convenient for everyone concerned.

STANDING ORDER VARIATIONS

Once a medication has served its purpose and is no longer indicated for the patient in his or her treatment, the doctor may cancel the order. Also, certain drugs being given to a patient may cancel automatically after a designated number of hours or days and must be renewed by the doctor if the patient should continue to receive them.

Sometimes the physician may wish to increase or decrease the dosage of a particular medicine or to change its route of administration or preparation. If so, the doctor will have to write a new order to that effect. You will learn how to transcribe medication orders for cancellations, renewals, and changes.

Cancellations

> *Discontinue order for Procaine Penicillin 600,000 U IM q8h p̄ 4 pm dose*
> *Cancel Aspirin gr x̄ po qid*
> *Discontinue Streptomycin 0.5 gm IM bid after today*

When the doctor writes an order for a specific medication to be canceled, several things must be done (Pharmacy will be notified by NCR copy or computer, and the nurse by NCR copy of orders or by health unit coordinator (Fig. 14.9)):

- First, the canceled order must be erased from the Kardex (or lined through).
- Next, the medication must be canceled on the medication record.
- If medicine tickets are used, they must be destroyed.

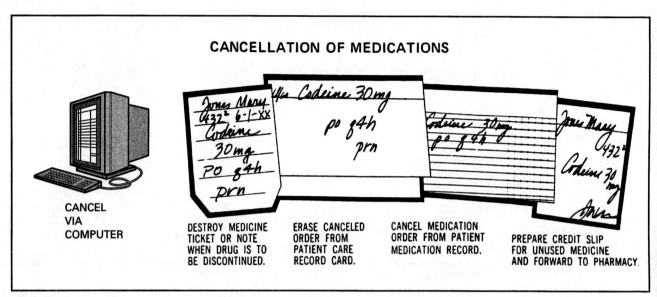

FIGURE 14.9

If the patient has been charged for more of the drugs than were used before the cancellation order, the remainder must be sent to the pharmacy, where it can be credited to the patient's account. In many hospitals this process is taken care of by the pharmacy.

Automatic Stops

In most hospitals, certain medications cancel automatically after being in use for a specified, generally limited, number of hours (48 to 72). The continued administration of hypnotics, narcotics, antibiotics, and anticoagulants might result in addiction, habituation, or serious side effects. Orders for such medications usually specify a limited number of times for administration. Many hospitals have established routines by which a patient's doctor is notified that an order for a particular medication has run out. If the doctor wishes the order to be continued, the doctor must write an order for renewal. Many hospitals use a stamp on the doctor's order sheet to indicate that an automatic-stop drug must be canceled or reordered (Fig. 14.10).

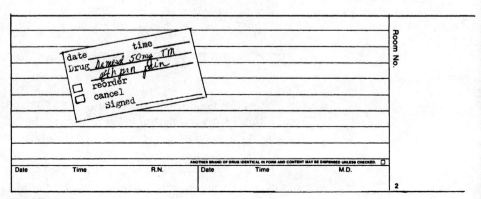

FIGURE 14.10

Renewals

If the doctor wishes an order to continue unchanged, the order may be written as follows:

> *Renew Streptomycin 0.5 Gm IM bid order*
> *Renew order for Codeine 30 mg po q4h prn*
> *Continue order for Aspirin gr x̄ po qid*

Other Variations

The amount of a drug can be changed in several different ways:

- The *dosage* of a drug can be directly increased or decreased.

> *Change Procaine Penicillin 600,000 U IM q8h order to read Procaine Penicillin 300,000 U IM q8h.*

- Or, the *same dosage can be given to the patient more or fewer times during the day.* Over a period of time, this method may have the same effect as an increase or decrease in dosage.

> *Change Procaine Penicillin 600,000 U IM q8h to Procaine Penicillin 600,000 U IM qd.*

The *route of administration* may also be changed.

- If the patient has difficulty swallowing large pills, the doctor may change the order to a liquid preparation. If the patient is nauseated and vomits medication given by mouth, the doctor may order that it be given by injection.

> *Dilantin 100 mg po tid. If pt refuses, give IM as ordered previously.*

The *type of medication* may be changed.

> *Change sleeping medication from Seconal 100 mg po hs to Nembutal 100 mg po hs prn.*

The *preparation of medication* may also be changed.

> *Change Aspirin gr x̄ po qid to EC Aspirin tabs gr x̄ po qid.*

In these kinds of situations, the doctor is always responsible for writing the order for a change in medication on the doctor's order sheet.

TRANSCRIBING SINGLE-DOSE AND STAT ORDERS

Procedures for handling single-dose and stat orders vary widely among hospitals, so specific guidelines will necessarily come to you from your instructor. Single-dose and stat orders must be brought to the immediate attention of the nurse. The medication should be obtained from the pharmacy quickly. These orders are very high priority and should be attended to at once.

CONTROLLED DRUGS

The manufacture, distribution, and utilization of medications is the subject of a large body of federal and state laws. The general regulation of drugs by the federal government started with the Food and Drug Act of 1906. Certain drugs have a high potential for abuse. The Controlled Substances Act of 1971 contains the laws regarding these drugs. **Controlled substances** are classified into five categories called **schedules.** Schedule I drugs are experimental. Schedule II drugs have the highest potential for abuse, and schedule V the least. Prescriptions of these drugs are regulated, and the containers are labeled with a *C* followed by the Roman numeral (II–V) indicating the schedule of the drug. As dispensers of controlled substances for medicinal purposes, hospital pharmacies are required by law to be registered with the Drug Enforcement Administration, and careful records must be kept on certain drugs.

Controlled substances are kept locked on the nursing unit, and the nurse or nurses who give medications carry the key to this locked cupboard or drawer of a medicine cart.

When a controlled substance from the locked cupboard is given to a patient, the nurse must record the patient's name and dosage on the sheet for that drug and sign the sheet. When the sheet is completed, it is returned to the pharmacy. The nurse responsible for medications must count each of the controlled drugs at the end of each shift with the nurse coming on duty, who receives the key and assumes the responsibility for the drugs during the next shift. Each drug must be accounted for. Any inaccuracy is serious and must be resolved. No controlled drug may go unaccounted for.

The pharmacy is responsible for the replacement of controlled drugs, which are delivered in person by pharmacy personnel. The nurse receiving the new supply of drugs must sign the sheet accompanying the drug at the time of delivery. Clearly, very strict controls of these drugs, mainly narcotics and barbiturates and other hypnotics, are maintained.

When transcribing orders for medications, the health unit coordinator must be aware that drugs in the category of controlled substances are already on the nursing unit in the locked cupboard or drawer. Learn the names of the controlled substances kept on the nursing unit of your hospital.

The transcription of medication orders demands great accuracy and attention to detail. The health unit coordinator must be familiar with the names of drugs frequently ordered and must recognize medication abbreviations. Doctors write many medication orders for their patients, and the health unit coordinator must recognize these orders, expedite their processing, and properly complete all forms and records as required by the hospital. Attention must be given to the automatic-stop requirements for certain drugs. In addition, the health unit coordinator must always remember to ask the nurse or doctor when in doubt about a medication order.

LEARNING ACTIVITIES

Complete the following classifications of medications.

   1. Drugs that destroy or render harmless microorganisms are called _____
       _____ drugs.

   2. Drugs that alter disease by stimulating or depressing normal body functions
       are called _____ drugs.

   3. Drugs that treat neoplastic disease are called _____
       drugs.

Match the category of antimicrobial drug in Column A with its description in Column B.

Column A	Column B
(a) Sulfonamides	____ Produced by microorganisms that prevent the growth of or destroy other microorganisms.
(b) Antiseptics	
(c) Antibiotics	____ Chemicals used on inanimate objects that kill or inhibit the growth of microorganisms.
(d) Disinfectants	
(e) Antituberculars	____ Drugs that inhibit the growth of the bacteria that cause tuberculosis.
	____ Commonly called *sulfa drugs*.
	____ Chemicals used on living tissue that kill or inhibit the growth of microorganisms.

Match the category of pharmacodynamic drug in Column A with its description in Column B.

Column A	Column B
(a) Anesthetic	____ Produces vomiting
(b) Stimulant	____ Lowers blood sugar
(c) Hypoglycemic	____ Increases urine output
(d) Emetic	____ Treats cancer
(e) Antitussive	____ Inhibits blood clotting
(f) Antacid	____ Relieves cough
(g) Anticonvulsant	____ Relieves allergic symptoms
(h) Antihistamine	____ Improves quality of heart action
(i) Cardiotonic	____ Produces loss of sensation
(j) Antineoplastic	____ Produces increased functional activity
(k) Diuretic	____ Lowers acidity of gastric secretions
(l) Anticoagulant	____ Suppresses seizures

Complete the following.

4. List two common anticoagulants.
    (a) _____
    (b) _____

5. Explain why anticoagulant drugs require careful monitoring.

    _____
    _____
    _____

6. Name two common laboratory tests for monitoring anticoagulants.
    (a) _____
    (b) _____

7. Define the term *sliding scale*.

    _____
    _____

8. List the four main categories of the medication order form.
    (a) _____
    (b) _____
    (c) _____
    (d) _____

9. What is the additional category? _____

    _____

10. Each drug has at least three names, which are:
    (a) _____
    (b) _____
    (c) _____

11. The generic name is never _____.

12. What does it mean when a medication is ordered IVP? _____
_____
_____

13. What is an IV heparin lock? _____
_____
_____

14. List the three main types of medication orders, identified by the time and frequency of administration.
    (a) _____
    (b) _____
    (c) _____

15. A special category of the standing order is the _____ order.

16. Give two examples of types of single-dose orders.
    (a) _____
    (b) _____

17. The factor that generally identifies an order as a single-dose order is the
_____ of administration.

18. Give two reasons why a medication may be canceled.
    (a) _____
    (b) _____

19. State two ways the dosage of a drug can be changed.
    (a) _____
    (b) _____

20. List two reasons why the route of administration of the medication may be changed.
    (a) _____
    (b) _____

21. The Controlled Substances Act of 1971 contains laws regarding those drugs that have a _____ for abuse.

22. Where are controlled substances kept on the nursing unit? _____
_____

23. Which schedule of controlled substances has the highest potential for abuse—II or V? _____

24. Define the following medical abbreviations:
    (a) ac _____
    (b) OS _____
    (c) bid _____
    (d) mEq _____
    (e) $\bar{s}$ _____
    (f) Gm _____
    (g) gr _____
    (h) gtt _____
    (i) H _____
    (j) hs _____
    (k) cc _____

(l)   U _____

(m)   tid _____

(n)   stat _____

(o)   sos _____

(p)   c̄ _____

(q)   qid _____

(r)   qh _____

(s)   qd _____

(t)   OD _____

(u)   prn _____

(v)   pc _____

(w)   IM _____

(x)   IV _____

(y)   PDR _____

(z)   AU _____

25. The following are drugs listed in this chapter. Circle the correct drug for each category.

   (a) **anesthetic** (local) (1) codeine (2) amoxicillin (3) ibuprofen (4) lidocaine (5) Flexeril

   (b) **emetic** (1) Imferon (2) ipecac syrup (3) Lasix (4) Lopressor (5) Proventil

   (c) **antiviral** (1) acyclovir (2) digitoxin (3) Zantac (4) Zocor (5) Mylicon

   (d) **antiemetic** (1) Hycodan (2) Haldol (3) Nitrobid (4) Premarin (5) Vistaril

   (e) **antihypertensive** (1) Dulcolax (2) phenobarbital (3) Vasotec (4) streptokinase (5) Theragran

   (f) **potassium replacement** (1) epinephrine (2) SSKI (3) Aldactone (4) atenolol (5) meperidine

   (g) **antidysrhythmic** (1) Colace (2) isoproterenol (3) Halcion (4) prednisolone (5) DES

   (h) **diuretic** (1) ephedrine (2) Retrovir (3) Tagamet (4) claritin (5) furosemide

   (i) **anti-infective** (1) Diamox (2) Versed (3) Levophed (4) Theolair-SR (5) tetracycline

   (j) **cardiotonic** (1) Coumadin (2) Prozac (3) digoxin (4) Humalin R (5) Mylicon

26. What kind of mistakes could you, as a health unit coordinator make when dealing with medication orders? In how many ways could your mistakes adversely affect the patient? _____

_____

_____

_____

_____

_____

_____

_____

_____

_____

_____

27. What is the purpose of therapeutic drug monitoring? What could happen if these orders were overlooked?_____

_____

_____

_____

_____

_____

_____

_____

28. It is a busy morning and the charts are stacking up. You now have 10 charts in front of you that have orders to be transcribed. Describe what steps you will take to make sure that all medication orders are expedited. How will you choose which orders must be taken care of first? What will you do about these orders?_____

_____

_____

_____

_____

_____

_____

29. Complete the following.
  (a) A _____ action of a drug occurs when it is applied directly to a certain area.
  (b) A _____ action of a drug is one that occurs when the drug is carried in the bloodstream and affects tissues and organs away from the site of entry.
  (c) A _____ is an action of a drug other than what was intended.
  (d) An _____ is an undesirable and harmful side effect.
  (e) A drug _____ occurs when a drug, food, or alcohol reacts with a drug.

30. Go to a web site such as MedicineNet.com (*http://www.medicinenet.com*). Select 10 drugs from different categories. Learn as much as you can about them. List the 10 drugs by brand and generic name below. Discuss with the class what you learned about the drugs.

	Brand	**Generic**
(a)	_____	_____
(b)	_____	_____
(c)	_____	_____
(d)	_____	_____
(e)	_____	_____
(f)	_____	_____
(g)	_____	_____
(h)	_____	_____
(i)	_____	_____
(j)	_____	_____

31. Once again you have a stack of charts in front of you. It seems as if every doctor made rounds at once. You go through each chart and tear off the NCR copies for the pharmacy. As you scan each set of new orders how do you identify medication orders from other kinds of orders? _____

_____

_____

32. What will happen if you do not tear off the NCR copies and route them to the pharmacy? _____

_____

33. Why is it so important that you regularly check charts for new orders? Can you always count on the doctor to bring new orders to your attention?

_____

_____

_____

34. What can happen to a patient who doesn't get his or her medications because the orders were missed? _____

_____

35. Why is it so important that medication orders be brought to the nurses's attention right away?

_____

_____

_____

36. What would you do with an order that says, "start IV c̄ 1000 cc D51/2NS"? Since there is no time attached to this order, when do you think the doctor wants it done?

_____

_____

_____

37. How would you feel if you had an NG tube or were catheterized and someone missed the doctor's order for "DC NG tube" or "DC Foley cath," and the order wasn't found until hours later?

_____

_____

_____

38. What would you do if a nurse asked you to stay with a patient and help him take his pills because the nurse was running late and had so much to do?

_____

CHAPTER 15

Nursing Procedure Orders

Blood pressure — Force of the blood exerted against the walls of the arteries when the heart contracts

Catheter — Sterile tube used to withdraw fluids and air from the body

Catheterization, urinary — Removal of urine from the body through a sterile tube

Consultation — Advice and services given by one physician at the request of another

Intake and output — Measurement of fluids taken into and those that come out of the body

Normal saline solution (NSS) — The physiological saline solution of the body; an 0.85% salt solution similar to that of serum

Pulse — The rhythmic expansion and contraction of arteries when the heart beats

Respiration — The process of inhaling and exhaling and bringing oxygen into the body and expelling carbon dioxide

Suction — The removal of fluid or air from the body through the use of tubes or catheters and suction machines or gravity drainage

Temperature — A measure of heat in the body

Traction — Exertion of a pull on the body by weights and pulleys

Treatment — A medical or nursing procedure done to improve or monitor a patient's condition

Vital signs — Temperature, pulse, respiration, and blood pressure; the signs of life

OBJECTIVES

When you have completed this chapter, you will be able to:

- Define the terms listed in the vocabulary.
- Describe nursing treatment orders for suction, bowel care, heat and cold applications, and urinary catheterization.
- Discuss monitoring orders for vital signs, circulation, neurological checks, and blood and urine tests done by nursing.
- Describe the various types of intravenous orders.
- Give examples of activity, positioning, comfort, and safety orders.
- Give examples of miscellaneous orders.
- Show knowledge of the abbreviations used in this chapter.
- Demonstrate the ability to transcribe treatment orders.

A **treatment** can be defined as any medical or nursing procedure intended to keep a record of, improve, or in any way treat a patient's condition. It would be impossible to describe every type of treatment a doctor might order for a patient; it is even difficult to categorize treatments effectively. You should be familiar with the treatments most frequently ordered. The following descriptions are given for that purpose. As you study this chapter, note the list of abbreviations and definitions for the various orders included in this chapter. Add to the list any other terms in general use in your hospital.

This chapter will include information regarding the following types of orders:

- Suction
- Bowel care
- Heat and cold applications
- Urinary catheterizations
- Vital signs
- Circulation checks
- Craniotomy or neurological checks
- Intake and output
- Capillary blood glucose testing

- Urine tests by nursing for glucose and acetone
- Intravenous therapy
- Activity
- Positioning
- Comfort and safety
- Miscellaneous orders
- Transcription procedure

*T*REATMENT ORDERS

*S*UCTION ORDERS

Fluids or air are removed from the patient's body through tubes or catheters. The methods used are either **gravity** or **suction.** When fluids are removed by **gravity,** the collecting container is placed near the patient at a level that is lower than the patient's body. The fluids drip into the container. Suction is most commonly ordered to remove fluids from the throat, stomach, intestines, chest, or wounds. Suction apparatus includes various tubes and machines. The doctor will write orders for the establishment, maintenance, and removal of the suction equipment. There may also be orders for irrigation of the various tubes in order to keep them **patent** (draining).

Throat suction is ordered when a patient's throat is blocked by mucus secretions. A catheter and a continuous type of throat suction machine are used.

Deep tracheal suction is a sterile procedure requiring sterile catheters and the use of sterile gloves. The instillation of sterile saline to loosen secretions precedes this procedure. If a patient has a **tracheostomy** (an artificial opening into the windpipe), suctioning is often ordered. This is also a sterile procedure.

Gastric suction is ordered to remove gastric fluids and air from the patient's stomach. This is a low, intermittent type of suction machine quite different from that used for throat suction. It may be portable (Gomco) or built into the wall at the patient's bedside (Fig. 15.1).

To accomplish gastric suction a *nasogastric tube* (also called *Levin tube* or just *NG tube*) is inserted through the patient's nose and into the stomach by the nurse or doctor. This is a single-lumen tube that comes in several sizes: 16 French (Fr) is used most commonly for adults, 6 Fr to 12 Fr for children. This tube is then attached to a tube leading to the gastric suction machine. The nurse will frequently milk and/or irrigate the NG tube with normal saline (NS) to keep the tube draining. An irrigation tray, usually disposable, is needed for this procedure (Fig. 15.2).

Another short tube is a *gastric sump tube* (e.g., *Salem* or *Ventrol*), which is a double-lumen tube. A special procedure that washes out the patient's stomach by use of the nasogastric tube is called *lavage* (feeding through the NG tube is called *gavage*).

Long tubes are used to decompress the bowel and are usually 6 to 10 feet long. The *Miller–Abbott tube* is a double-lumen tube with a balloon that, once inserted, is inflated with air, or partially filled with mercury, to help it pass into the small intestine.

FIGURE 15.1

FIGURE 15.2

The *Cantor tube* is a single-lumen tube with a small rubber bag at the distal (far) end that is filled with mercury before insertion.

Gastric suction may also be accomplished via a gastrostomy tube. This tube leads directly from the stomach and is sutured in place by a doctor. It is connected to the gastric suction machine.

Thoracic drainage is accomplished when chest tubes are inserted by the physician into the chest cavity to remove air or fluid. This is usually done in surgery, often as an emergency procedure. These tubes are then attached to a water-sealed bottle system or disposable plastic unit (e.g., Pleur-evac), and either gravity drainage or suction such as an Emerson pump is used to drain air and fluids from the pleural cavity.

> *Chest tube to Emerson pump c̄ 20 cm (centimeters) pressure*

Hemovac Suction A Hemovac is a small, disposable suction apparatus attached to a drain (tube) during surgery that leads from a patient's wound. It is used frequently with mastectomies. The throat, gastric, and chest suction machines must be plugged into an electrical outlet for operation. The Hemovac is *not electrical* and is manually compressed at intervals and allowed to expand to create suction.

The health unit coordinator should know that the tubes or catheters utilized in throat, gastric, and chest suction are disposable. The machines are not disposable. The kind of catheter and suction machine is different with each type of suction, and the machine is returned to central supply for cleaning and reissue. A licensed nurse (RN or LVN/LPN) carries out the various types of suction orders. In many hospitals deep tracheal suction is done by the inhalation or respiratory therapists.

Wound Reinfusion

In wound reinfusion or autoreinfusion, a drain from a wound (usually an orthopedic wound), instead of being attached to a Hemovac is put into a sterile collector where blood and other wound drainage is collected (usually about 100 to 200 cc). The fluid then drops into a sterile blood bag and reinfuses as an IV. The Stryker Autovac and CBC II are examples of these devices.

Bowel Care Orders

Doctors frequently write orders dealing with patients' intestinal elimination. Orders for enemas are often written prior to surgery, certain x-ray procedures, delivery, or during a patient's hospitalization to relieve flatus (intestinal gas) or constipation. Common types of enemas are the following:

- **TWE**—tap water enema
- **SSE**—soapsuds enema
- **NSE**—normal saline enema
- **OR enema**—oil retention enema
- **Fleet or Travad enema**—disposable enema (Fig. 15.3)

FIGURE 15.3

Disposable Enema Bag

Prepackaged Enema

Other Intestinal Elimination Orders

Harris Flush. An irrigation of the rectum in which water is run into and out of the rectum for about 10 minutes is called a Harris flush. The purpose of the Harris flush is to relieve the patient of uncomfortable intestinal gas.

A **rectal tube** (flatus bag) is a tube attached to a bag and inserted into the rectum for the purpose of removing intestinal gas.

Colostomy Irrigation. A **colostomy** is an artificial opening into the patient's large intestine to allow for bowel movements. This opening is created when the colon is diseased or injured. An order for a colostomy irrigation is an order for an enema. The difference between an enema and an irrigation is that the irrigating tube is inserted into the **stoma,** or surgically created opening, to change the path of the patient's feces from the rectum (Fig. 15.4).

SIGMOID COLOSTOMY

Stoma

FIGURE 15.4

A person with a stoma often must wear an ostomy appliance to collect fecal matter released through the stoma (Fig. 15.5).

FIGURE 15.5 Ostomy appliance in place over the stoma.

$\mathcal{H}$EAT AND COLD APPLICATION ORDERS

Heat may be applied to an area of the body to speed up the healing process or to ease the pain caused by inflammation and congestion. A **generalized application** is applied to the patient's entire body. A **localized application** is applied to a specific part or area of a patient's body (Fig. 15.6).

Cold applications are applied to prevent or reduce swelling and pain or to control bleeding. Cold may also be applied to a patient's entire body. This is usually done to lower a patient's body temperature in the case of a high fever. Orders for special equipment and procedures used to help lower the body temperature include those for the following:

- An oxygen tent with a temperature regulator
- Hypothermia blanket and refrigeration machine
- Alcohol sponge baths

$\mathcal{M}$OIST AND DRY APPLICATIONS

All applications are either moist or dry. A **moist application** is one in which water touches the skin. A **dry application** is one in which no water touches the skin (Fig. 15.7). There are several types of moist and dry application:

GENERALIZED APPLICATION
Applying warmth or cold to the patient's entire body

LOCALIZED APPLICATIONS
Applying warmth or cold to a specific part or area of the body

FIGURE 15.6

MOIST	DRY
■ Soak—warm or cold	■ Ice pack and ice collar
■ Compress—warm or cold	■ Heat lamp
■ Tub	■ Aquamatic K-pad

MOIST APPLICATION

DRY APPLICATION

Aquamatic K - pad

FIGURE 15.7

- Alcohol sponge bath
- Sitz bath
- Cool wet packs
- Commercial unit warm pack
- Thermal blankets
- Electric heat cradle
- Commercial unit cold pack

Two of these applications require further definition.

- A **sitz bath** is ordered when the doctor wishes warm water applied to the rectal and perineal area (genital area to anus). Special tubs and disposable units are used for this procedure (Fig. 15.8).

SITZ BATH

FIGURE 15.8 Sitz bath.

- **K-pads** (thermal units) are used for application of continuous dry heat to various parts of the body and especially to the limbs. In the K-pad the electrically heated water circulates throughout the pad. The pad comes in several sizes, and for safety, the temperature is preset in central supply.

Thermal Blankets or Hypothermia Machines

These are reusable pieces of equipment that circulate fluid through tubes in a patient-sized pad. They may be used for **hypothermia** (reduction of body temperature) or **hyperthermia**—elevation of body temperature. Patients receiving either of these treatments will be monitored very closely by the nursing staff.

URINARY CATHETERIZATION ORDERS

Urinary catheterization is ordered to remove urine from the body. A **urinary** catheter is a tube made of latex or silicon that is inserted through the patient's urethra into the bladder. This is a sterile procedure done by the doctor or nurse. Intermittent self-catheterization is taught to some patients when feasible. Urinary catheters vary in size and are designated by number. The higher the number, the larger the catheter. For adults, the catheter size is usually 14, 15, or 18 Fr. The two types of catheterization—nonretention and retention—are discussed in the next two paragraphs (Fig. 15.9).

The purposes of catheterization are

- To remove urine when the patient is unable to **void** (urinate);
- To obtain a **sterile urine specimen** to be sent to the laboratory; or
- To measure the amount of urine left in the bladder after a patient voids (**residual**).

The preceding types of catheterization are called **nonretention,** because the catheter is inserted and then removed. A nonretention catheter is sometimes called a *straight catheter.*

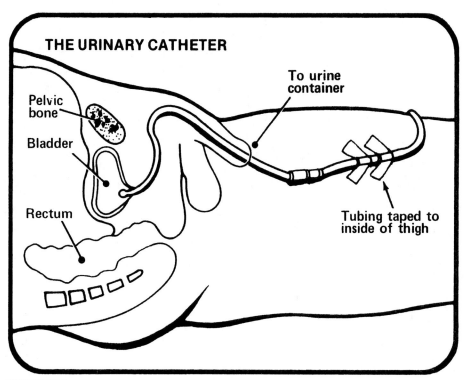

FIGURE 15.9

A **retention catheter** is ordered when a patient is unable to control his or her urine (**incontinence**) or when a patient is unable to void over a period of time. Retention catheters are also called **indwelling** or **Foley catheters,** which remain in the bladder and are connected to a tube that drains into a urine-collecting bag attached to the bed frame (Fig. 15.10). A urine meter, as part of the drainage system, makes hourly

PLASTIC URINE CONTAINER
HUNG ON BED FRAME

FIGURE 15.10

measurement of urine output possible. A smaller, leg bag may be worn by an ambulatory patient.

The health unit coordinator must know that the two types of catheterization require different types of catheters plus a catheterization tray. These items are disposable and are ordered from central supply or kept on carts on the nursing unit, which are stocked by central supply.

As with other types of tubes or catheters left in the patient's body, there may be orders for irrigation. This procedure requires another special disposable tray ordered from central supply and is always performed by a doctor or nurse.

Sometimes a doctor will order continuous or intermittent irrigation of an indwelling catheter. A Hoffman or Nesbit–Young irrigation setup may be ordered from central supply for this purpose. A three-way catheter and antimicrobial solution are used.

Normal saline solution (NSS) is most commonly ordered for catheter irrigation, although other solutions, such as acetic acid, may be ordered.

$\mathcal{M}$ONITORING ORDERS

Vital Signs

When the body is not functioning normally, changes happen in the measurable rates of the **vital signs: Temperature, pulse, respiration,** and **blood pressure** (Fig. 15.11). Common abbreviations for these signs follow.

Temperature (T)
The balance between the heat produced by the body and heat lost by the body

VITAL SIGNS

Blood Pressure (BP)
Force of blood pushing against the walls of the arteries

Pulse (P)
The rate at which the heart is beating

Respiration (R)
Process of inhaling and exhaling

FIGURE 15.11

- Temperature = T
- Pulse = P
- Respiration = R
- Blood pressure = BP
- Vital signs = TPR and BP

> *Average Normal Adult Rates*
> *Temperature: 98.6°F or 37°C*
> *Pulse: 72–80 beats per minute*
> *Respiration: 16–20 per minute*

Temperature

Body **temperature** is a measure of the amount of heat in the body. The body creates heat in the process of changing food into energy. The body can also lose heat—through perspiration, respiration (breathing), and excretion. The balance between the heat produced and the heat lost is the body temperature. The normal adult body temperature is 98.6° Fahrenheit or 37° Celsius. There is a normal range in which a person's body temperature may vary and still be considered normal (Table 15.1).

TABLE 15.1	*N*ORMAL RANGES OF BODY TEMPERATURE	
	Celsius	**Fahrenheit**
Oral	36.4 to 37.2°C	97.6 to 99°F
Rectal	37.0 to 37.8°C	98.6 to 100°F
Axillary	35.9 to 36.7°C	96.6 to 98°F

Types of Thermometers. The body temperature is measured by an instrument called a *thermometer*. There are several types of thermometers (Figs. 15.12 and 15.13):

- **Glass thermometers**—oral, rectal, and security for infant temperatures
- **Battery-operated electronic thermometers**
- **Chemically treated paper or plastic thermometers**

FIGURE 15.12

Battery-Operated Electronic Thermometer

Probe

Sheath

FIGURE 15.13

■ **Tympanic membrane thermometer**—also known as an aural thermometer, this device is fast becoming one of the most widely used. A disposable sheath is placed over the end of the thermometer, which is then inserted into the ear. In a matter of seconds an electronic reading is obtained (Fig. 15.14).

Pulse

Each time the heart beats, it pumps a certain amount of blood into the arteries. This causes the arteries to expand (get bigger). Between heartbeats, the arteries contract and return to their normal size. The heart pumps the blood in a steady rhythm. The rhythmic expansion and contraction of the arteries, which can be measured to show how fast the heart is beating, is called the **pulse.** Measuring the pulse is a simple method of observing how the circulatory system is functioning.

Normal Pulse Rates (per minute) for Different Age Groups	
Before birth	140–150
At birth	130–140
First year	115–130
Childhood years	80–115
Adult years	72–80
Later years	60–70

At certain places on the body, the pulse can be felt easily under a person's fingers. One of the easiest places to feel the pulse is at the wrist. This is called a **radial pulse**

FIGURE 15.14 The tympanic membrane thermometer.

because the nurse is feeling the radial artery (Fig. 15.15). You may hear the following terms used to describe a pulse:

- **Rate**—the number of pulse beats per minute
- **Rhythm**—the regularity of the pulse beats, that is, whether or not the length of time between the beats is steady and regular
- **Force** of the beat (weak or pounding)

The normal average rate of pulse for adults is 72 beats per minute. The range of normal rates for adults is from 72 to 80 beats per minute. Special notice will be taken of a pulse rate of under 60 or over 100 beats per minute.

MEASURING THE RADIAL PULSE

FIGURE 15.15

Sometimes the doctor will order that pulses be taken in the patient's lower extremities. This is often done when there is concern for the circulation to this area. Common orders include those for taking **popliteal pulses** (pulses in arteries behind the knee) and **pedal pulses** (from the artery on top of the foot) (Fig. 15.16).

MEASURING THE PULSE

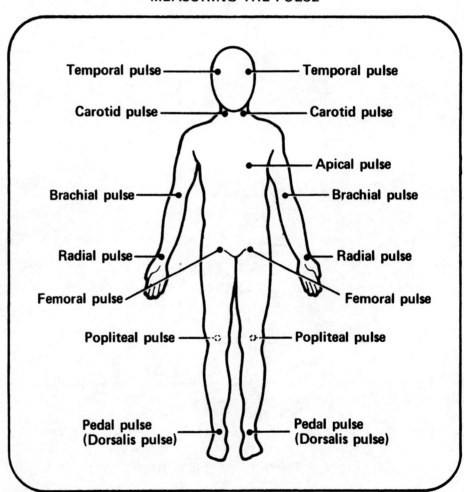

Temporal pulse — Temporal pulse

Carotid pulse — Carotid pulse

Apical pulse

Brachial pulse — Brachial pulse

Radial pulse — Radial pulse

Femoral pulse — Femoral pulse

Popliteal pulse — Popliteal pulse

Pedal pulse (Dorsalis pulse) — Pedal pulse (Dorsalis pulse)

FIGURE 15.16

The pulse rate should be the same as the heart rate. However, in some patients the heartbeats are not strong enough to be transmitted along the arteries. This may be because of some forms of heart disease. For these patients, an **apical pulse** is taken. An apical pulse is a measurement of the heartbeats at the apex of the heart, which is located just under the left breast (Fig. 15.17A).

FIGURE 15.17A

Sometimes the patient has a **pulse deficit.** This means that there is a difference between the apical heartbeat and the radial pulse rate. To determine this difference, the apical pulse (heart rate) is counted with a stethoscope over the apex of the heart. At the same time, the pulse rate is counted at the radial pulse. The two figures are compared. The difference between the apical heartbeat and the radial pulse beat is the pulse deficit (Fig. 15.17B).

MEASURING APICAL PULSE DEFICIT

FIGURE 15.17B

Pulse Oximeter. The pulse oximeter is a device that electronically measures the arterial blood oxygen saturation (SaO_2) and then, through careful calculation, closely estimates the patient's partial oxygen pressure (pO_2). It is attached most commonly to the tip of a finger and sometimes to the earlobe or the bridge of the nose. This test is performed at the patient's bedside by the nurse or respiratory therapist.

Respiration

The human body must have a steady supply of air. The body needs the oxygen in the air in order to change food into heat and energy. When you breathe in, air is drawn into the lungs. In the lungs, oxygen is taken out of the air. The oxygen is used to produce energy for the body.

Respiration is the process of inhaling and exhaling. One respiration includes breathing in once and breathing out once.

Normally, adults breathe at a rate of from 16 to 20 times per minute. Children breathe more rapidly. The elderly breathe more slowly. Exercise, digestion, emotional stress, disease conditions, some drugs, stimulants, heat, and cold all can affect the number of times per minute that a person breathes.

When the nurse counts the patient's respirations, he or she will observe and make note of anything about the breathing that appears to be abnormal. Descriptions of different types of respirations include (Fig. 15.18):

FIGURE 15.18

- **Stertorous respiration**—the patient makes abnormal noises like snoring sounds when breathing
- **Apnea**—absence of respirations
- **Abdominal respiration**—breathing in which the patient is using mostly the abdominal muscles
- **Shallow respiration**—breathing with only the upper part of the lungs
- **Orthopnea**—inability to breathe well when lying flat

- **Irregular respiration**—the depth of breathing changes and the rate of the rise and fall of the chest is not steady
- **Cheyne–Stokes respiration**—one kind of irregular breathing. At first the breathing is slow and shallow; then the respiration becomes faster and deeper until it reaches a peak. The respiration then slows down and becomes shallow again. The breathing may then stop completely for about 10 seconds and begin the pattern again. This type of respiration may be caused by certain cerebral (brain), cardiac (heart), or pulmonary (chest) diseases.
- **Dyspnea**—difficult breathing
- **Hyperpnea**—increase in depth of respirations
- **Tachypnea**—very rapid, shallow respirations. Hyperventilation.

Blood Pressure

Blood pressure is the force of the blood pushing against the walls of the blood vessels. When the nurse takes a patient's blood pressure, he or she is measuring the force of the blood flowing through the arteries.

There is always a certain amount of pressure in the arteries. This is because the heart, by pumping, is constantly forcing blood to circulate. The blood goes first into the arteries and then it circulates through the whole body. The blood pressure depends on

- The rate and strength of the heartbeat;
- How easily the blood flows through the blood vessels;
- The blood volume; and
- The elasticity of the arteries.

The heart contracts as it pumps the blood into the arteries. When the heart is contracting, the pressure is highest. This pressure is called the **systolic pressure.** As the heart relaxes between each contraction the pressure goes down. When the heart is most relaxed, the pressure is lowest. This pressure is called the **diastolic pressure.** When the nurse takes a patient's blood pressure, the nurse is measuring these two pressures—the systolic pressure and the diastolic pressure.

In young, healthy adults, the blood pressure range for systolic pressure is between 100 and 140 millimeters (mm) mercury (Hg). Diastolic pressure is between 60 and 90 millimeters (mm) mercury (Hg). These figures are written as follows:

$$120/80 \text{ or } \frac{120}{80} \begin{array}{l} = \text{Systolic} \\ = \text{Diastolic} \end{array}$$

When a patient's blood pressure is higher than the normal range for his age and condition, it is referred to as high blood pressure or **hypertension.** When a patient's blood pressure is lower than the normal range for her age or condition, it is referred to as low blood pressure or **hypotension.**

Instruments for Measuring Blood Pressure. When the nurse takes a patient's blood pressure, the nurse uses an instrument called a **sphygmomanometer** (Fig. 15.19). Sphygmomanometer is a combination of three Greek words:

- **Sphygmo**—meaning pulse
- **Mano**—meaning pressure
- **Meter**—meaning measure

This instrument, however, is usually called simply the *blood pressure cuff.*

FIGURE 15.19

CIRCULATION CHECK

A circulation check is most commonly ordered for patients with a limb in a cast. An order for **CMS** would require that the nurse check the patient's **circulation, motion, and sensation.** The nurse will check (among other things) warmth, color, and sensation in the patient's fingers or toes. If the nurse feels that the circulation check is abnormal, the nurse will notify the doctor, who may choose to adjust or remove the cast.

CRANIOTOMY CHECK (NEUROLOGICAL CHECK)

A craniotomy check is done to monitor the patient with injury, disease, or surgery of the head and/or brain. Because serious changes in the patient's condition may occur rapidly, the nurse will frequently check the patient's VS, level of consciousness, grip of each hand, orientation, ability to move, and pupils of the eyes reaction to light. Other reactions may also be included in the craniotomy or neuro check. The order **NVS** stands for **neurologic vital signs.** A special supplemental form is often added to the chart for this purpose.

PAIN ASSESSMENT

Patient's pain must be assessed and managed. To accomplish this a pain rating scale is used. Adult patients who are cognitively intact are regularly asked to rate their pain on a scale of 0–10 with 0 being no pain, and 10 being the worst pain. Faces of pain may be used for young children or cognitively impaired adults. The scale should also be translated as necessary into other languages. Once the pain level is determined and documented, pain management is instituted, often in the form of medication. A special form may be added to the chart for documenting pain assessment and management.

𝐼NTAKE AND OUTPUT

Water is essential to human life. Next to oxygen, water is the most important substance the body takes in (Fig. 15.20). A person can be starving—can lose half of his body protein and almost half of his body weight—and can still live, but losing only one-fifth of the body's fluid will result in death.

FIGURE 15.20

Through eating and drinking, the average healthy adult takes in about 3½ quarts of fluid every day. This is the **fluid intake.** The same adult also eliminates about 3½ quarts of fluid every day. This is the **fluid output.** Fluid is discharged from the body of a healthy person in several ways:

- Most of the fluid passes through the kidneys and is discharged as urine.
- Some of the fluid is lost from the body through perspiration.
- Some fluid is evaporated from the lungs in breathing.
- The remaining fluid is absorbed and eliminated through the intestinal system.

It is difficult to measure accurately the amount of fluid discharged through evaporation and breathing; therefore, a person may seem to have a greater fluid intake than output. There is, however, a fluid balance in the normally functioning body. Fluid balance means that just about the same amount of fluid taken in by the body is also eliminated.

An imbalance of fluids in the body occurs when too much fluid is kept in the body or when too much fluid is lost. In some medical conditions, fluid may be held in the body tissues and makes them swell. This is called **edema.** In other conditions, much fluid may be lost by vomiting, bleeding, severe diarrhea, or excessive sweating (Fig. 15.21).

When a patient's body loses more fluid than it is taking in or retains more than it is putting out, a doctor can treat the condition in various ways. A specific method is prescribed to meet the needs of the individual patient. Measuring a patient's intake and output helps the doctor know if the patient's body fluids are in balance. Therefore, it is very important for members of the nursing staff to keep accurate records of fluid intake and output. The record of the patient's intake and output is kept for a full 24-hour period.

The amounts of intake and output are written on a special sheet called the **Intake and Output (I&O) sheet,** kept near the patient's bed (Fig. 15.22). The patient's

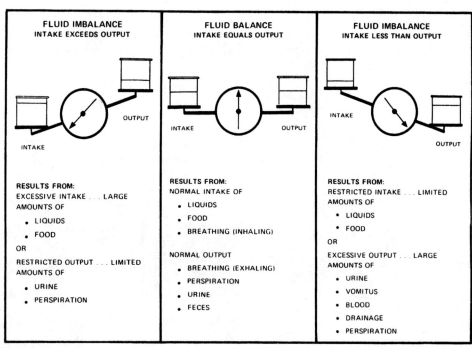

FLUID IMBALANCE
INTAKE EXCEEDS OUTPUT

RESULTS FROM:
EXCESSIVE INTAKE . . . LARGE
AMOUNTS OF
- LIQUIDS
- FOOD
OR
RESTRICTED OUTPUT . . . LIMITED
AMOUNTS OF
- URINE
- PERSPIRATION

FLUID BALANCE
INTAKE EQUALS OUTPUT

RESULTS FROM:
NORMAL INTAKE OF
- LIQUIDS
- FOOD
- BREATHING (INHALING)

NORMAL OUTPUT
- BREATHING (EXHALING)
- PERSPIRATION
- URINE
- FECES

FLUID IMBALANCE
INTAKE LESS THAN OUTPUT

RESULTS FROM:
RESTRICTED INTAKE . . . LIMITED
AMOUNTS OF
- LIQUIDS
- FOOD
OR
EXCESSIVE OUTPUT . . . LARGE
AMOUNTS OF
- URINE
- VOMITUS
- BLOOD
- DRAINAGE
- PERSPIRATION

FIGURE 15.21

INTAKE AND OUTPUT SHEET

Hospital # _____   Patient Name _____

Date _____   Room # _____

	INTAKE			OUTPUT			
				URINE		GASTRIC	
Time 7-3	BY MOUTH	TUBE	PARENTERAL	VOIDED	CATHETER	EMESIS	SUCTION
TOTAL							
Time 3-11							
TOTAL							
Time 11-7							
TOTAL							
24 HOUR TOTAL							
24 Hour Grand Total • Intake				24 Hour Grand Total • Output			

FIGURE 15.22

name, room number, the hospital identification number, and the date are recorded at the top of the page. The intake and output sheet is divided into two parts—intake on the left side and output on the right.

After measuring intake or output, the nurse will record the amount and time in the proper columns. At the end of each eight-hour shift, the amounts in each column are totaled and recorded.

*D*IABETIC TESTING

When a person who is diabetic is hospitalized, he or she is carefully monitored for the amount of glucose in the blood, and insulin is ordered based on the results of the tests. Two methods of testing done by nursing are capillary puncture and urine testing.

Capillary Puncture. This test requires that the nurse prick the patient's finger with a specially designed sterile needle or lancet. A drop of blood is then placed on a chemically treated strip of paper, and the paper is inserted into a device such as an Accu-Chek or Glucometer that electronically reads the blood sugar. The nurse then gives or does not give insulin based on the written orders of the physician (Fig. 15.23A).

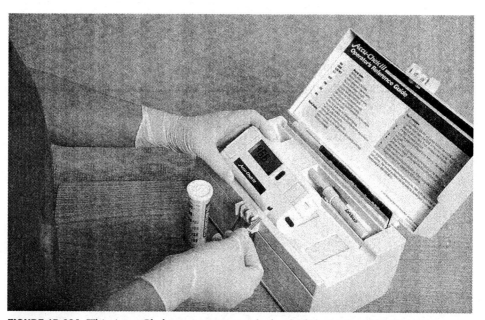

FIGURE 15.23A This Accu-Chek meter measures the level of glucose in a blood sample.

Urine Testing. This test for sugar and acetone (S&A) requires the nurse to place a chemically treated strip of paper into fresh urine and then compare the results with a color chart (Fig. 15.23B). These tests, called *fractionals,* are usually done four times a day, a half-hour before each meal and at bedtime. The capillary puncture previously described is considered a more accurate test.

An older test for sugar in the urine is called the *clinitest.* This test, which is rarely ordered any more, involves dropping tablets into urine, adding water, and observing any color change.

Remember, the foregoing are not considered laboratory tests and are done on the nursing unit, not by laboratory personnel. Other, more sophisticated tests for diabetic monitoring are ordered through the laboratory.

FIGURE 15.23B Test strips may be used to measure the sugar acetone level in a urine sample.

> *Urine Fractionals for Glucose and Ketones*
> *S&A qid ac and hs*
> *C&A qid ac and hs*

INTRAVENOUS ADMINISTRATION ORDERS

Orders for the administration of fluids by vein are extremely common and important forms of patient therapy. **Intravenous** orders are written for the following reasons:

- The patient, because of illness or surgery, is unable to swallow or tolerate fluids by mouth.
- The patient is unconscious.
- The patient is dehydrated (lacking in fluid intake).
- There is a need to replace electrolytes.
- Medications must be given into a vein.
- The patient's condition is such that he or she may require emergency medications by vein.
- The patient requires a blood or blood product transfusion.
- The patient's condition is such (e.g., shock) that the doctor wishes to measure the pressure in the venous system. This is called the **CVP (central venous pressure)** and is a special procedure requiring special equipment and often done in the Intensive Care Unit.
- The patient requires **parenteral nutrition therapy.** Parenteral nutrition support encompasses two modalities: peripheral parenteral nutrition (PPN) and total or central parenteral nutrition (TPN).

Three types of intravenous therapy are peripheral IV therapy, central venous pressure monitoring, and parenteral nutrition.

Peripheral Intravenous Therapy

Peripheral or **standard intravenous therapy** refers to the administration of fluids into a vein in the arm, leg, or, in babies, into a vein in the head. It is the most common type of IV order. The IV is typically started by the nurse using a needle or short indwelling IV catheter and then attached to IV tubing and the bag of fluid to be administered. The physician orders the type of fluid and the amount of fluid to be administered over a 24-hour period. The orders continue until they are changed or canceled (Fig. 15.24).

- IV Bag

- Drip Chamber

- IV Tube

- Clamp

FIGURE 15.24 Intravenous (IV) infusion.

Central Venous Pressure

To start central venous pressure monitoring, an IV catheter is inserted by the physician into a vein and then into the superior vena cava or right atrium of the heart. The catheter is connected to IV tubing that is attached to a manometer and a three-way stopcock. The CVP readings, usually taken with the patient lying flat, measure the pressure in the venous system and the efficiency of the right ventricle of the heart. Too low a reading may mean hypovolemia (not enough blood volume); too high a reading hypervolemia (too much fluid) or right ventricular failure. The changes indicate the blood volume, the need for more or less fluid replacement, and the effect of certain cardiac drugs on the heart.

When measurements are not being taken, the IV runs at a KVO (keep vein open) rate.

Parenteral Nutrition

Peripheral parenteral nutrition (PPN) is administered intravenously to provide nutrients. PPN is used often in conjunction with oral feedings or in the absence of gastrointestinal function for a shorter period of time. This therapy is limited in the amount of dextrose and amino acid concentration in the solution that can be administered, because the infusate may damage the blood vessel.

Total parenteral nutrition (TPN), on the other hand, is usually administered through the central vein via a catheter. The dextrose and amino acid solution concentrates can be higher, because the larger vein can dilute the infusate rapidly. Thus, greater amounts of nutrients can be given to meet the nutritional needs of the patient. Candidates for TPN are those patients who have a nonfunctioning intestine and require support for longer periods of time. Lipids are an important nutrient for preventing fatty acid deficiencies and can be given intravenously in TPN as fat emulsions that are calorie dense; they are a very useful energy source when volume is restricted. The amounts and types of additives may change frequently and are prepared by the pharmacist, based on the physician's orders. The dietitian works in conjunction with the pharmacist and other team members to assure that the nutritional needs of the patient are met.

Patients on TPN or hyperalimentation therapy generally have a surgically placed indwelling central venous catheter. An infusion-control device delivers the TPN at a controlled prescribed rate. The solutions are kept refrigerated until used.

Patients receiving TPN are monitored carefully and have their temperatures and fractional urines measured every six hours, as glucose imbalances and sepsis (infection) are potential risks (Fig. 15.25).

Note: If special procedures such as CVP or TPN are ordered, the health unit coordinator must check with the nurse to determine which special equipment will be needed.

IV Infusions of Analgesic via Syringe Pump with PCA Device

Patient-controlled administration (PCA) of an analgesic allows the patient to administer his or her own pain medication within limits prescribed by the physician. The infusion pump is obtained from central supply and the orders are written by the doctor and instituted and monitored by the nurse (Fig. 15.26).

IVs are started by doctors or registered nurses. The supplies required for this procedure include the bag of prescribed IV fluid (from the pharmacy), the tubing that is connected to the bag (IV tubing), and the needle or catheter that is inserted into the patient's vein (Fig. 15.27).

Types of Intravenous Fluid

There are many types of intravenous fluids supplied by the pharmacy. The doctor will specify the type to be administered. Some common orders include the following:

5% Dextrose in water—D5/W or D5W

5% Dextrose in 0.45% sodium chloride—D5/0.45NaCl or D5/½NS

5% Dextrose in Ringer's—(Ringer's has higher concentrations of Na and Cl than lactated Ringer's solution)

5% Dextrose in lactated Ringer's—D5/LR or D5LR (lactated Ringer's contains Na, K, Ca, Cl, and lactate)

Lactated Ringer's—LR or RL

TOTAL PARENTERAL NUTRITION "HYPERALIMENTATION"

1. ☑ PHYSICIAN TO PLACE CATHETER IN CENTRAL VEIN
1A. ☐ PERIPHERAL INFUSION   (CHECK ONE)

2. CHEST X–RAY FOR POSITION OF CATHETER. (CENTRAL LINE)

3. KEEP I.V. OPEN WITH D5W UNTIL INSTRUCTED TO BEGIN TPN INFUSION.

4. NOTE: STANDARD TPN SOLUTION CONTAINS; 8.5% FREAMINE 500 ml, 50% DEXTROSE 500 ml,
              (CENTRAL LINE)   5 mEq SODIUM, 10 mEq PHOSPHATE 36 mEq
                                              ACETATE AND 875 NON–PROTEIN CALORIES
                                              PER LITER.

5. SPECIAL ORDERS AS FOLLOWS:

BASE SOLUTION:
    DEXTROSE ___50___ %   _500__ ml
    AMINO ACIDS   8.5%   _500__ ml
ADD:
    NaCl   _50__ mEq
    KCl   _25__ mEq
    K PHOSPHATE   _10__ mEq
    Ca GLUCONATE   _4.6_ mEq
    MgSO₄   _8-1_ mEq
    MVI - 12   (1 amp. daily)
    TRACE ELEMENTS   (once daily)

STANDARD ADDITIVES

50 mEq NaCl
25 mEq KCl
4.6 mEq Ca Gluconate
10 mEq K acid phosphate
8.1 mEq MgSO₄

6. WEIGH PATIENT ___Daily_____

7. INTAKE AND OUTPUT   q̄ 8h.

8. TEST SUGAR/ACETONE OF URINE Q6H. CALL M.D. IF 3+ – 4+

9. TEMPERATURE Q6H. CALL M.D. FOR NEW FEVER OVER __101°__

10. SMA-14, EVERY MONDAY, WEDNESDAY AND FRIDAY.

11. CBC, Mg EVERY MONDAY.

12. START TPN WHEN INSTRUCTED AT INITIAL RATE OF __100__ ml/hr WITH INFUSION PUMP
    TPN SOLUTION SHOULD BE GIVEN AT A CONSTANT RATE THROUGHOUT 24-HOUR PERIOD.

13. CONSIDER ADDING IV LIPIDS PERIODICALLY IF PATIENT IS TO BE ON HYPERALIMENTATION
    FOR MORE THAN 2 WEEKS.

    10% 500 ml Q _____   INFUSE OVER _____ HOURS (550 KCAL/500ml)
    (20% 500 ml) Q 2 d.   INFUSE OVER __10__ HOURS (1000KCAL/500ml)

FOR FURTHER INFORMATION – CALL PHARMACY

Nurses Signature	DATE	TIME	TRANSCRIBER	PHYSICIA

TOTAL PARENTERAL NUTRITION
"HYPERALIMENTATION"

FIGURE 15.25

Normal saline (0.9% sodium chloride)—NS or NSS

½ Normal saline—0.45 NS or ½ NS

10% Dextrose in water—D10/W or D10W

Procalimine—provides extra nutrients

These various types of sterile fluids are supplied, as previously stated, in bottles or plastic bags and come in several quantities. Most commonly the doctor will order 1000 cc or 500 cc. Smaller quantities may be ordered in 250-cc, 100-cc, or 50-cc containers. These smaller amounts are most often ordered for children or infants.

I. Mainline IV Solution - Type
      Rate *per surgeon*

II. Select Mode
   1. PCA
   2. PCA/BASAL
   3. CONTINUOUS

Mode 1. Patient may self administer with PCA control device according to the following order:

   1. Check One
      Medication: _X_ Morphine Sulphate (1 mg/ml conc)
                  ____ Meperidine (10 mg/ml conc)
   2. PCA Dose: the amount administered each time patient activates the infusor _1.5_ mg (_1.5_ ml).
   3. DELAY the minute time interval between doses _12_ minute delay
   4. Dose Limit - maximum volume that will be delivered in 1 hr _9.5_ mg (_9.5_ ml).
      * Include PCA and Basal in Dose Limit Total.
   5. Bolus Dose: Initial amount of medication given at beginning of PCA treatment. *PRN, titrate to effect* _2.0_ mg (_2.0_ ml) *MRP X 6, to max 14mg.*
   6. If pain relief from PCA is inadequate notify MD
   7. If respiration rate below _8_ per minute and / or sedation level @ 5, give NARCAN ~~0.4~~ MGM IV _X_ IM ____ SQ ____ May repeat x 1 notify MD Stat. *0.2*

Mode 2. Patient may self administer with PCA control device according to Mode 1 orders plus a continuous IV infusion of: _2.0_ mg/hr (_2.0_ ml/hr)

Mode 3. Continuous IV infusion of:

   1. MS ____.____ mgm (1 mgm/ml conc)
     @ ____.____ ml/hr
     Meperidine ____.____ mgm (10 mgm/ml conc)
     @ ____.____ ml/hr
   2. If pain relief inadequate, notify MD.
   3. If respiration rate below ____ per minute and/or sedation level @ 5, given NARCAN 0.4 MGM IV ____ IM ____ SQ ____ May repeat x1. Notify MD Stat.

III. Automatic 48 hour stop — unless re-ordered by the physician
IV. Additional orders. *Compazine 10mg IM Q6° prn N&V*

Physicians Signature	Date	Time	Transcriber	Nurses Signature
			ADDRESSOGRAPH	

ORDERS FOR IV INFUSION OF
ANALGESIC VIA SYRINGE PUMP WITH PCA DEVICE

FIGURE 15.26

PHARMACY CHARGE SLIP

✓	DESCRIPTION	✓	DESCRIPTION	✓	DESCRIPTION	✓	DESCRIPTION
	ACCUSET		ANS SAFTISET		HEPARIN LOCK		
	ABBO CATH 22		BUTTERFLY		INTERCATH		SAFTI-TANDEM
	ABBO CATH 16		CATHETER PLUG		IV LOOP		SEC. ADD SET
	ABBO CATH 18		CHEX SET Y		PRIMARY ADD SET		SUBCLAVIAN
	ABBO CATH 20		EXTENSION SET		SAFTIFILTER		VOLUTROLE

DOSE	DRUGS DESCRIPTION	QTY	DO NOT USE	DESCRIPTION (TYPE & SIZE)	QTY	DESCRIPTION
						PLASMANATE 250cc
						PLASMANATE 500cc
						SALT POOR ALBUMIN 50cc
						SALT POOR ALBUMIN 100cc

DO NOT WRITE BELOW THIS LINE	PRICE OVERRIDE	MISC.	CODE 417	DO NOT WRITE BELOW THIS LINE	PRICE OVERRIDE
DRUGS TO DATE			417		
DRUGS CLOSING			417		

DEPARTMENT COPY

FIGURE 15.27

Types of IV Tubing

The tubing required for IV administration is usually ordered from the pharmacy. The tubing is a prepackaged, sterile, disposable item. One end is inserted into the container of the IV fluid and the other into the needle, which is inserted into the patient's vein.

Common types of IV tubing are the following:

■ **Straight tube**—tube without special modification that leads from bag or bottle to needle (Fig. 15.28).

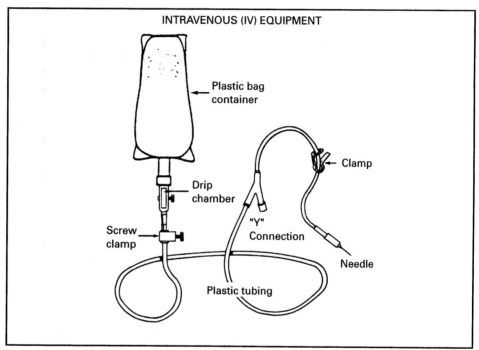

INTRAVENOUS (IV) EQUIPMENT

FIGURE 15.28

■ **Tube with minibag or volume control chamber**—modified straight IV tubing with addition of a small bag of its own. This is located several inches below the point of insertion into the IV fluid bag or bottle and can be filled and then shut off by a clamp from the main IV bag. The purpose of a minibag type of IV tubing is:
 1. To allow the nurse to carefully limit the amount of fluid a patient may receive at one time. Most minibags hold 100 cc. The nurse can fill the minibag from the 1000-cc bag with 100 cc, clamp the minibag off above the minibag, and then be assured that the patient will receive only 100 cc of fluid at a time. This is especially important when administering fluids to small children or to adults with conditions that may be seriously jeopardized by receiving too much fluid at one time.
 2. To provide a receptacle (container) for the administration of IV medications. Very often the doctor wishes the patient to receive medication into the vein. The minibag type of IV tubing is a safe and convenient method of administering many types of IV medication. The nurse allows some IV fluid to run into the minibag, clamps the bag off, and then injects the prescribed medication into the fluid in the minibag through a special portal, which slowly drips into the patient's vein and circulation. When the minibag with the medication is nearly empty, the nurse will open the clamp and

allow the IV fluid to flow again as prescribed by the physician. There are a number of secondary sets that can be attached to the primary IV tubing to allow for blood withdrawals, or intermittent injections.

- **Y tubing for blood administration**—a special type of IV tubing. One point of the Y tube is inserted into a bag of IV fluid (usually normal saline solution [NSS] or a variation of a saline solution), and the other point of the Y is inserted into the bag containing blood. Another important feature of blood tubing is that there is a special part that serves as a filter for the blood that will be transfused into the patient's vein.

The nurse or doctor always starts the blood transfusion by clamping off the part of the Y tube that leads to the bag of blood and opening the clamp that allows the other IV solution to run in first. When the IV is established, the clamp to the NSS is closed and the clamp on the Y tubing to the blood is opened to allow the blood transfusion to occur.

Types of Needles and Intravenous Catheters

IV therapy requires a container (most commonly sterile bag) of IV fluid, the proper tubing, and a means of piercing the skin and entering the vein. The latter requires the use of some type of needle. The most common types of needles include:

- **IV catheters**—sterile, prepackaged, disposable items from the pharmacy. IV catheters have a needle attached to a very narrow tube. The nurse or doctor inserts the needle into the vein and then threads the IV catheter through the hole of the needle. The plastic tube remains in the vein; the needle does not. The IV tubing leading from the IV bottle is attached to the IV catheter.
- **Butterfly or scalp vein needle**—a short, tiny needle with flaps resembling wings for taping to the skin that comes in various sizes. The higher the number, the thinner the needle. Common sizes are #18, 20, 21, and 22 G (or gauge). A #18 needle is the thickest, #22 the thinnest. The length of the needle is usually ½ to 1 inches.
- **Indwelling central venous catheters**—these are more common than cutdowns (a small incision the doctor makes into the vein to insert an IV catheter) and do away with the need for repeated venipunctures.
  - **Peripheral inserted central catheter**—PICC or PIC is inserted by the physician or specially trained nurse into the arm and to the superior vena cava.
  - **Subclavian** line or percutaneous central venous catheter is inserted by the physician through the skin and into the subclavian vein and superior vena cava. PICCS and subclavian lines require a signed consent and an x-ray to confirm proper placement.

Rate of Flow

In order to ensure that the patient will receive the proper amount of IV fluid, the doctor will order the rate of flow of the solution.

If a pump is not used, the nurse controls the rate by adjusting the clamp on the IV tubing to regulate the flow of drops from the drip chamber. A tape is often placed vertically on the IV bag with calibrations that tell the nurse where the fluid level should be each hour. The nurse checks the IVs frequently and adds bags as necessary so that the patient will receive the fluids as ordered.

Often the patient's condition is such that exact fluid intake must be constant, or if certain medications must be infused (put into the vein) at an exact rate, an infusion-control device such as an **IVAC** is obtained from central supply (Figure 15.29).

The physician orders the rate of flow, the solution, and the medication to be infused. The nurse sets the machine so that a consistent and accurate amount is administered to the patient.

Remember, IVs are supplied most commonly in 1000-cc or 500-cc quantities. If the doctor wishes the patient to receive one liter, or 1000 cc of fluid in a specified number of hours, he or she will write 1000 cc or 1 L, the name of the solution, and the rate of flow (number of drops per minute or number of hours over which the IV is to be given).

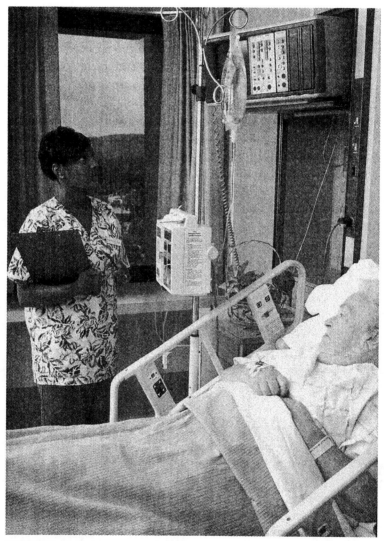

FIGURE 15.29 Infusion control device.

- To convert drops to minutes:
    Order: 1000 cc D51 /2S @ 100 cc/hr
        1 cc = 15 drops
        100 × 15 = 1500 drops/hr (60 min)
        1500 ÷ 60 = 25 drops/min

■ To convert number of hours to cc per hour:
   Order: 1000 cc 5% DW over next 8 hours
       1000 ÷ 8 = 125 cc/hr

Examples of doctor's orders:

> *1000 cc 5% DW over next 8 hrs*
> *1000 cc D5W @ 100 cc per hr*
> *1L 5% D/RL @ 50 gtts/min*
> *500 cc 0.45 NS over next 6 hrs*

The doctor may order several different IVs over a 24-hour period:

> *#1) 1000 D5W*
> *#2) 1000 cc D5/NS*
> *#3) 1000 cc D5/R*

Here each liter would run 8 hours, or 3 liters (1000 cc ea) per 24 hours. If the IV is only to keep the vein open, the order will read:

> *IV D5W TKO or KVO*

The nurse will set the drip at a very slow rate to accomplish this.

Sometimes the doctor wishes more than one IV to run at the same time. The common term for this is **piggyback.** One IV will be started and a second will be hung and run through the tubing of the first. This is usually done when special medications are contained in the piggybacked IV. It is not unusual for several IVs to be piggybacked.

IV Medications

Medications are discussed in Chapter 14. However, to understand IV orders, the health unit coordinator must know that when medications are to be added to the bottle of IV fluid, that order must be a part of the original IV order. The following example shows such an IV order:

> *1000 cc 5% DW c̄ 40 mEq KCl (potassium chloride)*
> *1000 cc 5% D½S. Add 1 amp MVI-12.*

When medications are to be added to the IV bag itself, this will be done by the nurse or, more commonly, in the pharmacy (IV Admixture). The admixture is then sent to the nursing unit for administration. This is not considered the same as an IV medication order, which was discussed in Chapter 14.

Heparin Lock

When the patient no longer needs intravenous fluids but there still needs to be access to a vein to administer IV medication, a heparin lock or VAD is established. In this way medications can be given intermittently without the need for the patient to be attached to IV tubing and solution. Heparin locks were also discussed in Chapter 14 (Fig. 15.30).

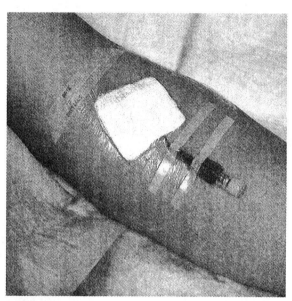

FIGURE 15.30

IV Team

Because of the importance of IV therapy, many hospitals have special teams of nurses whose main responsibility is starting, maintaining, and discontinuing IVs throughout the hospital.

As you can see, orders for intravenous therapy are complex. You must understand IV orders and be careful to transcribe these orders exactly as written by the physician. As always, when you have any question about an order, you must ask a nurse.

ACTIVITY ORDERS

The nursing staff must always know how much or how little activity doctors want their patients to have. A seriously ill patient may be confined to bed. A convalescent patient may be allowed out of bed at will, without restrictions. Some of the common phrases associated with patient activity and their abbreviations follow:

Order	Meaning
Out of bed (OOB)	No restriction
Ambulate ad lib. (Amb)	No restriction
Complete bed rest (CBR)	The patient is to remain in bed at all times
May use bedside commode (BSC)	May use a portable commode or toilet at bedside
Stand to void	Male on bedrest may stand at bedside to urinate

Order	**Meaning**
Bathroom privileges (BRP)	May go to bathroom only
May shower or take a bath	A doctor's order is necessary for this activity
Progressive ambulation (prog. amb.)	Ambulation allowed in following progressive stages:

- Dangle—sit on bed with feet dangling over side
- Stand—may stand at bedside
- Walk c̄ help
- Walk alone

Orders allowing increased activity may also specify the length of time and/or number of times per day this activity will occur:

> *Up in hall c̄ help 5 min bid*
> *May sit in chair 15 min tid*

Certain devices to aid ambulation may also be ordered, such as wheelchairs, walkers, and crutches (Fig. 15.31).

FIGURE 15.31 Walker.

POSITIONING ORDERS

If the doctor, for medical reasons, requires that a patient's body or body part be placed in a special position, orders will be written to indicate this. The patient's head may be elevated to facilitate breathing or as a position of choice following a head injury or certain diagnostic procedures, or kept flat because of other conditions or procedures. The patient may be turned to a specified side, or a limb may require elevation. Certain positions may be utilized for examinations or for comfort. Patients may require certain types of special beds to facilitate turning. There are endless reasons for orders that require special patient positions. Some examples follow:

- Elevate head of bed (↑ head of bed) and may include height (e.g., 20°–30° c̄ 2 pillows etc.)
- Fowler's position (patient is placed in a semisitting position and the patient's knees are slightly bent)
- Elevate rt. foot on 2 pillows (↑ rt. ft. on 2 pillows)
- Keep flat for 2 hrs—the patient is not allowed to raise head for specified time
- Turn, cough, and deep breathe (TCDB)—the patient is to do this activity under the supervision of the nurse; the frequency will often be ordered also, such as TCDB q 2° (Fig. 15.32).

Stryker Frame

A Stryker frame is a special device that is often used for patients with burns or injuries to the neck to facilitate turning and maintain body alignment when patients cannot be lifted or moved. It is used in place of the usual hospital bed.

A circle bed may be ordered for the same purpose (Figs. 15.33 and 15.34).

Traction

Traction is the exertion of pull by means of weights and pulleys. Traction is used to promote and maintain alignment of broken (fractured) bones and for other orthopedic conditions. It may be applied to the skin externally or to the bone internally through surgery. Traction is maintained by the use of a special frame on the bed. Buck's traction is frequently used for a fractured leg (Fig. 15.35). Common types of skin traction include Russell's and cervical traction.

COMFORT AND SAFETY ORDERS

Many devices are used to increase the patient's comfort or safety during hospitalization. Most of these require a doctor's order. Table 15.2 gives examples of some of those most commonly used.

REVERSE TRENDELENBURG

Head up

Feet down

FOWLER'S POSITION

45°

KNEE-CHEST POSITION

HORIZONTAL RECUMBENT POSITION (SUPINE POSITION)

DORSAL RECUMBENT POSITION

PRONE POSITION

TRENDELENBURG POSITION

Feet up

Head down

LEFT SIMS' POSITION

DORSAL LITHOTOMY POSITION

FIGURE 15.32

STRYKER FRAME

FIGURE 15.33

**CIRCULAR DOUBLE
FRAME ELECTRIC BED**
FIGURE 15.34

FIGURE 15.35 Buck's traction.

TABLE 15.2 *C*OMFORT AND *S*AFETY *D*EVICES

Device	Description
Air or rubber rings	Devices that look like small inner tubes, used to relieve pressure over the lower back or buttocks, to prevent or treat decubiti (bedsores).
Alternating-pressure (A-P) mattress	A device like an air mattress placed beneath the bedridden or elderly patient to prevent pressure on the shoulders, back, heels, and elbows.
Bed board	A large board placed beneath the mattress to provide additional support for patients with back or bone involvement.
Bed cradle	A device placed over the patient's body in bed to raise the bedclothes away to prevent pressure on sore or chafed areas.
Egg crate mattress	All-foam mattress that looks like the underside of an egg carton. To help prevent pressure sores.
Elastic bandages	Long strips of elasticized cotton, used for the same purposes as elastic stockings.
Elastic stockings	Elasticized stockings that extend from toes to knees to improve circulation or to provide support after strain or sprain at the ankle joint; also called TED or antiembolism hose.
Foot board	A small board placed perpendicular to the bed springs at the foot of the bed; used to keep the feet in proper alignment.
Sheepskins or lamb's wool	Wide strips of lamb's wool or soft synthetic materials used for the same purpose as air or rubber rings.
Restraints	Devices, generally made of cotton, that restrain a patient's arms, legs, or body to prevent self-injury.
Roto-Rest bed	Used to eliminate pressure points and prevent bedsores (Fig. 15.36).
Pneumatic hose or boots	Placed on patient's feet/legs to compress vessels by way of intermittent air pressure delivered by a device attached to boots.
Portable patient lift	A mechanical device used to move the patient from bed to chair and back again; used when the patient needs full assistance.
Sandbags	Reusable bags of sand made in various sizes to maintain a body part in a certain position.
Stretcher	A narrow table on wheels used to transport patients; also called a litter or gurney.
Slings	A disposable bandage used to support an arm (Fig. 15.37).
Walker	An aluminum frame used by the patient to help the patient ambulate.
Wheelchair	A specially designed chair with wheels used to transport patients (Fig. 15.38).

ROTO-REST BED

FIGURE 15.36

FIGURE 15.37 Sling.

EQUIPMENT

FIGURE 15.38

𝓜ISCELLANEOUS ORDERS, PERMISSIONS, RESTRICTIONS

Sometimes the doctor believes it necessary to place specific restrictions on the patient or to reinforce hospital regulations by written order (Fig. 15.39). These permissions and restrictions are all written on the doctor's order sheet and, with a few exceptions, must be transcribed only to the Kardex. Your instructor will tell you which section of the Kardex used in your hospital best suits the recording of orders like the following:

Limit visitors to one at a time.

Nurse may cut patient's fingernails.

May take shower.

Allow visitors at any time during day.

Patient may be discharged alone. Must go home by taxi.

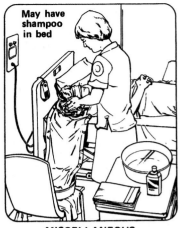

**MISCELLANEOUS
PERMISSION ORDER
FIGURE 15.39**

CONSULTATIONS

Consultations are ordered when a doctor wishes to obtain another physician's opinion about a case. A doctor's order is needed to initiate a consultation and the consultant's opinion and services must be documented in the chart.

The routine for arranging consultations may require these immediate steps:

- Filling out a requisition
- Telephoning the office of the consultant whose services are requested

Additional duties concerned with the transcription of orders for consultations are:

- Transcribing the order to the patient care record card
- Making an appointment if the consultation is to be with a department rather than with an individual physician

Typical orders for consultation follow.

> *G-U consultation — Dr. Biers.*
> *Physical therapy consultation.*
> *Contact Social Service.*
> *Consultation c̄ Dr. Ainsley on heart murmur and EKG abnormalities.*

CRITICAL CONDITION LIST

Patients, by hospital policy, are classified according to clinical status. When a patient's condition meets the criteria for being serious enough to be termed *critical* the patient is placed on the critical list for information purposes. A written order from the doctor is usually required to place a patient on the critical condition list or remove a patient from it. The orders are written and are generally transcribed only to the Kardex. The nursing office, information desk or switchboard, and the patient's family are notified of this change.

> *Place on Critical Condition List.*
>
> *Discontinue Critical Condition List.*

*I*SOLATION TECHNIQUE

The isolation of one patient from the others may also be referred to as *precautions*. The type of precaution varies with the patient's disease and the reasons for the isolation. Isolation is discussed in Chapter 6—Diseases and Diagnoses.

*T*RANSCRIPTION PROCEDURE FOR NURSING PROCEDURE ORDERS

*S*TANDING ORDERS

Step 1—Recognize

As is evident in all the preceding examples, the form of a treatment order is not as standardized as that of a medication order. Three factors will help you recognize a treatment order:

1. The order will always mention the treatment itself.

2. Usually, some sort of time schedule or limitation will be included.

3. Often, there will be fairly specific directions on how to carry out the order.

Step 2—Rip

Rip is always the second step if NCR copies are used.

Step 3—Prioritize

Step 4—Kardex

- **Kardex.** All standing orders for treatments must be transcribed exactly as written to the treatment section of the patient care record card.
- When done by computer, all orders will be printed on a computer-generated Kardex.
- **Treatment tickets.** Some hospitals provide treatment tickets similar to medicine tickets. They are not ordinarily used for all standing-order treatments but only for those to be repeated at specific intervals during the day. Compare the two orders shown in Fig. 15.40.

The first order is a continuous one; the nurse caring for the patient is responsible for changing the soak whenever necessary. The second order is to be carried out

> *Hot soaks to right elbow continuously.*
> *Irrigate Foley catheter c̄ 10 cc saline qid.*

PATIENT'S NAME
Jones, Mary

ROOM
432²

TIME
9-5-1-9

TREATMENT
Irrigate Foley

Catheter c̄
10cc. Saline
q.i.d.

FIGURE 15.40

only at specified intervals throughout the day. The time schedule on a treatment ticket serves as a reminder to the nurse that this task must be performed.

Step 5—Requisition

For many treatments, specialized equipment must be requisitioned. You should already be familiar with frequently used patient-care equipment. By now you should know where different types of equipment are stocked in your hospital. If a treatment order requires equipment *not* available on the nursing unit, a requisition form may be necessary. A sample request-charge slip for equipment is shown in Fig. 15.41. Items are increasingly requisitioned by computer.

CENTRAL SUPPLY DEPARTMENT		IMPRINT SPACE	
REQUEST-CHARGE SLIP			
Description of Service			
Requested by:	Chg. by:		$

FIGURE 15.41

- **Special records and forms.** Treatment orders may need to be transcribed to certain other chart records or special forms. For example, a patient with diabetes being tested for blood and urine glucose throughout the day requires the addition of a diabetic summary sheet to his chart.

 Also, many nursing units compile daily lists of patients for whom blood pressures or temperatures have been ordered on a special basis. In such cases, a new order might require that the patient's name be transcribed to these records.

Step 6—Symbols

Utilize the symbols used in your hospital.

Step 7—Nurse Checks

A nurse must check the treatment orders after you have completed the transcription process. Use the same methods that were described or decided on for checking medication orders.

STAT AND SINGLE-TIME ORDERS

A stat treatment order is a fairly rare occurrence. When encountered, it must be carried out without delay as in the case of stat medication orders.

 A few treatments—e.g., enemas—are ordered on a single-time basis. These are transcribed differently than standing orders. One-time orders frequently require high priority. Bring them to the nurse's attention right away. Your instructor will describe the procedure to be used for transcribing single-time orders.

ORDER VARIATIONS

The preceding orders are concerned solely with starting a treatment. Like medication orders, orders for treatments can also be canceled or altered according to the patient's needs and the doctor's wishes.

CANCELED TREATMENT ORDERS

Canceled treatment orders usually read in the straightforward way shown in the following example:

> *Discontinue nasal oxygen or 5/min prn.*
> *Discontinue hot soaks continuously elbow.*
> *Remove NG tube in AM.*
> *Discontinue qid temperature.*

Qualified Canceled Treatment Orders

However, sometimes a canceled order will include additional instructions, requiring notification and transcription, as described next:

> DC IV—Call Dr. Smith if unable to tolerate oral fluids.
> Remove Foley catheter in AM; replace if pt has not voided within 8 hrs.

CHANGED TREATMENT ORDERS

Sometimes the doctor will change the original treatment order. Changed treatment orders ordinarily can be considered and handled as new orders, since the original (or old) order has in effect been canceled. The following orders show changed treatment orders.

> Continue dressing change on leg qd, but omit wash and powder.
> Apply DSD (dry sterile dressing).
> Clamp Foley 1 hr on, 1 hr off × 24 hrs. Then clamp continuously, emptying at q4h intervals × 24 hrs, then remove.

CANCELED TREATMENT ORDER TRANSCRIPTION

Most of your duties in connection with canceled treatment orders are simply the reverse of the steps taken when the order was started.

- Reusable equipment must be removed from the patient, cleaned, and returned to the proper department.
- The order must be erased from the Kardex, shown as canceled in the computer, and all indications of it removed from special records.
- If tickets have been made out, they must be discarded.

The changing of an order may require that certain equipment be returned or other equipment be ordered. The order should be changed in the computer, on the Kardex, on the ticket (if any), and on all other pertinent record forms.

LEARNING ACTIVITIES

Complete the following.

1. A treatment can be defined as _____.

2. Define the following.
   (a) Gravity suction (or drainage)_____
   (b) Catheter _____
   (c) Patent _____
   (d) Throat suction _____
   (e) Gastric suction _____
   (f) Tracheostomy _____

    (g)   Nasogastric tube _____

    (h)   Lavage _____

    (i)   Gastrostomy tube _____

    (j)   Chest suction _____

    (k)   Hemovac suction _____

3. Give the meaning of the following terms and abbreviations relating to bowel care orders.

    (a)   TWE _____

    (b)   SSE _____

    (c)   NSE _____

    (d)   Harris flush _____

    (e)   Colostomy _____

    (f)   Stoma _____

4. List two purposes for the application of heat to an area of the body.

    (a)   _____

    (b)   _____

5. List two purposes for the application of cold.

    (a)   _____

    (b)   _____

6. A generalized application is applied to the patient's _____

_____.

7. A localized application is applied to _____.

8. Define the following.

    (a)   Sitz bath _____

    (b)   K-pad _____

    (c)   Thermal blanket _____

    (d)   Hypothermia _____

    (e)   Hyperthermia _____

9. List three purposes of urinary catheterization.

    (a)   _____

    (b)   _____

    (c)   _____

10. The insertion and removal of a urinary catheter is called a nonretention or _____ catheterization.

11. Urinary catheters vary in size and are designated by number. The _____ _____the number, the larger the catheter.

12. Urinary catheters sized 14, 16, and 18 Fr are available on the unit. Which is the smallest (in diameter)? _____

13. Retention catheters are also called _____

or _____ catheters.

14. Give the common abbreviation for each of the following vital signs.

    (a)   Temperature _____

    (b)   Pulse _____

    (c)   Respiration _____

    (d)   Blood Pressure _____

15. The temperature measures _____, and the average normal adult temperature is _____.

16. The pulse measures _____, and the average normal adult rate is _____.

17. The respiration measures _____, and the average normal adult rate is _____.

18. The blood pressure measures _____ and in young healthy adults is between _____ and millimeters of mercury systolic pressure and _____ to _____ mm Hg diastolic pressure.

19. The patient's BP is 134/82. Is the top reading the systolic or diastolic pressure? _____

20. Define the following.
    (a) Radial pulse _____
    (b) Apical pulse _____
    (c) Hypertension _____
    (d) Hypotension _____
    (e) Sphygmomanometer _____
    (f) Dyspnea _____
    (g) Apnea _____

21. Define the following.
    (a) Circulation check _____
    (b) Craniotomy check _____
    (c) Intake and output _____
    (d) Consultation _____
    (e) Traction _____

22. List two devices used by nursing to measure the glucose in the blood.
    (a) _____
    (b) _____

23. The doctor will often write an order for the medication _____ based on the results of the tests referred to in question 22.

24. Define the following abbreviations.
    (a) CVP _____
    (b) TPN _____
    (c) D5W _____
    (d) D5½NS _____
    (e) D5 0.45 NaCl _____
    (f) D5/R _____
    (g) D5 0.45 NS _____
    (h) D10W _____
    (i) TKO _____

25. Explain the following IV orders.
    (a) 1000 cc D5½S @ 100 cc per hour _____
    (b) 1L D5W at 60 gtts/min. _____
    (c) 1000 cc 5% DW c̄ 20 mEq KCl TKO _____
    (d) 1000 cc D5W @ 40 gtts/min. Add 1 amp MV/12
        _____

True or False. Circle T if the statement is true and F if it is false.

    (a)   T   F   All IV tubing is the same.

    (b)   T   F   IV catheters are sterile tubes inserted into the vein for IV fluid administration.

    (c)   T   F   When an IV order includes the statement "with" or "add," and a medication and dosage, it means this medication is to be added to the IV bottle or bag.

    (d)   T   F   The term *piggyback* means a second IV is running in conjunction with the existing IV.

    (e)   T   F   A PCA device allows patients to administer an analgesic to themselves by IV.

Match the item in column A with its description in column B.

Column A

(a)   Slings

(b)   Bed board

(c)   Egg crate mattress

(d)   Elastic bandages

(e)   Sheepskins or lamb's wool

(f)   Sandbags

(g)   Air or rubber rings

(h)   Bed cradle

(i)   Elastic stocking

Column B

_____ Foam mattress that looks like the underside of an egg carton

_____ Wide strips of soft synthetic material used for the same purpose as air or rubber rings

_____ Reusable and made in various sizes to maintain a body part in a certain position

_____ Devices that look like small inner tubes, used to relieve pressure over the lower back or buttocks, to prevent or treat decubiti (bedsores)

_____ A device placed over the patient's body in bed to raise the bedclothes to prevent pressure on sore or chafed areas

_____ Elasticized stockings that extend from toes to knees to improve circulation or provide support after strain or sprain at the ankle joint; also called TED hose

_____ A disposable bandage used to support an arm

_____ A large board placed beneath the mattress to provide additional support for patients with back or bone involvement

_____ Long strips of elasticized cotton, used for the same purpose as elastic stockings

CHAPTER 16

Diagnostic and Therapeutic Department Orders

VOCABULARY

Cerebrospinal fluid (CSF)	Fluid that protects the brain and spinal cord
Chemistry	Division of laboratory that analyzes a specimen for its chemical components
Critical values	Test results so far outside normal range that they pose a serious risk to the patient
Culture	To grow microorganisms or living tissue cells in a culture medium that encourages their growth
Cytology	Division of laboratory that studies cells
Diagnostic order	Order for tests to determine the cause of a disease or monitor its progress
Endoscopy	Examination of the body organs or cavities by the use of an instrument called an endoscope
Hematology	The division of the laboratory that examines the blood for its basic physical properties
Histology	Division of laboratory that examines tissue samples
Microbiology	Division of laboratory that analyzes specimens to identify pathogenic microorganisms
Nutrients	Substances that supply the body with the nourishment necessary for life
Point-of-care (POC) testing	Simple laboratory tests done by nursing on the nursing unit
Therapeutic diet	A diet modified from the hospital's regular diet to treat or accommodate a patient's condition
Therapeutic order	Order for procedures that will provide treatment or improve the patient's condition
Urinalysis	Examination of the physical, chemical, and microscopic properties of the urine

OBJECTIVES

When you have completed this chapter, you will be able to:

- Define the terms listed in the vocabulary.
- Understand how to work with the following departments:
    Laboratory
    Radiology
    Cardiology
    Respiratory Therapy
    Physical Therapy
    Endoscopies
    Electroencephalography
    Dietary
- State the general purpose of each of the departments discussed.
- Recognize abbreviations and define the tests and procedures listed specific to each department.

- Discuss the health unit coordinator's responsibilities to each department.
- Demonstrate an ability to transcribe orders relating to each department.
- Describe a well-balanced diet and the four basic food groups.
- Define and describe the therapeutic diets.

In this chapter you will be introduced to some of the most important **diagnostic** and **therapeutic** departments in the hospital. You will learn the names of many tests and treatments ordered for patients by their doctors and will learn about your responsibilities as a health unit coordinator in relation to these orders.

This is a complicated study, and you will continue to add to your knowledge throughout your career. As technology advances, new diagnostic examinations are developed, and others are discarded. New forms of therapy are constantly being devised to improve patient care. Be alert and inquisitive as you come across orders for tests and treatments that are new to you, and make an effort to learn about them.

*T*HE LABORATORY

*P*URPOSE OF LABORATORY TESTING

There are several important reasons why a doctor orders laboratory tests.

1. **To help in making a diagnosis.** The doctor may suspect a certain diagnosis but needs the results of the laboratory tests to confirm it.

2. **To evaluate the success of certain medications or other treatments.** For example, a patient receiving an anticoagulant such as heparin will have a blood test called a PTT done daily to assess the need for more, less, or the same amount of the drug.

3. **To establish a normal baseline for an individual patient.** Individuals will have somewhat different normal levels based on such factors as age, sex, race, and geographic location. It is important to know what is normal for each patient.

4. **To provide early detection of disease and thereby reduce its severity.** Diabetes and anemia are examples of diseases that can be detected by routine blood examination. Prompt and proper treatment are required to control these conditions and help prevent serious complications.

5. **To meet the requirements of the law.** Many states require premarital screening for syphilis. Most also require that this test be done on pregnant women. The scope of AIDS screening is yet to be determined.

Laboratory tests may be ordered as routine, meaning the specimen may be obtained during the regular schedule of the laboratory. Laboratories usually draw blood early in the morning, so an order for a routine CBC written one day will normally be carried out in the morning of the next day. If the test is urgent, the doctor will write stat, now, or today, and the specimen must be obtained and analyzed immediately or just as soon as possible.

*C*RITICAL VALUES

Critical values are test results that are too low or too high, and potentially dangerous to the patient. They must be brought to the immediate attention of the nurse and physician.

In most hospitals, the tests performed in laboratories are divided into several broad categories.

*H*EMATOLOGY

The **hematology** division performs tests that analyze **specimens** of blood for its basic physical properties. For example, the number, size, shape, and microscopic appearance of red blood cells may be important to know when a patient has anemia. This department also performs tests related to clotting and bleeding disorders and coagulation studies to monitor patients on anticoagulant therapy.

Hematology Orders

Complete Blood Count (CBC) The CBC is done routinely on most admissions preoperatively and at any other time the doctor deems it necessary. Actually, the CBC is a combination of many tests. Any of these tests can be ordered separately. It is important that you recognize certain terms, listed in Table 16.1, related to the results of the complete blood count.

Hemoglobin (Hgb) The hemoglobin is the oxygen-carrying portion of the blood and is found within the red blood cells. The Hgb is frequently ordered to determine the need for blood following injury, surgery, or disease to diagnose anemia. *Critical values:* <5.0g/dl and >20g/dl

Hematocrit (Hct) or Packed Cell Volume (PCV) The Hct or PCV is a measurement of the volume percentage of red blood cells in the blood. In anemias and in polycythemia after hemorrhage the hematocrit reading is lowered, and in dehydration it is raised. *Critical value:* <15% and >60%

White Blood Cells (WBC) This test examines and counts the number of white blood cells (leukocytes) in the blood. WBC increase (*leukocytosis*) indicates the presence of

TABLE 16.1 *T*ERMS USED IN CONNECTION WITH COMPLETE BLOOD COUNT TEST

Examination	Abbreviations	Normal Value
Erythrocytes (red blood cells)	Eryths, RBCs	M, 4.6 million–6.2 million/mm^3 F, 4.2 million–5.4 million/mm^3
Leukocytes* (white blood cells)	Leukos, WBCs	4,000–10,000/mm^3
Lymphocytes	Lymphs	20–40%
Monocytes	Monos	2–8%
Neutrophils (polys, segs.)	Neutros	55–70%
Eosinophils	Eos.	1–4%
Basophils	Basos	0.5–1%
Reticulocytes	Retics	0.5–2%
Bands (stabs)		2–6%
Platelets		150,000–400,000/mm^3
Erythrocyte sedimentation rate	ESR Westergren method	M, up to 15 mm in 1 hr F, up to 20 mm in 1 hr
Hemoglobin	Hb, Hgb	M, 14–18 g/dl F, 12–16 g/dl
Hematocrit	Hct	M, 42–52% F, 37–47%
Mean corpuscular hemoglobin	MCH	$20 \pm 2 \ \mu\mu g$
Mean corpuscular hemoglobin concentration	MCHC	$34 \pm 2\%$
Mean corpuscular volume	MCV	$87 \pm 5 \ \mu m^3$
Red blood cell distribution	RDW	11–14.5%

Note: Normal values vary somewhat with different laboratories. M = male; F = female.

infection. A decrease (*leukopenia*) is seen in many forms of bone marrow failure. *Critical values:* <2500 and >30,000/mm^3. There are different kinds of white blood cells. The **differential** identifies and counts the number of each type of WBC.

The different WBCs in order of their frequency of occurrence are as follows:

- Neutrophils
- Lymphocytes
- Monocytes
- Eosinophils
- Basophils

Red Blood Cells (RBC) This test counts the number of erythrocytes in the blood. The size and shape (morphology) of the RBC are also studied.

Reticulocytes (Retics) This test is a count of the reticulocytes (immature red blood cells) to determine bone marrow activity.

RBC Indices These values indicate the amount of Hgb and help diagnose anemia. Results may be stated as:

- MCH—**mean corpuscular hemoglobin,** the hemoglobin content of the average red blood cell. Is reported in micromicrograms ($\mu\mu$g).
- MCHC—**mean corpuscular hemoglobin concentration,** the average hemoglobin concentration per 100 ml of packed red cells; reported as a percentage.
- MCV—**mean corpuscular volume,** the average volume or size of individual red cells; reported in cubic microns (μm^3).
- RDW—**red blood cell distribution width,** the variation in the size of red blood cells.

Sedimentation Rate (ESR or Sed Rate) This test determines how fast red blood cells settle out of the liquid portion of the blood and is used to determine the progress of inflammatory diseases. The sed rate is usually markedly increased during pregnancy.

Platelet aggregation Platelet aggregation (clumping) is the first step in hemostasis. This test examines that part of the clotting process.

Platelets (Thrombocytes) Platelets are a type of cell in the blood necessary for blood coagulation (clotting). This test counts the number of platelets in the blood. *Critical values:* <50,000/mm^3 and >1 million/mm^3

Thrombin Time (TT) This test is used to monitor the effectiveness of thrombolytic therapy.

Prothrombin Time (Pro Time or PT) This test measures the clotting ability of the blood. This test may be ordered daily when a patient is receiving anticoagulant therapy—usually Coumadin—so the doctor may be sure the correct dose is being administered. The normal value is 11.0–12.5 seconds, or 85–100%. The International normalized ratio (INR) is 2–3.5. *Critical value:* >20 seconds

Many hospitals now report both the prothrombin time and the INR. The World Health Organization recommends such reporting as an attempt to standardize prothrombin time results throughout the world.

Activated Partial Thromboplastin Time (APTT) and Partial Thromboplastin Time (PTT) These tests are other examples of coagulation studies. These tests are often used when a patient is receiving an anticoagulant such as heparin. The normal value for APPT is 30–40 seconds and for PTT 60–70 seconds. *Critical values:* APPT > 70 seconds PTT > 100 seconds.

Clotting or Coagulation Time This test measures how long it takes the blood to clot.

Clot Retraction This test is used to evaluate bleeding disorders.

Bleeding Time This is a test to determine how long it takes a capillary puncture (fingerstick) to stop bleeding. The normal value is 1–9 minutes. *Critical value:* > 12 minutes

Iglycosylated Hemoglobin (GHb) This test is used to monitor the treatment of diabetes. The GHb shows the amount of glucose to which a certain type of hemoglobin has been exposed over the past 120 days (the life span of the RBC). An advantage of this test is that it can be drawn randomly and does not require fasting.

An example of the hematology laboratory results sent from the lab to a nursing unit to be filed on the appropriate patient's chart is shown in Fig. 16.1.

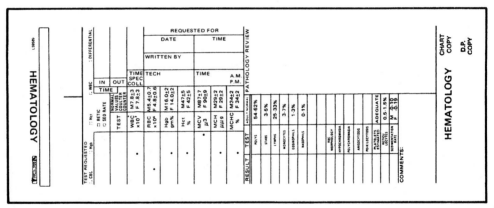

FIGURE 16.1

Urinalysis

The **urinalysis** is often done by the hematology division of the laboratory, although it is not a blood test. A urinalysis is ordinarily done on every hospital admission and consists of a physical, chemical, and microscopic examination of the urine. A sample chart showing results is given in Table 16.2.

The **physical examination** includes a determination of the color, transparency (clarity), and specific gravity (weight of the urine compared with the weight of an equal volume of distilled water). There may also be a comment regarding the odor of the urine.

The **chemical examination** of the urine includes tests for pH, glucose, protein, ketone bodies, blood, bilirubin, urobilinogen, and perhaps nitrite.

The **microscopic examination** studies the urine sediment (solid materials contained in the urine). RBCs, WBCs, epithelial cells, casts, and crystals may be seen during the microscopic portion of the urinalysis. Other structures that may be reported include mucus threads, bacteria, yeast cells, parasites, and spermatozoa.

TABLE 16.2	*S*AMPLE CHART SHOWING RESULTS OF A ROUTINE URINALYSIS	
Examination	**Abbreviation**	**Normal Values**
Color		Yellow/amber
Characteristics		Clear
Reaction	pH	4.6–8.0
Specific gravity	Sp gr/SG	1.025–1.035
Protein (albumin)	Prot/Alb	0–trace
Glucose		None
Acetone		None
Blood		None
Microscopic:		
Red blood cell casts	RBC casts	None
White blood cell casts	WBC casts	None
Hyaline casts		Few, possibly
Crystals	X1s	None
Renal tubular casts		None

There are several types of urine specimens, including the following:

- **Voided**—The patient urinates into a clean container.
- **Clean catch or midstream**—Nursing uses a special cleaning procedure and the patient starts his or her urine stream to wash away germs on the outside of the urinary tract. The urine is then collected "midstream."
- **Catheterized**—A sterile specimen is obtained through urinary catheterization and is sent to the lab in a sterile container.

The health unit coordinator should know that the requisition for a urinalysis is not sent to the laboratory until the specimen is obtained.

Urine specimens must be sent *directly* to the laboratory. If the urine is allowed to stand over 30 minutes, several changes can take place that may alter the true results of the urinalysis.

After the requisition and labeled urine specimen are received in the lab, the urinalysis is run, and the results are sent to your nursing unit to be filed in the patient's chart. An example of a urinalysis laboratory report is shown in Fig. 16.2.

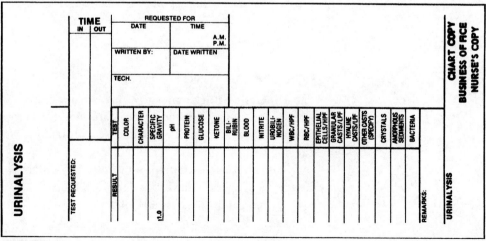

FIGURE 16.2

Miscellaneous Specimen Examinations

In addition to the routine urinalysis, many other tests may be performed on the patient's urine (see Table 16.3). Analysis of the urine for a particular chemical or mineral

TABLE 16.3	COMMON TESTS PERFORMED ON URINE SPECIMENS		
Specimen	**Examination**	**Abbreviation**	**Normal**
Urine for:	Ammonia	NH$_3$	0.8 Gm
	Bence Jones protein		Negative
	Catecholamines		80 mcg/24 hr
	Culture & sensitivity	C & S	Negative
	Hemoglobin	Hgb	Negative
	Porphyrins		20 mcg
	Urobilinogen		2 mg
	17-Hydroxycorticosteroids		5 mg/24 hr
	17-Ketosteroids		15 mg/24 hr

element, such as chlorides or ammonia, may be made on a single specimen or on a 24-hour collection of the patient's urine. The doctor usually indicates the type of specimen necessary for a test when writing the order.

Note: The tests shown in Table 16.3 are *urine chemistries, not routine urinalysis* (refer to the following section on chemistry). When a 24-hour urine specimen is ordered, it may be the health unit coordinator's responsibility to obtain a container from the laboratory to be used for the collection of the specimen. The urine container may contain a special additive or be kept on ice to keep the urine from deteriorating during the collection period. Nursing will save all the patient's urine for 24 hours and will then bring the container to the nurses' station. You will send the labeled container and the requisition you prepared when the original order was transcribed to the laboratory (Fig. 16.3).

24-Hour Urines

*Aldosterone
Amylase
Bence Jones protein
BUN
Calcium
*Catecholamines
*Coproporphyrins
*Cortisol
Creatinine clearance
Estrogen
Follicle-stimulating hormone
Glucose
Heavy metals
*5 HIAA
Hydroxyproline
17-Hydroxycorticosteroids
17-Hydroxysteroids
17-Ketogenic steroids
17-Ketosteroids
LDH
*Metanephrine
Oxalates
Phosphorus
*Porphyrins
Porphobilinogen
Potassium
Pregnanediol
Pregnanetriol
Quantitative HCG
Sodium
Uric acid
Urine total protein
*Uroporphyrins
*VMA

Specimens that require preservative.

FIGURE 16.3

Chemistry

The **chemistry** division of the laboratory analyzes specimens of body fluids for chemical constituents. Blood and urine are the specimens most commonly collected for study in the chemistry division of the laboratory; however, chemistry tests may be performed on other body materials (e.g., vomitus or gastric—stomach—contents). Many tests of the same name can be performed on either blood or urine, so the word **serum** will often be added to the order and will be your clue that the order is for blood rather than for urine.

Table 16.4 shows only a partial list of blood chemistry examinations. There are a vast number of additional chemistry exams the doctor may order. By studying the requisitions for chemistry supplied by the laboratory and by learning the lists of chemistry exams your instructor may provide, you will increase your knowledge of the types of chemistry examinations the doctor will order for his patients.

Because they are so commonly ordered, special mention is made of several blood chemistry orders:

- **Alkaline phosphatase (ALP)**—This test has many uses, but its major purpose is to diagnose liver and bone disease.
- **Electrolytes (lytes)**—The electrolytes help the body maintain a balance between acidity and alkalinity. This test may be called an electrolyte panel and include sodium (Na), potassium (K), chlorides (Cl), and carbon dioxide (CO_2).

These tests may be ordered separately.

- **Acid phosphatase**—aids in diagnosis of cancer of the prostate gland.
- **Amylase**—aids in diagnosis of pancreatic disease, abdominal obstructions, diseases of salivary glands and ducts. *Critical value:* >3 × upper limit of normal
- **Total bilirubin**—helps identify liver disease, gallstones, and extrahepatic duct obstruction.
- **Blood urea nitrogen (BUN)**—kidney function test. *Critical value:* >100 mg/dl
- **Calcium**—one of the essential ions of the body; decrease called hypocalcemia occurs in alkalosis, celiac disease, sprue, hypoparathyroidism, and some kid-

TABLE 16.4	*T*YPICAL BLOOD CHEMISTRY EXAMINATIONS	
Examination	**Abbreviation**	**Normal Values**
Acid phosphatase	Acid P'tase	0.11–0.60 U/L
Albumin	Alb.	3.5–5.0 Gm/dl
Alkaline phosphatase	ALP	30–85 ImU/ml
Amylase		56–190 IU/L
Antinuclear antibody	ANA	Negative
Antistreptolysis titration	ASO titer	160 Todd u/ml
Asparate aminotransferase	AST	5–40 IU/L
Bilirubin (total)	Bili	0.1–1 mg/dl
Blood urea nitrogen	BUN	10–20 mg/dl
Calcium	Ca	4.5–5.6 mg/dl
Carbon dioxide	CO_2	23–30 mEq/L
Chlorides	Cl	90–110 mEq/L
Cholesterol	chol	<200 mg/dl
Creatinine	creat	0.7–1.3 mg/dl
Creatinine phosphokinase	CPK	F, 30–135 U/L M, 55–170 U/L
Electrolytes (see Na, K, Cl, and CO_2)	lytes	
Glucose	FBS, BS	70–110 mg/dl
Glucose tolerance test	GTT	70–115 mg/dl Fasting and at 4 hours
Lactate dehydrogenase	LDH	115–225 IU/L
Lipase		0–110 U/L
Lithium		0.5–1.0 mEq/L
Nonprotein nitrogen	NPN	20–35 mg/dl
Phosphorus	Phos	2.5–4.5 mg/dl
Potassium	K	3.4–5.0 mEq/L
Protein-bound iodine	PBI	4.0–8.0 μg/dl
Prostate specific antigen	PSA	4.0 ng/ml
Serum glutamic pyruvic transaminase or ALT	SGPT	5–35 IU/L
Sodium	Na	135–145 mEq/L
T_3 uptake		40–205 mg/dl
Total proteins		5.9–8.0 Gm/dl
Triglycerides		10–150 mg/dl
Uric acid		F, 2.0–7.0 mg/dl M, 2.5–8.0 mg/dl

ney diseases; increase (hypercalcemia) is found in acidosis, hyperparathyroidism, multiple myeloma, and some respiratory diseases. Too low calcium concentration can result in tetany, too high calcium, in coma. *Cricital values:* <6 mg/dl and >14 mg/dl

■ **Carbon dioxide (CO_2)**—measured in cases of suspected respiratory insufficiency; higher-than-normal concentration of CO_2 may indicate that gas exchange is inadequate; provides information regarding patient's acid–base balance. *Critical value:* <6 mEq/L

■ **Cardiac enzymes (AST, LDH, and CPK)**—When a patient has had a heart attack (myocardial infarction or MI), the enzymes found in the cardiac muscle are elevated. They rise and fall in the blood at different times following an MI. By comparing these changes against normal enzyme levels a diagnosis of myocardial infarction can be made. These tests may also be ordered separately and may aid in the diagnosis of other disease conditions, such as liver disease, pulmonary disease, and skeletal muscle injury.

AST—This test is useful in diagnosing an MI. It typically becomes elevated about 6 to 10 hours after heart injury, reaches peak levels at 12 to 48 hours, and then drops to normal levels in about 3 to 4 days if there is no further heart injury. The AST is also elevated with liver, acute kidney, and pancreatic disease.

LDH—These levels rise in an MI in 24 to 48 hours, peak in 2 to 3 days, and generally returns to normal in 5 to 10 days.

CPK—This is the main cardiac enzyme tested in an MI. The CPK is done on admission and typically at 12 and 24 hours. An electrophoresis is also ordered to identify three CPK isoenzymes: CPK-MM, CPK-MB, and CPK-BB. These tests are specific for heart muscle injury.

- **Chemistry screen (chem. screen) or SMA**—A special machine in the laboratory performs a number of tests on one sample of blood. An SMA 12 performs 12 tests; an SMA 20 performs 20 tests, and so on.

- **Cholesterol**—Cholesterol is measured to determine whether a patient is at risk for arteriosclerotic heart disease. Cholesterol testing is usually part of a lipid profile, which includes testing the lipoproteins. *HDLs* carry cholesterol away from the tissues for excretion from the body. They are the "good cholesterol." *LDLs* are the "bad cholesterols" and carry lipids to the tissues.

- **Chlorides**—measured to help diagnose disorders in the maintenance of normal osmotic relationships, acid–base balance, and water balance of the body; usually performed together with measurement of other ions of the blood. *Hyperchloremia* is too much chloride in the blood; *hypochloremia* is too little. *Critical values:* <80 mEq/L and >115 mEq/L

- **Creatinine**—increased quantities are found in advanced stages of renal (kidney) disease. *Critical value:* >4 mg/dl

- **Lipase**—test for damage to the pancreas.

- **Lithium**—test to monitor the lithium dosage (a medication) in the treatment of manic–depressive psychosis (bipolar affective disorder).

- **Potassium (K⁺)**—essential ion found in large concentrations in all cells; alterations in serum potassium levels may produce serious changes in body function, or even death.

    Marked decrease (*hypokalemia*) may cause cardiac arrhythmias and muscle weakness. Causes include severe vomiting and diarrhea and chronic kidney disease.

    Marked increase (*hyperkalemia*) also produces arrhythmias; there may also be lethargy and coma. Causes include severe cell damage, adrenal cortical deficiency, and hypoventilation. *Critical values:* <2.5 mEq/L and >6.5 mEq/L

- **Prostate specific antigen (PSA)**—The PSA is a test for prostate cancer and to monitor the response to cancer treatment. It is considered more sensitive than the prostatic acid phosphatase (PAP), another prostate cancer test.

- **Serum glutamic oxaloacetic transaminase (SGOT)**—elevated especially in liver disease, or coronary occlusive disease.

- **Sodium (Na)**—the main cation of blood and extracellular fluid. Increased serum sodium levels may be caused by markedly inadequate water intake or the administration of excessive amounts of sodium (*hypernatremia*).

    Decreased sodium levels (*hyponatremia*) occur in diarrhea, heat exhaustion, Addison's disease, and certain kidney disorders. *Critical values:* <120 mEq/L and >160 mEq/L

- **T₃ uptake, thyroxine index (free), T₃–T₄, T₄RIA**—tests for thyroid disease.

- **Total iron binding capacity (TIBC)**—useful in diagnosing iron deficiency anemia.

- **Total protein**—This test measures a patient's nutritional state. It studies the serum albumin and globulin, which make up most of the body's protein. The total protein is decreased in the presence of malnutrition and liver disease.

- **Uric acid**—usually performed to diagnose gout. Elevated uric acid is called *hyperuricemia*. *Critical value:* >12 mg/dl

The Blood Sugar Tests

- **Blood sugar (BS or glucose)**—determines the amount of sugar in the blood. Fasting blood sugar (FBS) determines the amount of sugar in the blood when the patient has not eaten for a period of time and so is done in the early morning. *Critical values:* <40 mg/dl and >400 mg/dl
- **Glucose tolerance test (GTT)**—This test is done over several hours when the patient has been fasting. The patient is given a large amount of glucose to drink. Blood and urine specimens are taken to determine abnormalities in glucose metabolism.
- **One-hour glucose screen**—for gestational diabetes.
- **Postprandial blood sugars (PP BS)**—This test is done to determine the patient's response to the intake of carbohydrates. It is most commonly ordered as a 2-hr PP BS, and the blood is drawn two hours after any meal. *Note:* You will be expected to notify the laboratory when a patient has finished eating so that the laboratory may plan to draw the blood in 2 hours.

  These tests are usually performed to aid in the diagnosis of and monitoring of diabetes. Results of these tests may be included on the supplementary chart form often called the **diabetic flow sheet.**
- **TORCH tests**—Tests for toxoplasmosis, other (such as syphilis) rubella, cytomeglavinus, and herpes. These are all infections that have a damaging effect on the fetus.

  Results of the blood chemistry examinations are sent to the unit to be filed on the patient's chart.

Sample Chemistry Requisitions Many hospitals order laboratory tests by computer. If your hospital does not, requisitions similar to the ones pictured in Fig. 16.4 are used.

Microbiology

Microbiology is concerned primarily with tests designed to isolate and identify disease-causing microorganisms. These microorganisms may be present in a specimen of any type of material from the patient's body. The most common are blood, urine, sputum, and wound drainage but may also include stool, vaginal secretions, cerebrospinal fluid, and others (Fig. 16.5).

Examples of some diseases that can be identified through microbiological examination of a body specimen include candidiasis, chlamydia, gonorrhea, meningitis, pneumonia, streptococcal infections, staphylococcal infections, and tuberculosis.

A division within the microbiology department is **bacteriology.** Bacteria found in body specimens are studied here. A frequent order for C&S is processed in this division.

The abbreviation C&S means **culture and sensitivity.** To determine whether bacteria are present in a particular specimen, a sample of the specimen is *cultured,* or placed under sterile conditions on a special medium that bacteria require to grow. If certain bacteria are present in a specimen (and are therefore at work causing disease inside the patient), *sensitivity* tests are performed. In these tests, the growths of bacteria from the specimen are mixed with certain antibiotics. The bacteria will be destroyed by the particular antibiotics to which they are sensitive. The doctor then knows which antibiotics to administer to cure the patient's bacterial infection.

The health unit coordinator should know that although a specimen for C&S may be *obtained* stat, the results will not be available immediately.

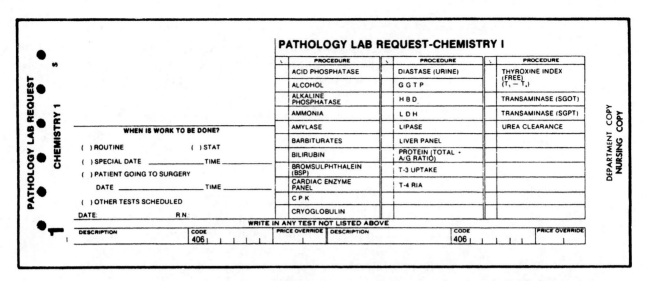

PATHOLOGY LAB REQUEST-CHEMISTRY I

PATHOLOGY LAB REQUEST — CHEMISTRY 1

WHEN IS WORK TO BE DONE?

( ) ROUTINE   ( ) STAT
( ) SPECIAL DATE _____ TIME _____
( ) PATIENT GOING TO SURGERY
    DATE _____ TIME _____
( ) OTHER TESTS SCHEDULED
DATE: _____ R.N. _____

PROCEDURE	PROCEDURE	PROCEDURE
ACID PHOSPHATASE	DIASTASE (URINE)	THYROXINE INDEX (FREE) (T₁ – T₄)
ALCOHOL	G G T P	
ALKALINE PHOSPHATASE	H B D	TRANSAMINASE (SGOT)
AMMONIA	L D H	TRANSAMINASE (SGPT)
AMYLASE	LIPASE	UREA CLEARANCE
BARBITURATES	LIVER PANEL	
BILIRUBIN	PROTEIN (TOTAL + A/G RATIO)	
BROMSULPHTHALEIN (BSP)	T-3 UPTAKE	
CARDIAC ENZYME PANEL	T-4 RIA	
C P K		
CRYOGLOBULIN		

WRITE IN ANY TEST NOT LISTED ABOVE

DESCRIPTION	CODE 406	PRICE OVERRIDE	DESCRIPTION	CODE 406	PRICE OVERRIDE

DEPARTMENT COPY   NURSING COPY

PATHOLOGY LAB REQUEST - CHEMISTRY 2

PATHOLOGY LAB REQUEST CHEMISTRY 2

WHEN IS WORK TO BE DONE?

( ) ROUTINE   ( ) STAT
( ) SPECIAL DATE _____ TIME _____
( ) PATIENT GOING TO SURGERY
    DATE _____ TIME _____
REQUEST DATE: _____ R N _____

PROCEDURE	PROCEDURE	PROCEDURE
ACETONE (SERUM)		OSMOLALITY, URINE
CALCIUM		OSMOLALITY, SERUM
CALCIUM (URINE)	GLUCOSE	PHOSPHORUS (PO₄)
CARBON DIOXIDE (BICARB CO₂)	GLUCOSE – 2 HR POST PRANDIAL	POTASSIUM (K)
CHLORIDE (CL)	GLUCOSE TOL 3 HR	CHEM SCREEN
CHOLESTEROL	GLUCOSE TOL 4 HR	SODIUM (Na)
CREATININE	GLUCOSE TOL 5 HR	UREA NITROGEN (BUN)
CREATININE CLEARANCE	GLUCOSE TOL 6 HR	URIC ACID
ELECTROLYTE PANEL	GLUCOSE TOL. 2 HR.	TRIGLYCERIDES
	MAGNESIUM	LITHIUM
	SALICYLATE	

WRITE IN ANY TEST NOT LISTED ABOVE

DESCRIPTION	CODE 406	PRICE OVERRIDE	DESCRIPTION	CODE 406	PRICE OVERRIDE

DEPARTMENT COPY   NURSING COPY

PATHOLOGY LAB REQUEST - CHEMISTRY 3

WHEN IS WORK TO BE DONE?

( ) ROUTINE   ( ) STAT
( ) SPECIAL DATE _____ TIME _____
( ) PATIENT GOING TO SURGERY
    DATE _____ TIME _____
( ) OTHER TESTS SCHEDULED
DATE _____ R.N. _____

PROCEDURE	PROCEDURE	PROCEDURE
CATECHOLAMINES (Urine)	IMMUNO ELECTROPHORESIS	RENIN
CORTISOL (PLASMA) Specify Time	IRON & IRON BINDING	SALICYLATE
	LDH ISOENZYMES	SEROTONIN (5-HIAA)
DILANTIN	LEAD (Blood Urine)	THYROXINE BINDING GLOBULIN (TBG)
DIGOXIN	LEUCINE AMINO PEPTIDASE	THYROID STIMULATING HORMONE (TSH)
D-XYLOSE TOLERANCE	LIPID PROFILE	TRIGLYCERIDES
ELECTROPHORESIS PROTEIN (SERUM)	LITHIUM	V M A VANILLYL MANDELIC ACID
ELECTROPHORESIS HEMOGLOBIN	MACROGLOBULIN (SIA WATER TEST)	VITAMIN A CAROTENE
ESTRIOL (PLACENTA) URINE	MAGNESIUM	VITAMIN B-12
FOLIC ACID (Folate)	ORINASE TOLERANCE	17 KETOSTEROIDS 24 HR URINE
GENTAMYCIN	QUINIDINE	17 KETOGENIC STEROIDS 24 HR URINE

WRITE IN ANY TEST NOT LISTED ABOVE

DESCRIPTION	CODE 406	PRICE OVERRIDE	DESCRIPTION	CODE 406	PRICE OVERRIDE

LAB COPY   NURSING COPY

PRINTED BY THE STANDARD REGISTER COMPANY U.S.A. 2PART

FIGURE 16.4

FIGURE 16.5

Blood Cultures

Multiple blood cultures must be ordered separately according to the number of times requested by the physician. For example:

- Order reads: Blood cultures × 2
  (Enter two separate orders for blood cultures.)
- Order reads: Blood cultures × 2, 15 minutes apart
  (Enter two separate orders for blood cultures and type "15 minutes apart" in remarks.)

Sputum Cultures

Obtained by having the patient expectorate into a sterile container, first thing in the morning if possible. Doctors often hold antimicrobial drugs until after the specimen is obtained unless the test is being used to evaluate the effects of medication. Initial results of sputum cultures typically take 24 to 48 hours to complete. Cultures for fungus and mycobacterium TB may take 6 to 8 weeks.

Cytomegalovirus Culture (CMV)

Culture of the mouth, urine, sputum, or blood to detect the presence of CMV, a frequent viral infection and the most common congenital infection of newborns.

Examples of orders for microbiology and serology are shown in Table 16.5.

TABLE 16.5 **COMMON TESTS RELATED TO PARTICULAR BODY MATERIALS**		
Specimen	**Examination**	**Abbreviation**
Stool for:	Culture & sensitivity	C&S
	Ova & parasites	O&P
Sputum for:	Culture & sensitivity	C&S
	Acid-fast bacilli (for diagnosis of TB)	AFB
Cerebrospinal fluid	Serology	CSF

- **Mycology**—analyzes specimens to identify fungi
- **Parasitology**—studies parasites, organisms that attach themselves to another organism and live off of that organism (e.g., helminths [worms] and the ova [eggs] of these parasites). Specimens from stool or fecal samples, the vagina, and the blood are studied for ova and parasites (O&P). Some human diseases caused by parasites include (but are not limited to) amebiasis, ascariasis, hookworm disease, tapeworm disease, pinworm disease, malaria, scabies, toxoplasmosis, trichinosis, and trichomoniasis.
- **Virology**—this division studies viruses.

Note: You as the health unit coordinator should know that specimens for microbiology should be taken to the laboratory immediately. Blood samples will be drawn by the laboratory; samples of urine, sputum, wound drainage, vaginal secretions, stool, and CSF will be obtained by the doctor or nurse and must be sent in the appropriately labeled container along with the requisition you prepared at the time the order was transcribed.

Immunosuppressant Laboratory Tests These are tests done to assess the effects of the body's diminished immune response as a result of disease (usually due to HIV).

- **Enzyme-linked immunosorbent assay (ELISA)**—A blood test that detects HIV antibodies. It is the most commonly used screening test for AIDS. It is confirmed by other testing such as the Western blot test. Normal results are negative.
- **Immunoglobulin electrophoresis**—tests used to diagnose and follow the course of a number of diseases such as immune and autoimmune deficiencies, chronic infections, intrauterine fetal infections, and hypersensitivity diseases. Test results include those for IgG, IgA, IgM, IgD, and IgE.
- **Western Blot Test**—confirmatory test for HIV. Normally negative.

Cytology

Cytology studies cells obtained from body tissues.

Pap smears, developed by Dr. George Papanicolaou, can be performed on various types of specimens to determine the presence of cancer. The most common type of "pap smear" or test is taken from the cervix during a pelvic examination. A pap smear can also detect estrogen–progesterone abnormalities that may be the cause of infertility or menstrual disorders through a test called the maturation index (MI).

Biopsies, or pieces of body tissues, taken from the skin or from internal body organs are examined by cytology. Tissues removed in surgery are examined by this department. **Histology** is the microscopic study of tissue (Fig. 16.6).

Bone marrow aspirations, samples taken from the center of certain bones where red blood cells are produced, are obtained through a special procedure performed by the doctor. If the specimen is obtained from the breastbone, the procedure is called **sternal puncture.** Other puncture sites include the posterior iliac crest, the iliac spines, or, in children, the proximal end of the tibia. This procedure may be done on the nursing unit using local anesthesia and the specimens sent to cytology for examination. **Ascites** (fluid formed in the abdominal cavity and withdrawn by an abdominal **paracentesis**) or fluid formed in the chest cavity and withdrawn by **thoracentesis** by the doctor may be examined.

Serology

The serology division studies blood serum and some other body fluids such as **cerebro-spinal fluid (CSF).** It deals with tests using antibody–antigen reactions which are the body's reaction to the presence of viral, bacterial, fungal, and parasitic infections. These types of diseases stimulate the body's production of antibodies in response to the antigens on the surface of the disease-causing organism. This reaction is studied in the laboratory tests listed (Fig. 16.7):

- **Antinuclear antibody (ANA)**—used to detect the presence of systemic lupus erythematosis (SLE), a serious chronic inflammatory disease involving multiple organ systems and producing widespread damage to connective tissue, blood vessels, and more. A negative result helps rule out SLE. This test also

HISTOLOGY

TISSUE SLICER

FIGURE 16.6

FIGURE 16.7

aids in the diagnosis of other rheumatic diseases. ANA has replaced LE Cell Prep as the test of choice for SLE with a correct result in about 95% of cases. Normal: negative.

- **Antistreptolysin titer (Asotiter)**—test used to determine if there has been a previous streptococcus infection that may be the cause of another condition such as rheumatic fever or glomerulonephritis.

- **Cold and febrile agglutinins**—tests to diagnose certain infectious diseases. Cold agglutinins are especially useful in diagnosing mycoplasma pneumonia, a type of bacterial pneumonia. Normal: negative.

- **C-reactive protein (CRP)**—used to detect inflammatory conditions and bacterial infections. Used postoperatively to diagnose wound infections. The test is also used to monitor the progress of an acute MI. The normal value is <0.8 mg/dl.

- **Hepatitis B surface antigen (HBsAg)**—test for hepatitis B. It usually indicates an acute and active infection. If the elevated level persists, the patient is a carrier of the virus. This is the test most often done for hepatitis B.

- **Heterophile antibody test (monospot test)**—used to diagnose infectious mononucleosis (IM), a disease that is caused by the Epstein–Barr virus (EBV). Normal: negative.

- **Rapid plasma reagin (RPR), Veneral Disease Research Laboratory (VDRL)**—test to diagnose syphilis, a sexually transmitted disease caused by the spirochete *Treponema pallidum*. Normal: negative.

Cerebrospinal Fluid Specimens of CSF are sometimes needed for laboratory analysis. A **lumbar puncture** (LP) is performed on the unit. A tray from central supply is requisitioned, and the doctor inserts a needle into the patient's lower spine below the level of the spinal cord. Fluid is withdrawn for laboratory analysis. An order for CSF might look this way:

> LP-Spinal fluid to lab for:
> #1—Cells
> #2—Protein
> #3—Glucose

The fluid removed is usually placed in vials labeled #1, #2, and #3; the doctor writes orders for tests for each vial number. You will note on your requisition which vial is for which test. The following tests may be ordered:

- C&S
- Cell count
- Chloride
- Colloidal gold
- Cytology
- Glucose
- Lactic acid
- LDH
- Protein
- Protein electrophoresis
- VDRL

An example of a requisition for CSF sent from the lab and filed on the patient's chart is shown in Fig. 16.8.

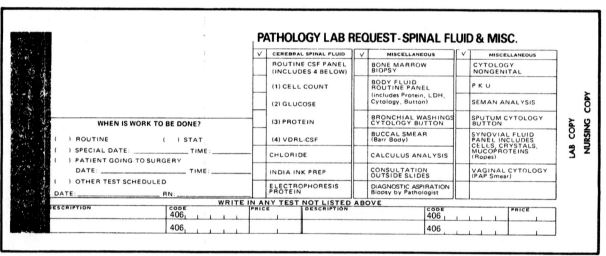

FIGURE 16.8

*T*HE BLOOD BANK

Blood transfusions are given to replace blood loss or to correct an anemic condition.

A reserve stock of whole blood and plasma (the fluid portion of the blood) is ordinarily kept at the hospital's blood bank. The blood must be obtained from suitable donors (*homologous* blood)—that is, people free of disease and in good health. Blood is stored, for a specific length of time, under refrigeration for emergency use when major blood loss occurs, as during surgery or in cases of severe injury. *Autologous* blood is a patient's own blood deposited for later use.

The blood bank is usually a part of the laboratory. Responsibilities of the blood bank include:

- Scheduling donor appointments to maintain an adequate supply of various types of blood
- Collecting the blood from the donors and processing it for future use

- Performing blood tests
- Keeping records pertaining to blood donations and transfusions

Execution of Forms

If you work in a surgical unit, you will probably have frequent contact with the blood bank. The services of the blood bank, however, are often required by nonsurgical patients as well. Examples of forms used in requesting the services of the blood bank are described on pp. 403 and 404.

Requisitions for Blood Grouping. Because different types of blood are not compatible, it is necessary to type the blood of the patient so that he or she can be given blood from a compatible donor (Fig. 16.9). Human blood is of four primary types (or groups): **O, A, B,** and **AB.** Additional factors, such as Rh (positive or negative), must also be compatible. Blood must therefore be typed for factors other than primary type. If two different types of blood are combined, dangerous reactions and sometimes the death of the patient will result. Some hospitals type all patients' blood routinely on admission (Figs. 16.10 and 16.11). Typing and crossmatching includes the following:

- ABO & RH type
- Antibody screen
- Units ordered

Requisition for Crossmatching It is not sufficient, however, simply to give a patient blood of his or her own type. When it is expected that a patient will need a transfusion, a sample of the patient's blood must actually be mixed with a sample from a potential donor, to ensure that the two bloods are definitely compatible. This process is called **crossmatching.** It is always done before whole blood from any donor is given to any recipient. After the blood has been crossmatched, the suitable blood is carefully labeled and held in reserve for the patient. The physician will indicate how much blood may be needed (Fig. 16.12).

DONOR'S BLOOD B Rh POSITIVE

METICULOUS ACCURACY IS REQUIRED
WHEN RECORDING INFORMATION
ABOUT A PATIENT'S BLOOD TYPE.

PATIENT'S BLOOD B Rh POSITIVE

FIGURE 16.9

REQUISITION FOR BLOOD GROUPING

BLOOD GROUPING				CIRCLE TEST DESIRED				
Date _____				Diagnosis _____				
Room No. _____								Units
Name _____								Charge No.
Hospital No. _____								Date
Doctor _____								
Group	O A B AB			Rh Factor	Pos.	Neg.	Classification	
Direct Coombs	Pos.	Neg.		Phenotype:	HR	Kell ☐		Duffy ☐
Rh. Antibody Titre: Neg.					Pos.in Titre	1:		
Isosensitization:								
Remarks:								

FIGURE 16.10

FIGURE 16.11

REQUISITION FOR CROSSMATCHING

BLOOD BANK—Crossmatch Request			
ONE UNIT ONLY ☐ Whole Blood ☐ Packaged Cells ☐ Fresh Blood (Specify Reason) _____ _____	Diagnosis _____ WHEN Date _____ REQUIRED: Time _____ am/pm By _____ RN	Name _____ Hospital No. _____ Room No. _____ Date _____ Doctor _____	

		FOR LAB USE ONLY	
Patient:	Donor:	Reactions:	
Group Rh	Donor No.		
Compatible yes no	Group Rh		
Saline ☐ ☐		Transfused by _____	
Protein ☐ ☐	VDRL:	Date _____ Time _____ am/pm	
Coombs ☐ ☐	Report by Date	Type & Crossmatch ☐ Transfusion ☐	Charge

FIGURE 16.12

Examples of doctor's orders for blood administration:

> *T & C 2 units WB (type and crossmatch units of whole blood)*
> *1 U PC now—(give one unit of packed cells immediately)*
> *Cryoprecipitates—1 unit*
> *2 U FFP—(2 units fresh frozen plasma)*
> *Give 1 U PRCs—(1 unit packed red cells)*
> *Platelets, 2 units*

Point-of-Care Testing

Point-of-care (POC) tests are laboratory tests that are done on the nursing unit by nursing staff. Therefore, it is not necessary to requisition point-of-care tests from the laboratory. Otherwise, the order is transcribed in the usual method. Results are immediately available and are recorded by the nurse.

Most point-of-care tests use automated analyzers or reagents (chemicals) and are relatively simple and inexpensive to perform. Tests that use reagents include pregnancy tests for the presence of human chorionic gonadotropin (HCG) such as the agglutination inhibition test (AIT), or the automatic clotting time (ACT) for blood clotting. Other POC tests include the one for blood glucose using the AccuCheck, those for glucose and acetone in the urine that use chemically impregnated dipsticks, and the one for occult blood in the stool, the Hemoccult.

Automated analyzers may be used for testing the hematocrit, hemoglobin, and various blood chemistries such as glucose, Na, K, Cl, CO_2, BUN, and cholesterol.

ORDERING TESTS

Health Unit Coordinator Responsibilities

When dealing with laboratory tests you should be most careful to:

- Recognize test names
- Use correct spelling

- Know and use the abbreviations in common usage
- Know the correct requisitions to use when applicable

Your primary concern with laboratory tests will be to order them correctly. It will be especially important for you to learn what tests are performed by each laboratory division. Your instructor will teach you the procedures for ordering as they are performed in your hospital. In most hospitals you will not send requisitions for specimens to be obtained by nursing (which the patient must produce—urine, stool, sputum) until the specimen has been taken. Therefore, appropriate stamped requisitions must be kept in a designated place at the nurses' station. All specimens must have the time of collection, date, and initials or name of the nurse clearly marked on the laboratory specimen slip. They must also have a correctly completed label attached to the specimen container. In some cases, you may be expected to notify the laboratory by telephone of an emergency test or a test requiring that an appointment be made.

The doctor may wish certain laboratory tests such as prothrombin times or PTTs done daily. Very careful attention must be given to these types of orders so that they are ordered, performed, and the results received on a daily basis as requested by the physician.

Most hospitals order laboratory tests by computer. You must be very accurate when performing this task.

Patient Preparations Some laboratory tests will require special preparation of patients on the night before or morning of the test. The most common type of preparation for routine laboratory tests is to withhold food from the patient until the test has been performed. The designation may be "NPO," that is, nothing by mouth after a certain hour, or simply a "hold breakfast." It may be part of your work to compile lists of patients for whom tests make special preparations necessary. Your instructor will provide you with information on such tests as well as your duties in connection with the necessary preparations.

Receiving Telephone Reports Often, when a laboratory test has been ordered stat, now, today, and so on, the laboratory will telephone the results to the unit before sending them in written form. This may also occur if a result is abnormal and the laboratory wishes to bring it to the immediate attention of the doctor and nurse.

Always repeat laboratory results and write them down with the patient's name, date, time of day, and your signature. Tell the nurse and affix the telephone report to the front of the chart holder.

Computer Retrieval of Laboratory Results If your computer is interfaced with the laboratory, it is possible to retrieve results as soon as the laboratory test is done. The laboratory will immediately generate a printout, so it is not necessary for you to call the laboratory or for them to call the unit. Laboratory results can be reviewed at any time using the computer.

Standard Precautions

You should avoid handling a laboratory specimen container unless it is inside a protective container (such as a plastic bag) or unless you are wearing gloves.

ℛADIOLOGY

Rapid advances are occurring in the field of radiology. A new breed of imaging devices is enabling doctors to view organs at work and identify blockages and growths—all without surgery (Fig. 16.13).

FIGURE 16.13

X-rays were discovered by Wilhelm Konrad Roentgen, a German physicist, in 1895. They have since been renamed Roentgen rays and serve as a diagnostic aid to visualize internal structures and organs. X-rays are high-energy, invisible electromagnetic waves. They are able to penetrate solid materials because of their short wavelength. Differences in density or thickness of various body structures exposed to x-rays produce shadows on the radiographic film.

Contrast medium is used when the densities of two structures or organs next to each other are similar and cannot be distinguished on the radiograph.

The simplest kind of radiographs are those that do not require preparation or use of a contrast medium.

Examples include the following:

- **Bone density studies**—x-rays to detect osteoporosis as early as possible and monitor patients receiving treatment for osteoporosis. The patient lies under a photon generator that is slowly passed across the lumbar spine, hip at the neck of the femur, and radius. This x-ray takes about 30 to 45 minutes in the radiology department. It should not be done for approximately ten days following barium studies.

- **Chest x-rays**—Used to examine the cardiac and pulmonary systems. Posterior anterior x-rays (PA) pass through the back to the front of the body; anterior posterior views (AP) from the front to the back; lateral views pass through the patient's side. In the oblique view the patient is positioned halfway on the side. In the decubitus view the patient is completely lying on the side.

    Most chest x-rays are done in the radiology department, but there are also portable units that can be brought to the patient's bedside if the patient's condition is such that he or she should not be transported to the x-ray department.

- **Extremity x-rays**—x-rays of hands, arms, feet, and legs. They are usually done to detect a fracture.

- **Flat plates**—show bony structures, foreign bodies in tissue, or determine the position of other organs.
- **Kidneys, ureters, bladder**—a plain film or "scout film" of the abdomen that shows the size, shape, and any deformity of these organs including calculi (stones). This x-ray can also show intestinal obstruction, rupture of organs, or the presence of masses.
- **Mammogram**—uses low doses of x-rays to image inside of the breast. Mammograms are used to diagnose lesions of the breast before they can be felt. A preoperative mammogram localization of a lesion is performed by inserting a wire into the lesion to guide the surgeon to the spot for the biopsy. Stereotactic biopsy with needle or mammotomy uses a computer to guide a biopsy needle into a lesion. With activation of the equipment a biopsy is obtained without the necessity of surgery.
- **Obstruction series of abdomen**—identifies internal obstructions, paralytic ileus (absence of peristalsis in the intestine), abdominal visceral tears, and abscesses; may be done as a scout film before a GI series that uses contrast medium; is usually done in radiology but can be a portable film.
- **Skull x-ray**—visualization of bones of skull and nasal sinuses to identify skull fracture, metastatic tumors, and other skull and nasal sinus abnormalities.
- **Spinal x-ray**—done to diagnose fractures of vertebra.

The following are examples of orders for nonpreparation x-rays:

- Flat plate of abdomen in A.M.
- Chest x-ray on admission
- XR L-S spine tonight (x-ray lumbosacral spine)

Radiographs Requiring Preparation and the Use of Contrast Media

Many x-ray procedures of nonbony structures require the use of special *radiopaque* substances to increase the contrast in the film, which is necessary because there is so little difference in the density between some body parts and their surrounding organs or vessels. This substance is called **contrast medium** and, depending on the x-ray procedure, is usually organic iodine or a barium preparation. Contrast medium may be swallowed, injected into a vessel, or inserted into the rectum. The contrast medium shows up on the x-ray film, outlines the organ, and indicate any abnormalities to the physician (Fig. 16.14). Some patients may have an allergic reaction to the dye—usually when it is administered intravenously. Patients with allerties to iodine and shellfish are likely to be allergic. In that case, alternative dyes must be used. Some dyes turn the urine a blue color.

The following four radiographic studies are commonly ordered and require contrast medium. You must remember that some of these radiographs cannot be done on the same day. Because this scheduling varies among hospitals, you should learn the proper sequence for ordering these radiographs in your hospital.

- **Intravenous pyelogram IVP**—the kidneys, ureters, and the bladder are outlined on the x-ray after an injection of radiopaque dye into the patient's veins. This test should be scheduled before tests that use barium because stool, flatus, and barium interfere with this study.
- **Gallbladder series (GB series)**—the gallbladder and its tubular connections to other body organs are outlined after radiopaque dye is taken by mouth and absorbed from the intestinal tract.

Ureter   Kidney

FIGURE 16.14

■ **Gastrointestinal series (GI series)**—the stomach and intestinal tract are outlined on the x-ray after barium is swallowed by the patient. An upper GI is a series of x-rays of the esophagus, stomach, and duodenum after the patient has swallowed barium. A barium swallow is an x-ray of the esophagus and is considered more useful than the upper GI in determining abnormalities of the esophagus.

■ **Barium enema (BE)**—barium is given to the patient in enema form and the rectum and large intestine are outlined on the x-ray film. It is done to identify polyps, tumors, and anatomical abnormalities. In an air-contrast barium enema, air is forced into the large intestine after the instillation of barium.

Preparation of patients who are to receive radiographs utilizing contrast media usually begin the afternoon or evening before the procedure is to take place. Such preparations may include enemas, tablets, changes in diet, orders for NPO p̄ midnight. Many hospitals utilize small cards or tickets on which are written the procedure to be followed in preparing the patient for each of the various special radiographic procedures. These preparation tickets are simply reminders to nursing concerning the preparation procedures. The tickets are placed in the patient's Kardex until the x-ray is completed.

Important Considerations

■ Generally, the following studies may be ordered as outlined.
  ■ Gallbladder series and upper GI
  ■ Gallbladder series and BE
  ■ Gallbladder series and IVP
  ■ IVP, gallbladder series, and BE
■ The nurse will notify radiology and the physician if the bowel preparation has been unsatisfactory.
■ Barium studies should follow other x-rays, sonograms, or scans, since barium in the gastrointestinal tract can distort the other studies.
■ The patient may be away from the unit for some time when undergoing these x-rays.

Other x-ray procedures requiring contrast media include the following:

- **Angiogram**—x-rays of the vascular structures within the body after injection of a contrast medium.
- **Arteriogram**—an x-ray picture of an artery after injection of a contrast medium. A catheter is most often inserted into the femoral artery in the groin area and then advanced into the artery to be examined. Contrast medium is rapidly injected. This x-ray is done to diagnose arterial tumors, obstructions, and other abnormalities. A technique called *digital subtraction angiography (DSA)*, which uses an advanced type of computerized fluoroscopy, can be used to hide bony structures from the picture. After contrast dye is injected, images are made, and the computer then subtracts or removes all the images such as bone that would confuse the image. This leaves a clear image of the artery being studied. Arteriography involves some risk. Hemorrhage, allergic reactions, and the dislodging of atherosclerotic plaque to produce an ebolus (piece circulating in bloodstream) are dangers of this procedure. An arteriogram may be identified according to the anatomic location (e.g., femoral arteriogram or carotid arteriogram).
- **Arthrogram**—an x-ray picture of an internal joint surface after injection of a contrast medium.
- **Bronchogram**—following the introduction of a contrast medium into the bronchi, an x-ray examination of the lungs and bronchial tree is made.
- **Cystogram**—a contrast medium is introduced into the bladder by x-ray personnel through a Foley catheter for the purpose of outlining the organ. A retrograde pyelogram is a visualization of the urinary tract following ureteral catheterization. The ureters are catheterized during a cystoscopy, dye is injected into the ureters, and x-rays are taken. In a voiding cystourethrogram, after the catheter is removed, the patient is asked to urinate while x-rays are taken of the bladder and urethra.
- **Esophagram (barium swallow)**—performed at the same time as an upper gastrointestinal x-ray study; the patient swallows the barium while the esophagus is studied by fluoroscopy and x-ray.
- **Hysterosalpingogram**—fluoroscopy and x-ray pictures of the uterus and fallopian tubes made after injection of a contrast medium.
- **Lymphangiogram**—fluoroscopy and x-ray pictures of the lymph channels and lymph nodes made after injection of a contrast medium. This test aids in diagnosis of metastasis to lymph nodes from lymphomas and Hodgkins disease.
- **Myelogram**—x-ray picture of the spinal cord after a contrast medium has been injected between the vertebrae into the spinal canal.
- **Percutaneous transhepatic cholangiography (PTC or PTHC)**—visualization of the biliary ducts after the injection of contrast medium.
- **Sialogram**—an x-ray picture of the salivary ducts made after injection of a contrast medium.
- **T-tube cholangiogram**—x-ray pictures of the bile ducts after a contrast medium is injected into a surgically placed T-tube.
- **Venogram**—x-ray picture of the veins made after injection of a contrast medium.
- **Ventriculogram**—x-ray picture of the cerebral ventricles taken after injection of a contrast medium.
- **Fluoroscopy**—a procedure used to observe the form and motion of internal structures of the body and to detect the presence of foreign bodies. The image, instead of being recorded on a film, is focused on a radiosensitive plate and can be studied "in action" by the doctor. A radiopaque medium is often

used to outline the body parts. During the procedure radiographs can also be taken for further study and as a permanent record.

■ **Computed** or **computerized tomography** or **CT Scan**—A CT scan is a special kind of x-ray that produces three-dimensional pictures of a cross section of a part of the body. Developed in 1972, CT scans are able to detect some conditions that conventional x-rays cannot and are used for many diagnostic procedures, including head scans, which are used to detect tumors, blood clots, enlarged ventricles or openings in the brain, and other abnormalities of the brain structure and nerves or muscles of the eye. Body scans are used for many reasons and are especially important in diagnosing pancreatic disease, enlarged lymph nodes, back problems, and various types of cancer. A CT portogram is a CT scan of the liver in which the dye is injected through a catheter that is placed in the splenic artery. It is useful in diagnosing liver metastasis in patients with cancer (Fig. 16.15).

Patients may be NPO for 4 to 8 hours before the test if contrast medium is to be used. The test may be done with or without contrast medium and may be given orally or by injection immediately or after the first set of scans.

The patient is placed in the scanner gantry (chamber), and the table moves. As the equipment scans, the patient hears a whirring sound of the motor.

FIGURE 16.15 Computed tomography.

CT scans should always be done before barium studies. Because contrast medium may be given, a check will be made for allergies to seafood or iodine.

Ultrasound (Sonography) Ultrasound is not an x-ray. Rather, it is a procedure that uses sound waves at very high frequencies to produce images of internal body structures and organs. It can also image internal movements such as the heart beating or blood flowing through the veins as it measures and records the reflection of these pulsed or continuous high-frequency sound waves.

It is considered safe and painless because it does not involve the use of x-rays and has reduced the need for invasive procedures such as surgery and cardiac catheterization.

A transducer (transmitter and receiver), which is often handheld, is placed against the body and slowly moved over the area to be examined. As the sound waves pass through the skin into the body they strike various organs and send echoes back to the transducer. The echoes differ based on the structures they strike and are separated and identified by the transducer.

The transducer then changes the sound waves into electrical energy and forms an image on a TV screen that represents a cross section of the organ being studied. Films of the images are taken, and the results are sent to the physician. Names of ultrasound tests include abdominal, thyroid, testicular, and scrotal ultrasound; prostate, renal, transesophageal, and transrectal ultrasonography; breast sonogram; and echocardiography.

- Ultrasound is used widely in medicine and is particularly valuable for diagnosis during pregnancy.
- An ultrasound **Doppler** is useful in detecting diminished blood flow through the heart and arteries. A shift in the frequency of the sound waves produced by the flow of the blood reveals faulty valves and vein and artery blockage. In venous Doppler studies a conductive gel is applied over areas above and on the lower extremity such as the groin, thigh, calf, or ankle. Normally a "swishing" sound is picked up by the Doppler ultrasound detecter. Absence of this sound indicates venous occlusion. Arterial Doppler studies can be either single-mode nuclear scans or duplex Doppler scanning.
- Patients having gallbladder scans are placed on a fat-free diet the day before and they are NPO after midnight before the procedure.
- Pelvic scans require a full bladder, and patients have to drink several glasses of water and not void before the study.
- Barium studies should be done after ultrasonography.

Imaging

Magnetic resonance imaging (MRI) is a noninvasive procedure that uses a huge electromagnet, a radio-frequency generator, and a computer to image structures in the body by measuring the release of energy by hydrogen atoms in tissues when they are subjected to changes in their magnetic environment. When the body is subjected to a magnetic field, the hydrogen atoms align themselves with the field. When pulses of radio waves are aimed at the tissues, the atoms change the alignment of their nuclei. When the radio waves are turned off, the nuclei of the hydrogen atoms realign themselves and give off energy in the process. This energy is converted to electrical signals that form an image that is clearer than any seen by conventional x-ray or a CT scan. Patients are questioned about the presence of metal plates, pins, and the like in the body; they are asked if they have a metal splinter embedded in their eye; or they are asked if they work with metal because the magnet may pull the metal object in the body and injure the patient. Patients with pacemakers are excluded from this procedure. The MRI is a unique procedure in that it does not require the patient to be exposed to ionizing radiation. However, claustrophobic, agitated patients or those on life support equipment are usually not good candidates for this procedure (Fig. 16.16).

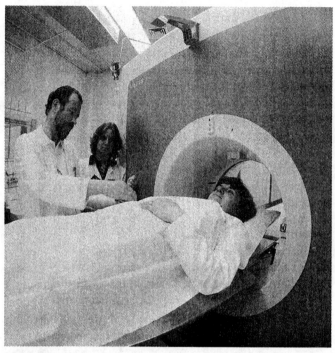

FIGURE 16.16 Magnetic resonance imaging.

Patient Positioning

The doctor often orders that the patient be placed in certain positions during x-ray to obtain the best view of the area being x-rayed.

When writing the x-ray order on the requisition, the health unit coordinator must be sure to transcribe the order exactly as written by the doctor. The doctor will always include R or L when a limb is to be x-rayed to indicate right or left.

Portable X-rays When a patient is unable to go to the radiology department, a portable x-ray is ordered. A mobile x-ray machine is taken to the patient's bedside. This is often not the procedure of choice because of the limitations in good patient positioning. The word *portable* must always be included when ordering.

𝒩UCLEAR MEDICINE

The nuclear medicine department uses radioactive materials called **radionuclides** that are injected into a vein or are ingested by the patient. These radioactive materials give off radiation in the form of gamma rays from the specific organ where the radionuclide is taken up. These tests are often called **radioisotopic procedures.**

An instrument called a *gamma scintillation camera* images the concentration of the radioactive material and produces a picture called a **scan.**

Scans may be ordered of many body organs including the bones, brain, heart, kidneys, liver, lungs, pancreas, and spleen. They may be done to evaluate the performance of an organ such as a thyroid uptake or to help determine the presence of cancer.

You should be aware that the patient will remain in Nuclear Medicine for at least an hour when a scan is ordered (Fig. 16.17).

Positron emission tomography (PET) is a procedure that uses radioactive substances, either inhaled or injected, that through combination of positively and negatively charged particles emit gamma rays. The gamma rays are detected and converted into color-coded images that measure metabolism and many of the body processes. The PET technique studies blood flow and metabolism of the heart as well as various kinds of cancer and the biochemical activity of the brain.

Single photon emission computed tomography (SPECT) shows the blood flow by imaging trace amounts of radioisotopes after a radionuclide is administered intravenously. This procedure has improved the quality of liver scanning.

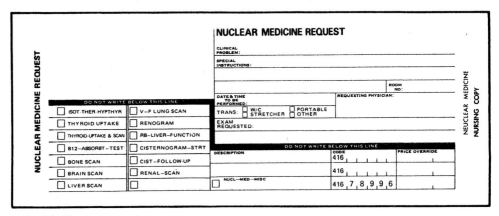

FIGURE 16.17

- **Gallium scan**—Following a tracer dose of gallium, a radioactive isotope of gallium is injected intravenously. Gallium concentrates in areas of tumors, abscesses, inflammation, and infection. These studies are useful in detecting lymphomas and certain metastatic tumors.

- **MUGA (multigated acquisition scan)**—cardiac nuclear scanning or thallium scan. After an injection of a radionuclide, a gamma-ray scanner is placed over the heart and a scan is taken.

- **Thallium exercise stress test**—Following an injection of radioactive thallium the patient exercises to the maximal heart rate and then lies down and the scan is done.

- **Gastroesophageal reflux scan (GE reflux scan)**—After the patient ingests a tracer radionuclide, images are taken over the esophageal area. The addition of an abdominal binder increases pressure on the abdominal area. This test is used to diagnose gastroesophageal reflux and evaluate symptoms of heartburn, regurgitation, and difficulty swallowing.

- **Radioactive iodine uptake (RAIU)**—After the patient ingests radioactive iodine a gamma-ray detector is used to analyze the percent iodine taken up by the thyroid gland over a given amount of time. This test is useful in evaluating thyroid function.

$\mathcal{R}$ADIATION THERAPY

The radiation therapy division of radiology is highly specialized and utilizes radiotherapy to bombard malignant growths (cancer) with doses of radiation. The radiation is given in doses calculated to destroy malignant tissues without harming normal cells.

Usually a requisition form is utilized for the initial order, and the radiation therapy department arranges the subsequent visits and notifies the nursing unit of that schedule (Fig. 16.18).

FIGURE 16.18

Execution of Forms

The numbers and types of forms to be used in ordering procedures from radiology will vary depending on the extent of use of computers, the size of the hospital, and the complexity of the radiological facilities. All hospitals do not provide all the services mentioned in this chapter; some will provide more. Your instructor will tell you about the services and method of ordering in your hospital or the hospitals in your community.

Health Unit Coordinator Responsibilities

- Order by computer or complete the proper requisition. If the addressograph plate does not include the patient's room number, be sure it is always written in. This is true of all requisitions. Radiology requires it so they will know where to go to pick up the patient.
- Telephone radiology with the order so that the x-ray may be scheduled in the appointment book in that department if your hospital requires that you do so.
- Prepare the appropriate consent form as required by your facility.
- Record the *clinical problem* on the radiology requisition if required. This is not always the same as the diagnosis and indicates the *reason* for the x-ray. For instance, a patient with a diagnosis of diabetes with an order for an IVP (intravenous pyelogram) may have a clinical problem such as urinary infection. If the doctor does not indicate the reason for the x-ray or the patient's clinical problem, you will often have to consult the nurse for this information. The routine chart form, called the progress notes, will often aid the nurse in making this decision. You would also communicate this information by computer.
- Communicate with the nursing staff concerning patient preparation, and communicate with the dietary department regarding diet changes. These are prime responsibilities. Errors in any phase of patient preparation may affect

the outcome of the x-ray and may result in additional costs and discomfort to the patient.

■ Be aware of the time the patient leaves on the day of the x-ray and when he or she returns so that postexamination procedures may be instituted or the regular regimen resumed.

CARDIOLOGY

The cardiology or cardiovascular department is responsible for many important tests and procedures within the hospital. Most hospitals also provide cardiac rehabilitation on an outpatient basis. Some of the important tests follow:

■ **Electrocardiogram (ECG, or EKG)**—a mechanical tracing of the heart's action made by a special machine called an *electrocardiograph*. The ECG is an important aid in the diagnosis and treatment of patients with heart disease. Electrocardiograms are usually taken at the patient's bedside with a portable unit. The routine 12-lead ECG examines the heart through 12 perspectives— a rhythm strip is 1 lead (Figs. 16.19, 16.20, and 16.21).

■ **Echocardiogram**—a picture produced by sending sound waves through the body. A routine echocardiogram includes an *Echo M-Mode,* which traces the activity and functioning of each chamber of the pericardium. *Echo-2-D* refers to a two-dimensional study and is performed with deeper ultrasound to show the valves and interior of the heart for diagnosis of abnormalities.

■ **Phonocardiogram**—a study that shows a graphic representation of a patient's heart sounds and heart murmurs.

■ **Treadmill stress test**—records the patient's heart activity while the patient's blood pressure is monitored. The electrodes attached to the patient's chest transmit the electrical activity from the heart to a monitor in the form of a heart tracing. The angle of the slant on the treadmill walker and the rate of the walk are increased to the patient's tolerance. Certain changes in the tracing on the

FIGURE 16.19

FIGURE 16.20

ECG TRACING

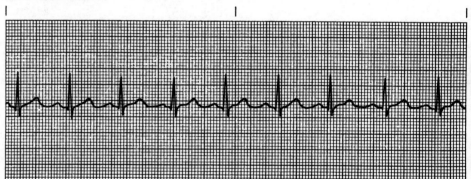

FIGURE 16.21

monitor are danger signals and that will cause the test to be discontinued. The treadmill stress test helps the physician determine the patient's tolerance to activity and aids in planning an appropriate exercise regimen (Fig. 16.22).

■ **Holter monitor**—a small device worn by the patient on the nursing unit that provides a continuous ECG recording for a prescribed amount of time (often 12 to 24 hours) while the patient goes about usual activities. Usually, three leads (small buttons) are attached to the chest, and wires are connected to the pack worn by the patient via a shoulder strap. A diary is kept by the patient during the time the Holter monitor is worn so that the physician may correlate abnormalities in the tracing with the activity of the patient at that time.

■ **Cardiac monitors**—continuous ECG tracings shown on an instrument called an *oscilloscope* or screen. In the critical or subintensive care units oscilloscopes are located at the nurses' station and in ICU and CCU at the patient's bedside as well. An ECG tracing on paper can be printed at will or will be printed automatically when abnormalities occur.

■ **Telemetry**—Patients on the nursing unit may be connected to cardiac monitors that are viewed via oscilloscopes in the ICU/CCU units. Health unit coordinators in the units often receive special training in cardiac monitoring and learn to recognize common abnormalities in the ECG tracings.

■ **Cardiac catheterization**—an invasive diagnostic procedure in which a radiopaque catheter is passed through a vein and into the heart. The catheter, because of its special coating, can be followed on a special screen (*fluoroscopy*).

FIGURE 16.22 Treadmill stress test.

Samples of blood are taken and dye may be injected for visualization of the vessels. Cardiac catheterizations are done to diagnose heart diseases or defects. This is a serious procedure and orders will include a surgical consent, careful monitoring of the vital signs, IV fluids, pressure devices to the area if an artery was entered, and permission or restriction orders regarding diet and activity. This test is done in a cardiac catheterization lab or in radiology (Fig. 16.23).

Although not "done" by the cardiology department, the following procedures affect the heart:

■ **Swan–Ganz catheter**—This procedure is highly specialized and is mentioned because of its frequent use in critical care units. The catheter is inserted into a vein called the subclavian vein and through the heart to the pulmonary

FIGURE 16.23 Cardiac catheterization laboratory.

artery. This procedure is always done by the physician. The readings obtained by the Swan–Ganz help show the function of the heart, measure the pressure within the circulatory system, and help maintain the fluid balance of the critically ill patient.

■ **Pacemaker implants**—Pacemakers are mechanical devices that automatically stimulate the heart's activity when the heart is unable to do this on its own (Fig. 16.24).

■ **Temporary pacemakers**—connected by wires that lead from the patient's body to a control apparatus.

■ **Permanent pacemakers**—implanted under the muscle of the chest surgically. A catheter leads to the heart and stimulates heart activity.

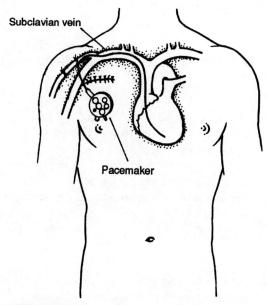

FIGURE 16.24 Pacemaker.

By far the most common test you as the health unit coordinator will order through cardiology is the ECG. The ECG is ordered at least once on the majority of adult hospitalized patients.

Health Unit Coordinator Responsibilities

Cardiology requisitions usually ask for the clinical impression or reason for the ECG. Again, this may not be the admitting diagnosis, and you must consult the nurse for this information.

Certain medications may affect the cardiologist's interpretation of the tracing. Many requisitions question medications the patient is receiving such as digitalis preparations, other heart medications, diuretics, and potassium. You should consult the nurse about these questions.

The requisition (Fig. 16.25) or computer may ask for the patient's height, weight, and blood pressure. The height and weight are taken on admission, and in some cases, the weight is measured more frequently. The blood pressure is measured at regular intervals. You will learn where to find this information.

CARDIOLOGY REQUEST

DATE FOR STUDY		TIME FOR STUDY		ROOM NO

ADMITTING DIAGNOSIS OR CLINICAL IMPRESSION

CIRCLE MEDICATIONS   DIGITALIS   PRONESTYL   INDERAL   DIURETICS   KCI   QUINIDINE

OTHER MEDICATIONS

HT: WT: BP:

SPECIAL COMMENTS OR INSTRUCTIONS:

SPECIAL PROCEDURES
PHONE SPECIAL PROCEDURES TO EXT. 183 or 184 BEFORE SENDING REQUISITION

DEPARTMENT COPY

CHECK EXAM REQUESTED

☐ TREADMILL STRESS (INCLUDES RESTING ECG)	☐ 2-D ECHOCARDIOGRAM	☐ E C G ROUTINE 12 LEAD	☐ E C G CODE BLUE RHYTHM STRIP	☐ E C G PACEMAKER EVALUATION
INSTRUCTIONS PATIENT TO BE FASTING FOR AT LEAST 6 HRS. BEFORE TEST (NO SMOKING). PATIENT SHOULD NOT RECEIVE SEDATION PRIOR TO TEST.	☐ HOLTER MONITOR	☐ E C G RHYTHM STRIP	☐ E C G TELEMETRY	☐ E C G CARDIOVERSION RHYTHM STRIP
	☐ PHONO CARDIOGRAM	MISC DESCRIPTION	DO NOT WRITE IN THIS SPACE CODE 411	PRICE OVERRIDE
	☐ TREADMILL THALLIUM		411	

FIGURE 16.25

$\mathcal{R}$ESPIRATORY THERAPY OR INHALATION THERAPY

$\mathcal{A}$DMINISTERING OXYGEN

Oxygen and other gases are used in inhalation therapy as a treatment for pulmonary (lung) difficulties. Oxygen is essential to life. When given by artificial means it can be harmful if used incorrectly, and so it must be given as prescribed by the doctor. To monitor the effectiveness of oxygen administration, special tests called **arterial blood gases (ABGs)** are often done. An oximeter measures the degree of oxygen saturation in the blood. Oxygen is most commonly administered to an adult by face mask or by nasal prongs (Fig. 16.26). Very occasionally a nasal catheter may be ordered.

FACE MASK
FIGURE 16.26

When a patient has a tracheotomy a *T-tube* or surgically designed tracheotomy mask is used. Oxygen may be administered to children by isolette, tent, or plastic hood.

Any time oxygen is being used, a card will be hung on the door stating "No Smoking—Oxygen in Use" (Fig. 16.27).

FIGURE 16.27

Oxygen is measured in liters per minute (L/min) or by percentage. Oxygen flowmeters are inserted into wall outlets in the patient's room, and oxygen is carried to the flowmeter through a central delivery system (Fig. 16.28).

FIGURE 16.28

Nasal Cannulas

Nasal cannulas, or tubes inserted into the patient's nostrils, are used to give oxygen to a patient. They are used when the patient needs extra oxygen, not when equipment must provide a patient's total supply of oxygen. The cannula, which is made of plastic, is a half-circle length of tubing with two openings in the center. It extends about half an inch into the patient's nostrils. Nasal cannulas are held in place by an elastic band around the patient's head and are connected to the source of oxygen by a length of plastic tubing (Fig. 16.29).

Nasal Cannula

FIGURE 16.29

Nasal Catheter

The nasal catheter (Fig. 16.30) is a piece of tubing that is longer than a cannula. It is inserted through the patient's nostril into the back of the mouth. The nasal catheter is a more effective but less comfortable way to give oxygen to the patient than the nasal cannula. The nasal catheter is used when the patient must have additional oxygen at all times. The nasal catheter is fastened to the patient's forehead or cheek with a piece of adhesive tape that holds it steady.

$\mathcal{R}$ ESPIRATORY EQUIPMENT

Other equipment provided by the respiratory therapy department may include the following:

- **Vaporizers**—humidifying devices with a heating element to produce steam.
- **Isolette**—a type of crib that has controlled temperature, humidity, and oxygen into which an infant is placed. An **oxygen hood** is often used with this method.
- **Humidifiers**—produce a mist that fills the patient's room and helps keep the respiratory secretions moist.
- **Nebulizers**—reduce liquids and medications to small droplets so that they will go deep into the respiratory tract. *Ultrasonic nebulizers* do this by sound vibrations. The droplets produced are smaller than those of the ordinary nebulizer and therefore provide more humidity.

NASAL CATHETER

FIGURE 16.30

- **Partial rebreathing mask**—a mask with a reservoir bag fitted tightly to the patient's face. With a prescribed flow of oxygen running, the patient rebreathes approximately 33% of the air that is expired or breathed out because of the reservoir bag.
- **Nonrebreathing mask**—similar to partial rebreathing mask but delivers a more concentrated supply of oxygen.
- **Venturi mask**—maintains a constant mixture of air and oxygen without using a reservoir bag.
- **T-tube**—a special tube attached to a tracheostomy or endotracheal tube. The air is both warmed and moistened.
- **Intermittent positive pressure breathing** (IPPB)—a machine that causes the patient to breathe more deeply, helps open the small bronchial tubes, and aids the patient to cough up sputum. Medications may be added and are nebulized by the machine.
- **Respirators or ventilators**—machines that assist patients to breathe when they are unable to do so on their own. A patient on a ventilator, will have a tube in his or her trachea (intubation or endotracheal tube or ETT) or will have a tracheostomy. The respirator is attached to the tube leading to the airway.

    Assist/control—With this setting, each time the patient inspires, he or she receives a preset machine breath.

    Control—With this setting, the respirator breathes for the patient. Therefore, the patient is ventilated regardless of respiratory effort.

- **Positive end expiratory pressure (PEEP)**—therapy that is used when the patient is in serious respiratory distress as a result of some condition such as shock, prematurity, surgery, or trauma, and respirations are inadequate. The patient is intubated and a respirator is attached that cycles air through the endotracheal tube. With PEEP, positive airway pressure is added to the mechanically assisted breathing. During this procedure the patient is usually sedated, and vital signs and arterial blood gases are monitored carefully.

- **Intermittent mandatory ventilator (IMV)**—a machine that gives the patient a set number of breaths at a set volume in addition to whatever spontaneous breaths are generated. If the machine is set for 5 breaths a minute and 1000 cc TV (**tidal volume** or the amount of air exchanged during a normal breathing cycle), the patient will get 5 machine breaths at 1000 cc TV in addition to their own number of breaths. The order would read IMV_5 q1h.

- **Microprocessor ventilators**—machines that offer advanced ventilation techniques such as jet ventilation and extra corporeal lung assist, which require specialized ventilation equipment.

- **Incentive spirometer (IS)**—devices designed to cause the patient to breathe deeply. After surgery, it helps the patient get rid of the anesthetic from the lungs. Patients are usually taught to use these bedside devices by the respiratory therapy department before surgery.

OTHER FUNCTIONS OF RESPIRATORY THERAPY

- **Arterial blood gases (ABGs)**—ABG samples are drawn from a patient's artery by respiratory therapy or the nurse by inserting a heparinized needle into an artery. The specimen is placed on ice and taken to the laboratory labeled with the appropriate requisition if used, and analyzed for its content of O_2 (oxygen), CO_2 (carbon dioxide), pH, pCO_2, pO_2, T_{40}, and percent of saturation.

The doctor may order ABGs on R/A (room air) on when the patient is receiving oxygen as a treatment.

The ventilator is adjusted based on the results of the arterial blood gases.

ARTERIAL BLOOD GASES

Gas	Normal Values (at Sea Level)	Critical Values
O_2 saturation	95–100%	<75%
pO_2	80–100 mm Hg	<40
pCO_2	35–45 mm Hg	<20, >60
HCO_3	21–28 mEq/L	<15, >40
pH	7.35–7.45	<7.25, >7.55

- **Chest physiotherapy** (CPT)—a procedure done to loosen secretions. The respiratory therapist cups the back (produces percussion with the hands) while the patient is placed in a position with the head lower than feet. This is called **postural drainage.** Following CPT, the patient coughs and expectorates (spits out) secretions.

■ **Suctioning**—Patients who are unable to cough and bring up their secretions or patients who are intubated or have tracheostomies may require tracheal suctioning. This is a sterile procedure often done by respiratory therapy as well as by a licensed nurse (Fig. 16.31).

RESPIRATORY THERAPY REQUEST

DOCTORS ORDER:_____

PATIENT DIAGNOSIS:_____

DO NOT WRITE BELOW THIS LINE

QTY.	TREATMENT	QTY.	TREATMENT	QTY.	TREATMENT	QTY.	TREATMENT
	I P P B		SPEC. THERP ½ HR		HEATED MIST SU		OXYGEN USE
	I P P B SET UP		VOL VENT ¼ DAY		AERSOL TREAT		OXYGEN STAND BY
	I P P B / USN		VOLUME VENT SU		ULTRASONIC NEB SET UP		OXYGEN CONNECT TUBE
	I P P B / USN SU		INC SPIROMETRY SU		ULTRASONIC NEB		OXYGEN CANNULA
	CHEST PT		INC SPIROMETRY		OXYGEN SU		OXYGEN MASK
MISC. DESCRIPTION		CODE 418	PRICE OVERRIDE	MISC. DESCRIPTION		CODE 418	PRICE OVERRIDE

RESPIRATORY THERAPY COPY / NURSING COPY

FIGURE 16.31

■ **Pulmonary function tests (PFTs)**—analyze the state of the respiratory system through a variety of different measurements. These tests may be done with or without ABGs. They include spirometry, measurement of the rate of airflow in the lungs, and calculation of lung capacities and lung volumes (Fig. 16.32).

PULMONARY FUNCTION LAB REQUEST

ROOM: _____ DATE: _____

R.N.: _____ ☐ PHONE REPORT

☐ COMPLETE PULMONARY FUNCTION TEST c̄ A B G
☐ COMPLETE PULMONARY FUNCTION TEST w/o A B G
☐ FLOW VOLUME LOOP
☐ MEDICAL SCREEN (LOOP – SPIRO – PLETHYSMOGRAPHY)
☐ SPIRO B/A BRONK
☐ SPIRO SIMPLE
☐ PREOPERATIVE PULMONARY EVALUATION (SPIRO & A B G)

☐ ARTERIAL BLOOD GAS

ROOM AIR: _____ OXYGEN _____ LITERS

VENTILATOR: _____

SKIN TEST

☐ BATTERY   ☐ HISTOPLASMOSIS
☐ P P D   ☐ CONTROL
☐ COCCIDIOIDOMYCOSIS ☐

DO NOT WRITE IN THIS BLOCK

			PRICE OVERRIDE
☐ O₂ ACID BASE MON	408	6 1 0 0 7	
☐	408		
☐ MISC.	408		

PULMONARY FUNCTION LAB REQUEST / PULMONARY FUNCTION LAB NURSING

FIGURE 16.32

$\mathscr{E}$XECUTION OF FORMS

A patient requiring therapy from one of these departments will usually need a series of appointments. You will generally be responsible for making the first appointment; later ones may be arranged by the therapist. You should be notified of all appointments so that you can keep a record of the times at which the patient will be receiving treatment.

When it is necessary that special equipment be brought from one of these departments to a patient's room, you may be expected to requisition it. When the patient no longer needs the equipment, you will call the department from which it came so that it can be returned.

Typical orders for inhalation therapy follow.

> Oxygen by nasal cannula at 4L/min
> Nasal O₂ at 2 liters/min prn
> IPPB with aerosol detergent 10 cc qid

PHYSICAL THERAPY

Orders for physical therapy treatments may be very general in nature if nursing personnel are to carry them out; they may be more specific and precise if qualified physical therapists are on hand or if special facilities are available. Examples of physical therapy orders under any of these circumstances follow.

> Teach crutch-walking.
> Measure for crutches and begin 2-point gait.
> Whirlpool bid.
> Complete passive ROM (range of motion) exercises tid.
> Start patient on walker in AM.
> Begin ADL (aid to daily living) instruction.

When an order is received for physical therapy, you will order by computer or fill out the appropriate requisition and may telephone the department. Because the patient may require a series of treatments, physical therapy will then arrange the schedule of appointments based on the frequency of the treatment ordered by the doctor (Figs. 16.33 and 16.34).

FIGURE 16.33

FIGURE 16.34 Physical therapy.

Occupational Therapy

Occupational therapy consists of directed activities, such as games and work projects. These activities aid in the treatment and rehabilitation of patients confined to the hospital. The program is adapted to suit the particular needs of each patient to provide the sort of diversion and skills that will best contribute to his or her physical and emotional progress. In this department, partially disabled patients learn to develop and explore new vocational possibilities. In many instances, the activities of the occupational therapy department are coordinated with those of the physical therapy department, so that each patient may develop his or her skills both at work and in recreation.

ENDOSCOPIES

An **endoscopy** is an examination of the body with the use of an instrument having a light source. *Flexible fiber-optic endoscopy* (FFE) describes a technique using special plastic-coated endoscopes that are easy to move around and provide excellent visualization. They can send magnified images that can be viewed on a TV screen or a camera. The scopes contain openings into which other instruments can be passed, air inflated, suction employed, and biopsies taken.

These are diagnostic procedures done by the doctor. In larger hospitals endoscopies may be done in the endoscopy department. In others (depending on the type and complexity of the endoscopy) they may be done in an examination room on the nursing unit.

Some of the common endoscopies follow.

■ **Bronchoscopy**—visualization of the bronchi. FFE makes it possible to more completely view the bronchial tree than does the rigid bronchoscope.
■ **Esophagoscopy**—visualization of the esophagus.
■ **Gastroscopy**—visualization of the stomach.

- **Esophagogastroduodenoscopy (EGD)**—visualization of the esophagus, stomach, and duodenum (first part of the small intestine) using FFE. Ulcers, origins of bleeding, tumors, esophageal varicies, and other problems can be seen.
- **Proctoscopy**—visualization of the rectum by means of a proctoscope.
- **Sigmoidoscopy**—visualization of the sigmoid portion of the large intestine by means of a sigmoidoscope.
- **Colonoscopy**—visualization of the lower intestine by FFE as far as the cecum. Biopsies are taken and polyps (growths on stems) frequently removed.
- **Cystoscopy**—visualization of the bladder.
- **Mediastinoscopy**—visualization of the organs and lymph nodes in the mediastinum (a portion of the thoracic cavity in the middle of the chest). The instrument is inserted through a small incision.
- **Hysteroscopy**—visualization of the uterus through a hysteroscope inserted through the vagina and cervix into the uterus.
- **Laparoscopy/peritonoscopy**—visualization of the inside of the abdomen or peritoneum through a small incision in the abdomen.
- **Endoscopic retrograde cannulation of the papilla of Vater (ERCP)**—visualization of the pancreatic duct and biliary tree. Fluoroscopy is used, and if stones are seen they may be withdrawn using a basket adapter following electrocauterization.
- **Arthroscopy**—visualization of the interior surface of a joint, most commonly the knee.
- **Transesophageal echocardiography (TEE)**—Following the insertion of an endoscope a high-frequency transducer is inserted into the esophagus and an ultrasound is done.

Endoscopies require a signed consent and most require some preparation prior to the procedure.

- Laxatives and enemas are ordered in preparation for examinations of the bowel.
- Because bleeding is possible, the nurse or doctor must determine if the patient is taking anticoagulants or aspirin, and prothrombin times (PTs) and/or PTTs are often ordered.
- Prior to procedures in which the endoscope enters through the mouth, the patient will be NPO.
- Sedation is often given before the procedure.

When you receive an order for an endoscopy you will Kardex, requisition if necessary in your hospital, call the appropriate department, and if the procedure is to be done on the unit, check to see what equipment must be on hand. You will stamp an endoscopy consent (Fig. 16.35) if needed and prepare it for the nurse to obtain the patient's signature. You may communicate with the diet kitchen to hold meals until further notice.

Following the endoscopy, you will transcribe any postendoscopy orders written by the doctor.

The patient will be carefully monitored by the nursing staff. Possible complications include perforation and bleeding after biopsies or because of irritation of the mucosa. A patient who has undergone a procedure in which the scope has been passed through the mouth will not be allowed food or fluid until his or her gag reflex has returned (about 2 hours) because the throat was anesthetized.

MEMORIAL HOSPITAL

1. I, _____ , hereby request and authorize
_____ , M.D. and such assistants as may participate
with her/him for the following procedure (s): _____
_____

2. The nature and purpose of the procedure, the risks involved and the possibility of complications, possible perforation, hemorrhage, infection or drug reactions and even death, have been explained to my satisfaction by my Physician.

3. I consent to the administration of such sedatives and other medications as may be necessary or advisable by the Physician responsible for this service.

4. The hospital Pathologist is hereby authorized to use his/her discretion in disposition of any tissue or foreign body removed from my person during the above-named procedure(s).

5. I hereby authorize Memorial Hospital to undertake its appropriate hospital service and care necessary in conjunction with the procedure which I have asked my Physician and assistants to undertake in their efforts to alleviate my condition(s).

6. Permission is given to the above named hospital and the attending Physician to photograph or permit other persons to photograph during the surgical process as the Physician may deem necessary.

_____   _____
Date   **Signature of Patient**

_____   _____
Time   **(Witness)**

If patient is unable to sign or is a minor, complete the following:

(a) Patient is a minor of _____ years of age.

(b) Patient is unable to sign because _____
_____

I certify that I have informed the patient of the purpose, procedure, and potential risks and complications of the above mentioned endoscopic procedure(s).

_____
Signature of Physician

MEMORIAL HOSPITAL

ENDOSCOPY CONSENT

FIGURE 16.35

*E*LECTROENCEPHALOGRAPHY (EEG)

Electroencephalography is the process of recording brain-wave activity. Sixteen or more electrodes are attached to various places on the patient's scalp and a recording is made of the electrical activity within the brain (Fig. 16.36). EEG is used to help diagnose seizure disorders, to detect brain lesions, trauma, cerebral blood flow during surgery, drug intoxication, and brain death.

EEG TRACING

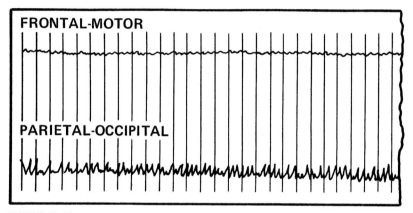

FIGURE 16.36

Prior to the test the patient should not have caffeine for 24 hours. The physician may withhold medications before the test. If the patient does take medication, the technician should be informed.

During the procedure, the patient remains quiet with the eyes closed. If being evaluated for seizure disorders, the patient will have been deprived of sleep, and then the EEG will be taken during sleep (which sometimes must be achieved by sedation). The procedure takes an hour or longer if the sleep study is done and does not cause pain. Your instructor will describe your hospital's method for ordering EEGs.

*E*LECTROMYOGRAPHY (EMG)

Electromyography is used to detect muscle disorders due to nervous and other system disease. A recording electrode (needle) is inserted into the muscle that is to be studied, and a reference electrode is placed on the skin. The EMG monitors the electrical activity of the muscle, which is displayed on an oscilloscope in a way similar to an electrocardiogram. The study is done in the EMG laboratory.

*T*HE DIETARY DEPARTMENT
*R*EGULAR AND SPECIAL DIETS

Eating properly is very important when a person is healthy and feeling well. Good nourishment is even more important when a person is ill. The food service department or dietary department in your institution prepares a well-balanced diet of nourishing meals for many different patients. This basic balanced diet is often called by different names:

- Normal diet
- Regular diet
- House diet
- Full diet

A well-balanced diet is one that contains a variety of foods from each of the four basic food groups at every meal.

The normal diet is sometimes changed to meet a patient's special nutritional needs. This modified diet is also known by several names:

- Special diet
- Restricted diet
- Modified diet
- Therapeutic diet

Therapeutic Diets

Therapeutic diets require the preparation of meals that differ from those regularly prepared for patients on the normal diet (Table 16.6). The special meals given to patients who cannot be on a normal diet are ordered by the doctor. They are planned by the dietitian according to the patient's illness and what is needed for his or her recovery. These special meals help the doctor in treating a patient. For example, a patient who has a disorder of the digestive system may be on a soft diet. A diabetic patient may be on a diet in which total calories are limited and the amounts of protein, fat, and carbohydrates are specified. A person with heart disease may be restricted to a low-salt (sodium) diet or a salt-free diet. The doctor may order changes in the normal diet for several reasons; including the following:

- To change the consistency of the patient's food, as in liquid or soft diets
- To change the caloric intake, as in high- or low-calorie diets
- To change the amounts of one or more nutrients, as in a high-protein, low-fat, or low-salt (sodium) diet
- To change the amount of bulk, as in a low-residue diet
- To change the seasonings in the patient's food, as in a bland diet
- To omit foods to which the patient is allergic
- To change the time and number of meals

Whenever the word *salt* is used it means "sodium," and when *sodium* is used it means "salt." Therefore, when we refer to a salt-free diet we mean a sodium-free diet, and when we refer to a low-sodium diet we mean a low-salt diet.

*A*DA OR AMERICAN DIABETIC ASSOCIATION DIETS

There are diets for diabetics that have been jointly agreed on by the American Diabetes Association and the American Dietetic Association. Hospitals purchase booklets from the ADA that contain exchange lists for diabetics based on the number of calories and amounts of carbohydrates, proteins, and fats the physician prescribes.

TABLE 16.6	$\mathcal{T}$YPES OF DIETS GIVEN TO PATIENTS	
Type of Diet	**Description**	**Common Purpose**
Normal regular	Provides all essentials of good nourishment in normal forms	For patients who do not need special diets
Clear liquid (surgical/liquid)	Broth, tea, ginger ale, gelatin	Usually for patients who have had surgery or are very ill
Full liquid (medical liquid)	Broth, tea, coffee, ginger ale, gelatin, strained fruit juices, liquids, custard, junket, ice cream, sherbet, soft-cooked eggs	For those unable to chew or swallow solid food
Light or soft	Foods soft in consistency, no rich or strongly flavored foods that could cause distress	Final stage for postoperative patient before resuming regular diet
Soft (mechanical)	Same foods as on a normal diet, but chopped or strained	For patients who have difficulty in chewing or swallowing
Bland	Foods mild in flavor and easy to digest; omits spicy foods, alcohol, coffee, tea	Avoids irritation of the digestive tract, as with ulcer and colitis patients
Low residue	Foods low in bulk; omits foods difficult to digest	Spares the lower digestive tract, as with patients having rectal diseases
High calorie	Foods high in protein, minerals, and vitamins	For underweight or malnourished patients
Low calorie	Low in cream, butter, cereals, desserts, and fats	For patients who need to lose weight
Diabetic (see ADA)	Precise balance of carbohydrates, protein, and fats, devised according to the needs of individual patients	For diabetic patients; matches food intake with the insulin and nutritional requirements
High protein	Meals supplemented with high-protein foods, such as meat, fish, cheese, milk, and eggs	Assists in the growth and repair of tissues wasted by disease
Low fat	Limited amounts of butter, cream, fats, and eggs	For patients who have difficulty digesting fats, as in gallbladder and liver disturbances
Low cholesterol	Low in eggs, whole milk, and meats	Helps regulate the amount of cholesterol in the blood
Low sodium (low salt)	Limited amount of foods containing sodium, no salt allowed on tray	For patients whose circulation would be impaired by fluid retention; patients with certain heart or kidney conditions

The six exchange lists or groups are milk, vegetables, fruits, starch, meat and meat substitutes, and fats. Foods in the same exchange list are interchangeable.

$\mathcal{T}$UBE FEEDINGS

A **tube feeding** is the administration of nutritionally balanced liquefied foods through a tube inserted into the stomach or duodenum, either by a tube passed through the nose (nasogastric or NG tube) or through one placed in the stomach in surgery—a gastrostomy tube.

The physician orders the number of calories, the amount of fluid over 24 hours, and the frequency of the feedings. The dietitian then prepares and blenderizes the feedings, which are sent to the nursing unit for administration.

Commercially prepared feedings may also be ordered. Ensure® is a brand name for a frequently ordered lactose-free nutritional supplement containing protein, carbohydrate, fat, vitamins, and minerals. Ensure Plus® is also available and has a higher caloric content (Fig. 16.37).

FIGURE 16.37A Gastrostomy tube feeding.

FIGURE 16.37B Gastrostomy tube.

𝒜 WELL-BALANCED DIET

The key to a healthful, well-balanced diet lies in eating a variety of foods and in no▮ eating too much. The foods that are essential for keeping the body well are divided intc six groups. Everybody needs the nutrients contained in all six groups. The number o▮ servings and the size of portions will depend on the age, size, and activities of the in- dividual. Following are the six basic food groups, along with suggestions for a goo▮

diet for the average person. Check your own eating habits to be sure you are eating a well-balanced diet (Fig. 16.38).

The food group pyramid is divided into six categories:

- **Dairy Products.** Milk or milk products are needed to supply protein, calcium, and other minerals, and to supply vitamins and carbohydrates. Every day a small child should have at least three to four 8-ounce glasses of milk. A teenager should have four or more glasses. An adult should have a glass or two daily, but pregnant women and nursing mothers need milk in greater quantity. Other acceptable forms of milk and milk products include concentrated, evaporated, skim, and dry milk, yogurt, buttermilk, and cream.

- **Vegetables.** Three to five servings from this group are needed every day to supply an adequate amount of certain vitamins and minerals and to provide roughage. At least four meals a week should include a dark green or yellow vegetable for vitamin A.

- **Fruits.** The U.S. Department of Agriculture (USDA) recommends at least three to five servings a day from this group. One of the servings should be from the citrus fruits—oranges, lemons, grapefruit—that are high in vitamin C.

- **Meat and Meat Substitutes.** These include meat, fish, poultry, eggs, cheese, dried beans, peas, and nuts. Two to three servings daily from this group are recommended for a good diet. At least one serving should be meat, fish, or poultry. One serving might be an egg, a slice of cheese, or a small serving of split peas or baked beans.

- **Breads, Cereals, Rice, and Grains.** Whole-grain or enriched bread and cereals are necessary for the body's nutrition because they provide carbohydrates

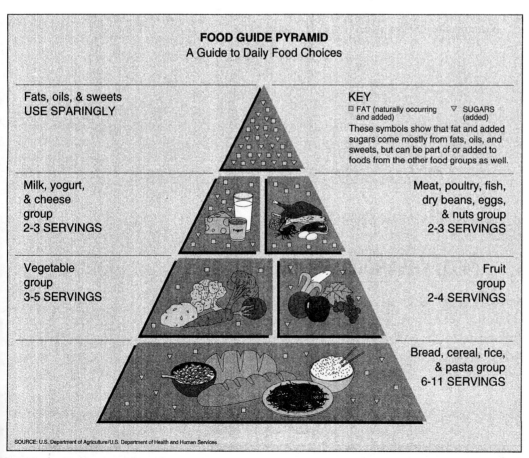

FIGURE 16.38 The food pyramid.

for energy. The USDA recommends six to eleven servings every day from this group.

■ **Fats and Oils, Sweets**—Should be used sparingly because of the high fat content and low nutritional value. They include butter, salad dressings, and desserts.

WHAT ARE NUTRIENTS?

Food is able to give nourishment to the body because it contains various chemical substances called **nutrients.** Some 50 individual **nutrients** are needed to build the body. Many others are useful although they may not be required. Scientists also have discovered that nutrients work better together than alone. For instance, you may get enough calcium from milk but it is wasted if you do not get enough vitamin C or D from other foods to help the calcium develop the bones.

Many foods we eat contain combinations of various nutrients that are responsible for body functions. For example, whole-grain cereals are high in carbohydrates, but they also contain some protein, minerals, and vitamins. Foods help the body perform its functions only if they contain the right nutrients.

How Nutrients Are Made

The first step in making nutrients takes place in green plants. They take water and minerals from the soil, and water and carbon dioxide from the air, and with the help of the sun's energy, turn these substances into nutrients.

How Nutrients Are Used

When people eat plants they get the nutrients from them. Also, when people eat meat they get the nutrients animals have taken from green plants and other food.

After food is eaten it enters the digestive tract where the nutrients are changed into simple forms. These simple forms then are transported by the blood to the body cells where the special functions of each are carried out.

There are five classes of nutrients: carbohydrates, fats, minerals, proteins, and vitamins. Water, although not a nutrient, is essential for the proper functioning of all the body's processes. Because there are several kinds of each class of nutrients, it is clearer to speak of the classes instead of the individual nutrients. Figure 16.39 gives a brief description of each nutrient class and its importance to the body.

EXECUTION OF FORMS

General Information

As a health unit coordinator you will notify the dietary department of the number and kinds of meals needed on your unit. You may also see to it that supplies of supplemental nourishments are stocked. Remember, however, that your first concern is to ensure that each patient's meal has been ordered. Being overlooked when meals are delivered is depressing and uncomfortable for any patient. Therefore, when a newly admitted patient arrives, or when a dietary change is ordered for a patient, you must notify the dietary department in plenty of time to make sure that the patient will receive the next meal. Although all dietary requests must be made by computer or requisition, you may find it necessary to call the dietary department; telephone if there is a possibility that the written request may be received too late.

Some typical forms used by many hospitals for requisitioning food from the dietary department are included in this chapter. Your instructor will show you samples of the forms used in your hospitals. It is likely this function will be done by computer

NUTRIENT CLASS	BODILY FUNCTIONS	FOOD SOURCES
CARBOHYDRATES	Provides work energy for body activities, and heat energy for maintenance of body temperature.	Cereal grains and their products (bread, breakfast cereals, macaroni products), potatoes, sugar, syrups, fruits, milk, vegetables, nuts
PROTEINS	Build and renew body tissues; regulate body functions and supply energy. Complete proteins: maintain life and provide growth. Incomplete proteins: maintain life but do not provide for growth.	Complete proteins: Derived from animal foods — meat, milk, eggs, fish, cheese, poultry. Incomplete proteins: Derived from vegetable foods — soybeans, dry beans, peas, some nuts and whole-grain products.
FATS	Give work energy for body activities and heat energy for maintenance of body temperature. Carrier of vitamins A and D, provide fatty acids necessary for growth and maintenance of body tissues.	Some foods are chiefly fat, such as lard, vegetable fats and oils, and butter. Many other foods contain smaller proportions of fats — nuts, meats, fish, poultry, cream, whole milk.
MINERALS Calcium	Builds and renews bones, teeth, and other tissues; regulates the activity of the muscles, heart, nerves; and controls the clotting of blood.	Milk and milk products, except butter; most dark green vegetables; canned salmon.
Phosphorus	Associated with calcium in some functions needed to build and renew bones and teeth. Influences the oxidation of foods in the body cells; important in nerve tissue.	Widely distributed in foods; especially cheese, oat cereals, whole-wheat products, dry beans and peas, meat, fish, poultry, nuts.

NUTRIENT CLASS	BODILY FUNCTIONS	FOOD SOURCES
MINERALS (continued) Iron	Builds and renews hemoglobin, the red pigment in blood that carries oxygen from the lungs to the cells.	Eggs, meat, especially liver and kidney; deep-yellow and dark green vegetables; potatoes, dried fruits, whole-grain products; enriched flour, bread, breakfast cereals.
Iodine	Enables the thyroid gland to perform its function of controlling the rate at which foods are oxidized in the cells.	Fish (obtained from the sea), some plant foods grown in soils containing iodine; table salt fortified with iodine (iodized).
VITAMINS A	Necessary for normal functioning of the eyes, prevents night blindness. Ensures a healthy condition of the skin, hair, and mucous membranes. Maintains a state of resistance to infections of the eyes, mouth, and respiratory tract.	One form of Vitamin A is yellow and one form is colorless. Apricots, cantaloupe, milk, cheese, eggs, meat organs, (especially liver and kidney), fortified margarine, butter, fish-liver oils, dark green and deep yellow vegetables.
B Complex B₁ (Thiamine)	Maintains a healthy condition of the nerves. Fosters a good appetite. Helps the body cells use carbohydrates.	Whole-grain and enriched grain products; meats (especially pork, liver and kidney). dry beans and peas.
B₂ (Riboflavin)	Keeps the skin, mouth, and eyes in a healthy condition. Acts with other nutrients to form enzymes and control oxidation in cells.	Milk, cheese, eggs, meat (especially liver and kidney), whole grain and enriched grain products, dark green vegetables.

NUTRIENT CLASS	BODILY FUNCTIONS	FOOD SOURCES
VITAMINS (Continued) Niacin	Influences the oxidation of carbohydrates and proteins in the body cells.	Liver, meat, fish, poultry, eggs, peanuts; dark green vegetables, whole-grain and enriched cereal products.
B₁₂	Regulates specific processes in digestion. Helps maintain normal functions of muscles, nerves, heart, blood — general body metabolism.	Liver, other organ meats, cheese, eggs, milk
C (Ascorbic Acid)	Acts as a cement between body cells, and helps them work together to carry out their special functions. Maintains a sound condition of bones, teeth, and gums. Not stored in the body.	Fresh, raw citrus fruits and vegetables — oranges, grapefruit, cantaloupe, strawberries, tomatoes, raw onions, cabbage, green and sweet red peppers, dark green vegetables.
D	Enables the growing body to use calcium and phosphorus in a normal way to build bones and teeth.	Provided by Vitamin D fortification of certain foods, such as milk and margarine. Also fish-liver oils and eggs. Sunshine is also a source of Vitamin D.
WATER	Regulates body processes. Aids in regulating body temperature. Carries nutrients to body cells and carries waste products away from them. Helps to lubricate joints. Water has no food value, although most water contains mineral elements. More immediately necessary to life than food — second only to oxygen.	Drinking water, and other beverages; all foods except those made up of a single nutrient, as sugar and some fats. Milk milk drinks, soups, vegetables, fruit juices. Ice cream, watermelon, strawberries, lettuce, tomatoes, cereals, other dry products.

FIGURE 16.39 How nutrients are used.

Diet Request

The diet request form is filled out for each patient soon after admission. It requests the kitchen to add a tray for the patient at the next meal and also indicates the type of diet required (Fig. 16.40).

```
                         DIET CARD

PATIENT'S NAME       George Thompson

ROOM NO.        437          FLOOR    2E

DIET                 Normal

NURSE                            DATE  11/20/XX
                  H. Brown HUC
```

FIGURE 16.40

Diet Change

Diet changes occur often in hospitals. Diets are canceled when a patient is discharged or expires. In all cases, dietary must be notified either by written notice or by computer. For example, a patient may have been on a normal diet before surgery, but after surgery he will need a postoperative diet, or the condition of a patient on a special diet may improve to the extent that she can resume a normal diet.

Stock Nourishments

Included on this form are all the standard nourishments routinely kept in supply in the unit. It may be your responsibility to check these supplies to see when reordering is necessary. In some hospitals, however, dietary personnel check and restock the supplies themselves.

Individual Patient Nourishments

This requisition is used to order special foods not included in the stock nourishments but required for a particular patient (Fig. 16.41).

```
              MISCELLANEOUS REQUISITION

ARTICLE DESIRED      Flavored Gelatin
PATIENT'S NAME       George Thompson
ROOM NO.             437
FLOOR                2E
DATE                 11/20/XX

              SIGNED   H Brown HUC
```

FIGURE 16.41

Extra Meals for Guests

This requisition is used for ordering an extra meal so that a friend or family member may eat with a patient. This form must usually be made out in duplicate; one copy is sent to the kitchen, the other to the cashier so that the meal can be charged to the patient's account (Fig. 16.42).

```
        REQUISITION FOR GUEST TRAY
DATE    11/14/XX    FLOOR  2E   ROOM NO. 437
ORDER TO BE BILLED TO:     George Thompson

   BREAKFAST
  ( DINNER )
   SUPPER                    H Brown HUC

   FLOOR NURSE         _____
   O.K'D BY HEAD NURSE _____

      SEND DUPLICATE SLIP TO CASHIER'S OFFICE.
      SEND FIRST COPY TO DIET KITCHEN.
```

FIGURE 16.42

*L*EARNING ACTIVITIES

*L*ABORATORY

Complete the following.

1. The division of the laboratory that analyzes the blood for its basic physical properties is _____.

2. The division that analyzes body fluids for chemical constituents is _____ _____.

3. The section concerned primarily with tests designed to isolate and identify disease-causing microorganisms is _____ _____.

4. The division that studies cells obtained from body tissues is _____ _____.

5. The urinalysis is often done by the _____ division of the laboratory, although it is not a blood test.

6. A urinalysis consists of a _____, _____, and _____ examination of the urine.

7. Urine specimens are obtained by _____, not by the laboratory.

8. When you receive an order for a Ua (urinalysis), what will you do?

_____

_____

_____

_____

9. How would you handle an order for a 24° urine?

_____

_____

_____

_____

10. List some of the responsibilities of the blood bank.
    (a) _____
    (b) _____
    (c) _____
    (d) _____

11. What is the purpose of crossmatching?

_____

_____

_____

_____

12. What is the purpose of blood typing?

_____

_____

_____

_____

13. List your greatest concerns regarding laboratory tests.
    (a) _____
    (b) _____
    (c) _____
    (d) _____

14. How would you handle a telephone laboratory report?

_____

_____

_____

_____

_____

15. What are critical values?

_____

_____

16. What is meant by POC testing?

_____

_____

_____

_____

Match the name of the hematology test or abbreviation in Column A with its definition in Column B.

Column A

(a) ESR
(b) Hct
(c) ANA
(d) APTT
(e) Bleeding time
(f) Hgb
(g) Reticulocytes
(h) RBC Indices
(i) Differential

Column B

_____ Measurement of the time it takes a fingerstick wound to cease bleeding

_____ Examination of the different kinds of WBCs

_____ Count of immature red blood cells

_____ Measures hemoglobin—the oxygen-carrying portion of the blood

_____ Measurements reported as MCH, MCHC, and MCV

_____ Diagnostic study for lupus erythematosus

_____ Determines rate at which RBCs settle out of liquid portion of blood; used to determine progress of inflammatory diseases

_____ A coagulation study

_____ Measurement of the volume percentage of erythrocytes in whole blood

Match the chemistry study term in Column A with its definition in Column B.

Column A

(a) Uric acid
(b) GTT
(c) Creatinine
(d) BUN
(e) Acid phosphatase
(f) Na, K, Cl, CO_2
(g) FBS
(h) AST, LDH, CPK
(i) Bilirubin
(j) SMA_{12-20}
(k) PP BS
(l) ELISA
(m) Western blot test

Column B

_____ Determines amount of sugar in the bloodstream after the patient has fasted

_____ Used in diagnosis of metastatic carcinoma of the prostate gland

_____ Test that detects HIV antibodies

_____ Chem screen

_____ Measures liver function

_____ Electrolytes

_____ Measures blood sugar *after* eating

_____ Blood test for kidney function

_____ Confirmatory test for HIV

_____ Cardiac enzymes

_____ Used principally to diagnose gout

_____ Done over several hours to measure glucose in urine and blood

_____ Increased quantities are found in advanced stages of kidney disease

Match the term in Column A with its definition in Column B.

Column A

(a) Biopsy

(b) Postprandial

(c) Cytology

(d) Differential

(e) Erythrocyte

(f) Mycology

(g) Paracentesis

(h) Serology

(i) Lumbar puncture

(j) Sternal puncture

(k) Electrolytes

(l) Virology

Column B

_____ The study of viruses and the diseases caused by them

_____ The removal of cerebrospinal fluid from the spinal canal

_____ Those body substances that help maintain a balance between acidity and alkalinity

_____ Tissue removed from a living body for examination

_____ The study of fungi that cause disease

_____ Removal of bone marrow from the breastbone cavity for diagnostic purposes

_____ After eating

_____ The study of blood serum for diseases such as syphilis

_____ Identification of the type of WBCs found in the blood

_____ The study of cells

_____ The puncture and drainage of a body cavity

_____ Red blood cell

Multiple Choice

1. A culture and sensitivity would be performed by which laboratory division?
   (a) Hematology
   (b) Biochemistry
   (c) Serology
   (d) Bacteriology

2. Histology means:
   (a) Study of blood
   (b) Study of cells
   (c) Study of tissues
   (d) Study of bacteria

3. A routine CBC would *not* include which of the following:
   (a) RBCs
   (b) WBCs
   (c) Platelets
   (d) Potassium

4. The greatest precautions for preventing contamination of urine may be taken by obtaining which kind of specimen?
   (a) Clean catch
   (b) Catheterized
   (c) Voided
   (d) Midstream

5. Lymphocytes are a type of:
   (a) Erythrocyte
   (b) Platelet
   (c) Reticulocyte
   (d) Leukocyte

6. An abnormal formation of fluid in the abdominal cavity is called:
   (a) CSF
   (b) Guaiac
   (c) Ascites
   (d) Urea

RADIOLOGY

Complete the following.

1. List the three major divisions of radiology.
   (a) _____
   (b) _____
   (c) _____

2. Preparations of patients who are to receive x-rays utilizing contrast media may include:
   (a) _____
   (b) _____
   (c) _____
   (d) _____

3. Why do many hospitals require that the health unit coordinator also telephone radiology with the order in addition to sending a requisition?
   _____
   _____
   _____
   _____

4. Why do many radiology requisitions have a space for the health unit coordinator to record the clinical problem? _____
   _____
   _____
   _____

5. Why must the health unit coordinator be aware of the time a patient leaves for radiology and when he or she returns? _____
   _____
   _____
   _____

6. Give the abbreviation and meaning of each of the following x-rays.

	Abbreviation	**Meaning**
(a) Barium enema	_____	_____
(b) Gastrointestinal series	_____	_____
(c) Gallbladder series	_____	_____
(d) Intravenous pyelogram	_____	_____

7. A barium enema, gastrointestinal series, gallbladder series, and intravenous pyelogram must be done in the sequence _____
   _____

Match the term in Column A with its definition in Column B.

Column A

(a) Thermogram
(b) Ultrasound
(c) Xerogram
(d) Tomogram
(e) Contrast media
(f) Angiogram
(g) Myelogram
(h) Scan
(i) Arteriogram
(j) Fluoroscopy
(k) Sialogram

Column B

_____ Substances introduced into the body that permit the radiologist to distinguish between different body densities

_____ Photograph of body surface temperature based on infrared radiation given off by body

_____ X-ray of vascular structures

_____ X-ray of salivary ducts

_____ Technique that utilizes photocopy paper instead of x-ray film to record pictures of soft body tissue

_____ The visible observation of internal structures "in action"

_____ Process of recording echoes of sound waves striking body tissues of different densities

_____ X-ray of arteries

_____ X-ray that studies selected levels of body

_____ X-ray of spinal cord after injection of contrast medium into spinal canal

_____ Picture produced by concentration of radionuclides in a specific organ

8. Define the following.
   (a) PEEP _____
   (b) Doppler _____
   (c) MRI _____
   (d) FFE _____
   (e) EGD _____

CARDIOLOGY

Complete the following.

1. The most common test the health unit coordinator will order through cardiology is the _____.

2. Where is the ECG or EKG usually taken? In the patient's room or in the department? _____

3. List the types of medications that may need to be included in the cardiology requisition.
   (a) _____
   (b) _____
   (c) _____
   (d) _____

4. List other information frequently requested on the cardiology requisition.
   (a) _____
   (b) _____
   (c) _____
   (d) _____

Match the term in Column A with its definition in Column B.

Column A

(a) Treadmill stress test
(b) Echocardiogram
(c) Holter monitor
(d) Swan–Ganz catheter
(e) Cardiac pacemaker
(f) Electrocardiogram
(g) Rhythm strip

Column B

_____ Small portable device worn by patient that provides a continuous ECG recording while the patient goes about usual activities

_____ Tracing of electrical activity of the heart

_____ Usually taken to establish regularity of heartbeat on one lead

_____ Catheter inserted by physician into pulmonary artery to measure pressure in circulatory system

_____ Measures heart's ability to tolerate increased activity

_____ Produced by sending sound waves through the body

_____ Mechanical device to stimulate heart activity

RESPIRATORY OR INHALATION THERAPY

Complete the following.

1. Oxygen is measured in _____ or _____.

2. List several different ways in which oxygen is administered.
   (a) _____
   (b) _____
   (c) _____
   (d) _____

3. What is a common method of letting others know, as a safety precaution, that oxygen is in use?

   _____
   _____
   _____

4. Machines that assist the patient to breathe when he is unable to do so on his own are called _____ or _____.

5. IPPB is the abbreviation for _____.

6. The machine that gives the patient a set number of breaths at a set volume in addition to whatever spontaneous breaths she can generate is the _____
   _____.

7. Patients are usually taught to use these bedside devices before surgery:
   _____

8. Percussion of the back to loosen secretions is called _____
   _____.

9. Tests that measure the state of the respiratory system are called _____
   _____ tests.

10. Samples drawn from arteries and analyzed by respiratory therapy are called
    _____.

11. Interpret the following orders:
(a) O_2 @ 6L/M _____
(b) IPPB qid _____
(c) IMV_2 q1h _____
(d) ABGs on R/A _____
(e) CPT qid _____

12. A patient requiring treatment from inhalation therapy will usually need a series of _____.

PHYSICAL THERAPY

Complete the following.

1. Physical therapy includes the use of
(a) _____
(b) _____
(c) _____
(d) _____
(e) _____
(f) _____
(g) _____

2. The physical therapy department will ordinarily have equipment such as
(a) _____
(b) _____
(c) _____
(d) _____
(e) _____
(f) _____

3. Through instruction and supervised practice, trained physical therapists help patients _____
_____.

OCCUPATIONAL THERAPY

1. Describe your understanding of the purpose of occupational therapy.
_____
_____
_____
_____
_____

ENDOSCOPIES

Complete the following.

1. An endoscopy is _____
_____

2. Endo means _____

3. -scopy means _____

4. Most endoscopies require a signed _____, and some require _____ prior to the procedure.

5. A patient who has undergone an examination of the upper gastorintestinal tract will not be fed until _____.

Match the type of endoscopy in Column A with its description in Column B.

Column A

Column B

(a)   Esophagoscopy
(b)   Sigmoidoscopy
(c)   Gastroscopy
(d)   Proctoscopy
(e)   Bronchoscopy

_____ Visualization of the bronchi through the mouth
_____ Visualization of the stomach
_____ Visualization of the sigmoid portion of the large intestine through the anus
_____ Visualization of the esophagus through the mouth
_____ Visualization of the rectum

*E*LECTROENCEPHALOGRAPHY

Complete the following.

1. The abbreviation for electroencephalogram is _____.

2. An electroencephalogram is a _____
_____.

*D*IETARY

1. Label each of the pictures in the food group pyramid with the food group listed here that it represents:
Dairy Products
Vegetables
Fruit
Meat and Meat Substitutes
Breads, Cereals, Rice, and Grains
Fats, Oils, and Sweets

2. Beside each of the following foods write the *letter* or *letters* of the food group to which it belongs:
D—Dairy Products
V—Vegetables
F—Fruits
M—Meat and Meat Substitutes
B—Breads, Cereals, Rice, and Grains
O—Fats, Oil, and Sweets

1. Peas _____

2. Onions _____

3. Milk _____

4. Macaroni _____

5. Broccoli _____

6. Rice _____

7. Bread _____

8. Dried beans _____

9. Yogurt _____

10. Cake _____

11. Nuts _____

12. Carrots _____

13. Potatoes _____

14. Cheese _____

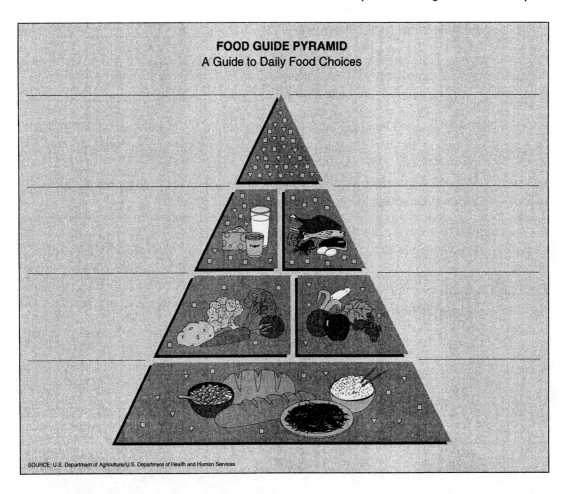

FOOD GUIDE PYRAMID
A Guide to Daily Food Choices

SOURCE: U.S. Department of Agriculture/U.S. Department of Health and Human Services

Complete the following.

1. Various chemical substances that give nourishment to the body are called

_____.

2. The process of taking food into the body to maintain life is referred to as

_____.

3. _____ diets help the doctor in treating a patient.

4. A diet containing a variety of foods from each of the basic food groups is called a _____-_____   _____.

Match the type of diet in Column A with its description in Column B.

Column A

(a) Bland
(b) Regular
(c) Soft
(d) Low residue
(e) Clear liquid
(f) Low fat
(g) Diabetic
(h) Sodium free

Column B

____ For patients who have difficulty chewing
____ For patients whose illness would be compounded by fluid retention
____ Broth, tea, gingerale, gelatin
____ For patients who are underweight or malnourished
____ Series of diets mild in flavor and easy to digest; omits spicy foods
____ Provides all essentials of good nourishment

Column A   **Column B**

(i)   High calorie   _____ Helps the growth and repair of tissues impaired by disease
(j)   High protein   _____ Foods low in bulk; omits foods difficult to digest
                       _____ Eliminates foods which would cause difficulty in digestion
                             as with gallbladder patients
                       _____ Precise balance of carbohydrates, protein, and fats planned
                             according to needs of individual patient

COMPUTER EXERCISE

Go to a web site such as MedicineNet.com. Click on Procedures & Tests. Choose 10 procedures (perhaps ones not discussed in this chapter). List the tests you researched below and their purpose, and be prepared to discuss with the class what you learned.

Test   **Purpose**

1. _____   _____
2. _____   _____
3. _____   _____
4. _____   _____
5. _____   _____
6. _____   _____
7. _____   _____
8. _____   _____
9. _____   _____
10. _____   _____

Complete the following.

1. What should you do if you find out that a patient who was supposed to be fasting for blood work ate his breakfast? _____
   _____
   _____

2. What is the same and what is different about an order for a CBC and a sputum specimen? _____
   _____
   _____

3. The orders on a new patient read "bld. culture stat. Give tetracycline 500 mg. Q4h." How should these orders be handled? _____
   _____

4. How is a 24-hr urine different from a routine Ua? _____
   _____

5. If you ever have to handle a laboratory specimen that is not already in a protective bag, why should you first put on gloves? _____
   _____

6. The order reads "2 hr PPBS." Other than the usual ordering process, what else will the laboratory need to know? When will they be notified?

_____

_____

_____

7. The order reads "blood culture × 3 when temp > 103." Why does this order require extra attention? What could interfere with the proper execution of this order? _____

_____

_____

_____

8. What mistakes could interfere with any of the tests in this chapter? List as many as you can think of. _____

_____

_____

_____

_____

_____

_____

9. If errors in ordering or in patient preparation occur, how will this affect the patient? How would you feel if someone made a mistake on an order for you or your loved ones? _____

_____

_____

_____

_____

_____

_____

10. If the laboratory calls with a critical value, describe how you will handle the situation. _____

_____

11. Patients often leave the floor for diagnostic and therapeutic procedures. How can you learn how long patients are usually gone for these procedures? Why do you need to know? What might delay a patient in another department longer than anticipated? _____

_____

_____

_____

_____

_____

12. You are asked by a nurse to transport a patient with IVs on a gurney to radiology because the floor is short-staffed. Why is this a problem? What might happen? What should you say to the nurse? Are there ever circumstances under which you, as an HUC with only unit coordinator education and not nursing assisting background, should assist with patient care? If no, why not? If yes, under what circumstances? _____

_____

_____

_____

_____

_____

_____

13. Answer the following by circling the correct answer.
  (a) Which is a blood test?
       (1) sed. rate   (2) AP & Lat Chest   (3) gastroscopy   (4) IVP
  (b) Which is a cardiology test?
       (1) PSA   (2) CPT   (3) Holter monitor   (4) liver scan
  (c) Which is an ultrasound?
       (1) upper GI   (2) chest sonogram   (3) Hubbard tank   (4) FBS
  (d) Which is an x-ray?
       (1) IPPB   (2) ELISA   (3) APPT   (4) BE
  (e) Which is a microbiology test?
       (1) PFT   (2) C&S   (3) LP   (4) MRI

CHAPTER 17

Health Unit Coordinator Procedures

Admission Set of procedures that provides a hospital bed for a patient who requires care for more than 24 hours

AMA discharge Departure from the hospital by a patient against medical advice

Autopsy The dissection of a corpse

Critical Pathways A plan developed by nursing on admission to provide for optimum consistency of patient care in difficult and complicated cases

Discharge Set of procedures that officially releases a patient from the hospital

Discharge Summary A chart form that must be completed by the physician when a patient is discharged

Intraoperative Period during the operation

Medical short stay Care given for less than 24 hours to a patient who would otherwise be admitted to the hospital

PACU Area where patients are taken after surgery to recover from the anesthesia; the recovery room

Postmortem care Procedures carried out after a patient has died

Postoperative After the operation

Preoperative Before the operation

Transfer A set of procedures that moves a patient from one bed to another, from one unit to another, or from one hospital to another

Transition Change

Valuables envelope A special envelope for a patient's valuables such as money and jewelry that is locked in the hospital safe for safekeeping

When you have completed this chapter, you will be able to:

Define the terms listed in the vocabulary.

Discuss the health unit coordinator's responsibilities as they relate to the following hospital procedures:

- Admissions
- Transfers
- Discharges
- Deaths
- The Surgical Patient

ADMISSIONS

A patient coming into a hospital is often frightened and uncomfortable and may or may not be seriously ill or in pain. This is a time when the health unit coordinator is very important to the patient. Being pleasant and courteous will make the patient's arrival easier for him or her. A warm welcome will create a favorable impression.

Introduce yourself. Learn the patient's name and use it often. Remember that the way you speak and behave will have a lot to do with the patient's impression of the institution. Smile, be friendly. Do not appear to be rushed or busy with other things.

As you efficiently perform your tasks as a health unit coordinator you can do much to facilitate a smoother transition for patients as they begin their stay in your hospital (Fig. 17.1).

There are two types of patient *admissions:*

1. Routine admissions that have been planned.
2. Emergency admissions that are unplanned and are due to a sudden illness or accident.

FIGURE 17.1

$\mathcal{R}$OUTINE ADMISSIONS

Appointments for routine admissions are arranged by the patient's doctor. Admissions of service patients are arranged by the clinic with the admissions office. A census of all empty beds is kept in the admissions office.

Patients entering for routine admissions must be processed through the admitting office before they are escorted to their rooms.

- The summary or face sheet, discussed in Chapter 11 is filled out by admitting office personnel, and the "release of liability" clause is signed by the patient at the same time. Patients are given the Patient's Rights form and Advance Directive to sign.
- The admitting office assigns a unit number to the patient that will be used to identify all records kept on the patient while he or she is in the hospital.
- The patient's name, unit number, and other identifying information will be transferred to an addressograph plate or imprinter card, which will be used by nursing personnel to stamp identification information on requisitions and chart forms.
- In most hospitals, the admitting office also makes out the patient's identification bracelet. This bracelet, usually make of plastic with a thin cardboard insert, is attached to the patient's wrist and must not be removed during hospitalization (Fig. 17.2).

PATIENT IDENTIFICATION

FIGURE 17.2

Sometimes patients will have completed their routine laboratory tests, such as chest x-rays and blood tests, which may be required on admission (preadmission testing or PAT), before they are escorted to the nursing unit or before they even enter the hospital. Today, managed care requires the use of patient preadmission testing whenever possible to keep down the cost of hospitalization.

When these preliminary procedures have been completed, the patient is ready to be taken to his or her room.

- A volunteer or an escort aide usually helps the patient by carrying luggage and directing the patient to the correct nursing unit. Family members often accompany the patient at this time.
- Some routine admission patients may walk to the nursing unit; most, however, including elderly or disabled patients, are transported to the nursing unit in a wheelchair or by gurney.

The escort may leave the patient in his or her assigned room and notify the health unit coordinator, or the escort may bring the patient to the nurses' station and introduce him or her to the health unit coordinator. In either instance, the escort will leave the summary or face sheet and the addressograph plate with the health unit coordinator.

ℰMERGENCY ADMISSIONS

The admitting procedure for emergency patients is often different from that for routine admissions (Fig. 17.3).

FIGURE 17.3

- Emergency patients are usually admitted through the emergency department, where immediate examinations take place.
- Emergency treatment may be initiated in the emergency room. If possible, identification information is requested from the patient or family.
- The admitting office must be notified so that a bed may be assigned to the patient. Ordinarily, the admitting personnel do not see the patient at this time, but they may come to the emergency room to complete the admission or may request that a member of the patient's family come to the admitting office.
- As soon as possible, the emergency patient and his or her belongings are transferred to the nursing unit, usually by gurney.
- Emergency admission patients are always taken directly to their rooms.
- Emergency patients may be admitted at any time of the day or night. The emergency patient or his representative must sign Conditions of Admissions or Release of Liability form. As with a routine admission, the admitting department will assign a unit number, prepare a face or summary sheet, and imprinter or addressograph plate, and if not made in the ER, an identification bracelet. You should be familiar with the ER record so that you will know which diagnostic tests and treatments were instituted there.

*A*DMISSIONS AND HEALTH UNIT COORDINATOR RESPONSIBILITIES

Your clerical duties with respect to a newly admitted patient are less likely to vary than your receptionist duties. Since you are primarily responsible for attending the desk at all times, you will generally give directions to the new patient and answer his or her questions only when it is impossible for someone else to do so. At the desk, however, you will be entirely responsible for getting the new patient's records in order. Listed next are the admitting procedures in which you may be expected to participate.

Clerical Duties

- Preparing the new chart by stamping all chart forms with the patient's identification plate and assembling them in the proper order.
- Locating old charts on the patient by calling the medical record room and requesting that the charts be sent to the nursing unit.
- Making available a *valuables envelope* and valuables control sheet if the patient wishes to have money and other items locked in the hospital safe. Figure 17.4 shows a valuables control sheet, and Figure 17.5 a valuables envelope receipt.
- Entering TPR, blood pressure, weight, and other pertinent information on the patient's graphic chart.
- Entering the patient's name in the TPR book, on the day's census report, and on other pertinent records.
- Transcribing all doctor's orders written on the new patient.
- If admitting still needs to see the patient, contacting them as soon as possible. Figure 17.6 shows a computer-generated notice to admitting.

Receptionist Duties

In a particular hospital, some of the receptionist duties may be the responsibility of nursing personnel. Learn the duties you will be expected to carry out. In general, receptionist duties will include the following:

- Greeting the patient at the nurses' station, introducing yourself, and welcoming the patient to the hospital.
- Notifying a member of the nursing staff that the patient has arrived on the floor and is awaiting admission instructions.
- Directing or guiding the new patient to his or her room and introducing the patient to his or her roommates, if any.
- Checking the application of or actually applying the patient's identification bracelet.
- Notifying the intern, resident, or attending doctor who will be responsible for completing the new patient's medical history and physical examination.

Orienting the patient to hospital personnel and routines are responsibilities that the nurse usually carries out. However, those that you may assist with include providing information about the following:

- Hospital smoking and noise control regulations
- Hours and regulations concerning meals and visitors
- Regulations concerning use of the day room and isolation unit
- Policies concerning radio and television rental
- The head nurse's name and introductions to other nursing staff members (Fig. 17.7).

PATIENT BELONGINGS RECORD

TRANSFERRED   TO: _____ FROM: _____
ADMITTED   TO: _____ FROM: _____

CLOTHING   NONE _____   SENT HOME WITH: _____
JEWELRY   NONE _____   RELATIONSHIP: _____
                        DATE: _____ TIME: _____

DESCRIPTION COLOR	WITH PT	SENT HOME
BELT		
BLOUSE		
BRA		
COAT		
DRESS		
HAT		
JACKET		
NIGHTGOWN		
PANTIES		
PANTS		
PAJAMAS		
ROBE		
SCARF		
SHIRT		
SHOES		
SKIRT		
SLACKS		
SLIP		
SLIPPERS		
SOCKS		
STOCKINGS		
SWEATER		
TIE		
T – SHIRT		
UNDERSHORTS		
MISC.		

MEDICATIONS:	LIST BY NAME	TO PHARM	SENT HOME

DESCRIPTION COLOR	WITH PT	SENT HOME
BRACELET		
EARRINGS		
NECKLACE		
RING		
WATCH		
RAZOR		
DRYER		
RADIO		
OTHER		

PROSTHESIS NONE _____	WITH PT	SENT HOME
DENTURES:		
UPPER ____ FULL ____ PARTIAL ____		
LOWER ____ FULL ____ PARTIAL ____		
HEARING AID LT __ RT __		
GLASSES		
CONTACTS		
WIG / HAIRPIECE		
AMBULATORY AID: TYPE ____		
OTHER		

MISCELLANEOUS TO SAFE	WITH PT	SENT HOME
CREDIT CARDS		
KEYS		
PURSE		
WALLET		
SUITCASE		
INSURANCE / MEDICARE CARD		
OTHER		
CASH		

SAFE ENVELOPE # _____ AMOUNT $ _____
AMOUNT WITH PATIENT $ _____

THIS IS A CORRECT LISTING OF MY BELONGINGS AND THEIR
DISPOSITION.

PT. OR
RESP. PARTY _____

WITNESS _____

CHART COPY White - PATIENT COPY Yellow

FIGURE 17.4 Valuables control sheet.

VALUABLES ENVELOPE

No. <u>00012</u>

CONTENTS

TOTAL NUMBER OF ITEMS

This envelope MUST be signed by the depositor. Valuables will be surrendered ONLY to the person whose signature appears below.

Signature of Depositor _____

Signature of Custodian _____

Date _____

NOTE: The hospital is not responsible for items which you retain in your possession.

- -

RECEIPT   No. <u>00012</u>

Signature of Depositor _____

Signature of Custodian _____

Date _____

FIGURE 17.5

```
                        MEMORIAL HOSPITAL
                   **************************
                      S P E C I A L
                      MAIL MAN MESSAGE
                   REGARDING THIS PATIENT'S
                 CONFIDENTIAL ADMITTING INFORMATION
                   **************************



PATIENT: EXAMPLE, IMANOTHER           AGE: 20 SEX: F   DOB: 12/12/19XX

MED REC NUMBER: 000000000             ADMITTING MD: FINEDOCTOR, MARY

PATIENT NUMBER:  0000000              NURSING UNIT: M   ROOM/BED: M202

SOC SEC NUMBER: 00000000000           FC: SP    ADMIT DATE: 04/21/2XXX

ADMIT DX: BRONCHITIS                  CURRENT DX: pneumonia



    ENTRY DEPARTMENT NO:     077
    ENTRY DEPT. MNEUMONIC:   XXX




    TO ADMITTING - ADMITTING INFO FORM




    ADMITTING CLERK MAY COME & SEE PATIENT NOW



    FAMILY IS HERE TO INTERPRET




                      SENT BY:   SUSIE SECRETARY
                      PH/EXT#:   1212




    ORDER NO.   716
    ORDER DATE: 05/30/2XXX
    ORDER TIME: 16:09
    ENTERED BY:                          PATTERN NO:
```

FIGURE 17.6 Computer-generated notice to admitting.

FIGURE 17.7

$\mathcal{A}$DMISSION ORDERS
$\mathcal{T}$YPES OF ADMISSION ORDERS

In most hospitals, nothing beyond the routine admission procedure is permitted to be done for the patient until the doctor has written the admission orders. These orders include all the general instructions pertaining to the patient's care. In most cases, you will find at least one order from each of the following categories:

Doctor's Admission Orders

- Diet
- Activity
- Diagnostic tests
- Treatment
- Medications

Diet

Every patient must have a dietary regimen, whether it be a regular diet, a therapeutic diet, or a complete restriction on intake (as when emergency surgery is anticipated).

Activity

All patients ordinarily have orders written to indicate the amount of activity they are allowed. In some hospitals, doctors may not be required to write an order if their patients are permitted movement *ad lib,* that is, without restriction.

Diagnostic Tests

Most hospital admissions must have at least two diagnostic tests: a CBC and a urinalysis. These and other tests must be ordered by the doctor. Other common admission diagnostic tests are ECGs and chest x-rays, although the physician may order a number of diagnostic tests on admission to the hospital.

Treatments

Except in cases where the patient has been admitted to the hospital only for diagnostic reasons, some treatment will probably be started to make the patient more comfortable or to improve his or her condition.

Medications

Admission orders usually include an order for medications. In some cases, the doctor may simply continue a medication the patient has been taking at home. In others, new medications intended to treat the patient's condition will be ordered. Sleeping medications (sedatives) are often ordered prn, as many people find it difficult to sleep in the hospital.

A sample of orders written at admission follows.

Complete bedrest.
Low Na diet.
Routine CBC & UA.
Serum electrolytes.
ESR & SGOT.
Stat ECG.
Digitoxin 0.2 mg po qd
Meperidine 75 mg IM q4h prn for chest pain
Secobarbital sodium gr i ss hs po prn
VS q2h Call Dr. Green for P > 120 or < 60

Admission orders.

Critical Pathways

Critical or **clinical pathways** are developed on admission by nursing for patients who have complicated high-risk, multiple, problem-likely diagnoses. They provide a guide for the health care team to ensure optimum interdisciplinary communication, and consistency in patient care.

R OUTINE ORDERS

Some physicians have their orders printed because they routinely order many of the same things for different patients. The doctor then adds or deletes as necessary to meet the needs of the individual patient. These orders are called *routine orders* and are

usually kept in the nursing unit and may be put into effect when the patient arrive
Changes are made or additional orders are given by the doctor by telephone or wri
ten when he or she visits the patient. Routine orders (and all orders) must be signe
by the doctor.

$\mathcal{M}$EDICAL SHORT STAY OR LESS THAN 24-HOUR ADMISSIONS

The purpose of **Medical Short Stay** is to provide treatment on a short-term basis t
patients who would otherwise be admitted to the hospital. This is a cost-saving al
ternative to hospitalization. Patients cannot remain in the MSSU for more tha
23 hours 59 minutes, and patients who are still in the MSSU after 12 hours must b
evaluated by the physician. If the patient requires hospital admission, those order
must be written.

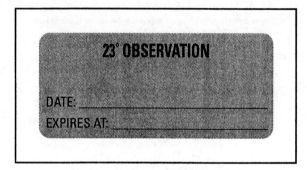

- Medical records—All patients in the MSSU require a medical record, which
  includes physician's orders for treatment, a history and a physical, and criteri
  for discharge, signed by the physician.
- Scheduling—Patients requiring specialized procedures are preschedule
  through the designated scheduling office such as Outpatient Admitting
  Those admitted through the emergency room may be registered through tha
  department, depending on hospital policy.

The following is an example of common criteria for admission to the Medica
Short Stay Unit:

- Diabetes mellitus
  - Blood sugar should be below 600.
  - No evidence of significant ketoacidosis (bicarbonate greater than 20).
- Congestive heart failure
  - Illness should be chronic rather than acute.
  - Require modest diuretic efforts and not complex cardiac drugs.
  - A response to treatment should be expected within 8 to 12 hours.
- Acute bronchitis
  - Patient should have symptoms capable of response to brief treatment wit
    respiratory therapy techniques, and chest x-ray should show no acute disease
- Pneumonia
  - Acute pneumonias not requiring IV therapy, rather, two courses of IN
    therapy to which a response is expected within 12 hours.
  - A diagnosis of pulmonary embolus is not considered.
  - Blood gases should be near normal values.

- Asthma
  - Patient should be without severe bronchospasm.
  - Patient should be without serious hypoxemia or CO_2 retention.
- Gastroenteritis
  - Patient should not have GI bleeding.
  - Patient should have no serious abdominal pain.
- Dehydration
  - Patients who are considered to be responsive to brief IV therapy.
- Ambulatory surgical care (ASC) patients
  - Patients who have had a surgical procedure and are experiencing prolonged pain.
- Surgical work-up
  - Patients requiring extensive testing prior to a surgical procedure.

Categories of Patients

- Patients admitted to the unit for antibiotic, chemotherapy, and blood transfusion will be Category I. The procedure shall be prescheduled.
- Patients admitted for stabilization shall be Category II.
- Patients admitted for special procedures shall be Category III. The procedures are prescheduled.

Patients Not Eligible for MSSU

- Patients requiring intensive care or special equipment
  - Cardiovascular monitoring
  - Suctioning of airways
- The patient who is unconscious, who demonstrates a deteriorating sensorium (ability to experience sensations and the world around him or herself)
- Suspected MI/chest pain
- Unstable angina/chest pain
- Life-threatening arrhythmias
- Suspected pulmonary embolus
- GI bleeders
- Vaginal bleeders
- Possible ectopic pregnancies
- Quadriplegics
- Patients who require a heparin infusion
- Patients requiring isolation for infectious disease
- Patients being observed for a seizure disorder
- Patients suffering from symptoms of alcohol or drug withdrawal, or patients requiring psychiatric disposition
- Patients less than 13 years old
- Patients who need hospital admission
- Patients scheduled for surgery
- Patients who require a sitter
- Patients who require social service disposition

Transcription

Sample admission orders have been provided at the end of this chapter. Use the symbols and methods you have been taught to transcribe each order.

SURGICAL ORDERS

Surgical patients require an operation illness or injury (Fig. 17.8). Surgical patients can be divided into three groups

1. **Preoperative** . . . before the operation.
2. **Intraoperative** . . . those in the process of having an operation.
3. Postoperative . . . after the operation.

FIGURE 17.8

*T*YPES OF SURGERY

Surgery may be divided into several categories:

- **Optional** (Elective)—done totally at the patient's request.
- **Required**—must be performed with a certain time frame (usually no more than two weeks).
- **Urgent**—needs surgery within one or two days.
- **Emergency**—immediate intervention is necessary.

Surgery may also be performed on an outpatient or inpatient basis.

Outpatient (Ambulatory) Surgery

Outpatient surgery provides care for patients scheduled for selected diagnostic procedures surgical intervention, and other specified treatment modalities of an elective nature. Patient are not admitted overnight. It is designed for the type of surgery that is of short duration where risk and probability of complications are low, and recovery is minimal (Fig. 17.9).

Figure 17.10 shows an example of an outpatient surgery record.

FIGURE 17.9

The following is a list of surgeries and procedures that might be scheduled on an outpatient basis:

Procedures

- Gynecological
  - Bartholin cystectomy
  - Dilation and curettage
  - Examination under anesthesia
  - Hymenotomy
  - Laparoscopy, diagnostic
  - Laparoscopy with tubal ligation
  - Removal of IUD
- **Neurosurgical**
  - Carpal tunnel
  - Alcohol injection of nerve and coagulation of nerves for control of pain
  - Intercostal neurectomy
  - Excision of neuroma
  - Morton's neuroma
- **Orthopedic**
  - (Without use of image intensifier)

- Closed reduction—fracture
- Ganglion
- Removal of orthopedic appliance (e.g., screws, Steinham pins)
- Tenotomy, hand or foot
- Excision of foreign body
- Exostosis excision (small)
- Release of tendon sheath
- Debridement, irrigation, and closure (small)
- Hand surgery
- **Plastic Surgery**
  - Augmentation mammoplasty
  - Dermabrasion
  - Otoplasty
  - Skin graft
  - Face lift
  - Face list with blepharoplasty
  - Blepharoplasty

ADMITTING RECORD Rm. No. _____ DATE _____ TIME _____ Procedure _____

Nickname _____					
Y N Heart Disease	Y N Dentures	TEMP. ____ P. ____ R. ____ B.P. ____	Allergies _____		
Y N Lung Disease	Y N Contact Lenses	N.P.O. _____ Hct. ___ U/A ___			
Y N Liver Disease	Y N Jewelry				
Y N Kidney Disease	Y N Smoke	RIDE _____			
Y N Diabetes/ Hypoglycemia	Y N Cough/Sob	DRUGS _____			
Y N Bleeding	Y N Mot. Sickness				
Y N G.I. Disease Height ____	Y N Dizzy Faint	_____	C of A _____ H & P _____		
Y N ↑ B.P. Weight ____		When Drugs Taken Last:			

Prev. Surgery, Hospitalizations and / or Same Procedure:

Prev. Problems With Medication and / or Same Procedure:

I.V. Sol.	Size	Site	Rate	Patent ☐	DSG ☐	HEP. LOC ☐

MEDICATIONS:

Admitted By _____

PROCEDURE RECORD

Procedure _____ | Dressings | Medications
Doctor _____
Procedure Time:—Start ____ Finish ____ Total ____
Diagnosis: _____ | Supplies Used
Nurse: _____ R.N.

RECOVERY ROOM RECORD   **REMARKS AND TREATMENTS**

TIME / 280 260 240 220 200 180 160 140 120 100 80 60 40 20 15 10 5

Total Recovery Rm

Time _____

P.O. Intake:	Voided:	I.V. Intake:

Start ____ Finish ____
Time Of Discharge ____ BY: _____

**OUTPATIENT PROCEDURES
NURSING ASSESSMENT**

FIGURE 17.10 Outpatient procedures nursing assessment.

- Scar revisions
- Rhinoplasty and septoplasty
- Excision of skin tumors (small)
- **Urological**
    - Circumcision
    - Dorsal slit
    - Meatomy
    - Prostate biopsy (needle)
    - Urethral dilation
    - Cystoscopy
    - Retrograde pyelogram
    - TURP (M.D. discretion—minor)
- **Dental**
    - Periodontal
    - Extractions
    - Impacted wisdom teeth, removal
- **Ear, Nose, and Throat**
    - Antral puncture
    - Arch bars, removal
    - Closed reduction, nose or zygoma
    - Interior Turbinates fracture
    - Myringotomy
    - Nasal polypectomy
    - Septal reconstruction, submucous, resection
    - Adenoidectomy
- **Endoscopy**
    - Bronchoscopy
    - Cystoscopy
- Cystocopy and retrograde
- Esophagoscopy
- **Eye**
    - Cataract
    - Muscle surgery
    - Chalazion
    - Discission
    - Plastic surgery of the eyelids
    - Eye examination under general anesthesia
    - Lacrimal duct probing
    - Pterygium
    - Insertion of glass tube into lacrimal duct
    - Laser beam
- **General Surgery**
    - Breast biopsy (only)
    - Removal of foreign body
    - Hernioplasty
    - Node biopsy
    - Muscle biopsy
    - Soft tissue tumors
    - Scalene node biopsy
    - Umbilical hernia
    - Rectal polypectomy
    - Excision of sebaceous cyst
    - Excision of skin lesions
    - Evacuation of hematoma
    - Liver biopsy—Menghini needle

The health unit coordinator working in outpatient surgery will be responsible for many of the clerical and receptionist duties described on the pages that follow. However, because the patient does not stay overnight (unless a change of condition warrants admission to the hospital), certain procedures will be modified based on hospital policy.

Following is a list of responsibilities of a same day, outpatient surgery, or ambulatory surgical center (ASC) health unit coordinator:

1. Keeps office in order and well supplied.

2. Greets physicians, offers assistance, and calls nurse in charge/nurse manager when needed.

3. Is aware of physicians and other personnel on the floor.

4. Answers telephone promptly and courteously. Gives name, position, and location. Relays messages promptly and accurately.

5. Relays telephone calls concerning patient's condition and physician's orders to the nurse in charge.

6. Answers patients' and visitors' questions promptly and courteously.

7. Handles communications daily and during emergencies.

8. Assists RN in obtaining central and pharmacy supplies and maintenance repairs.

9. Operates the computer.

10. Enters surgery, recovery, and special nursing procedures data in patient operative log.

11. Completes monthly utilization reports and distributes to medical records, surgery, utilization, and finance departments.

12. Collects scheduling slips from operating room and enters into outpatient surgery scheduling book/computer log.

13. Calls each patient for preadmitting information and instructions, and verifies time of surgery.

14. Arranges with patient when to come in for laboratory work, ECG, and x-rays.

15. Performs admitting functions to gather all pertinent information prior to or on patient's arrival.

16. Obtains proper signatures on all necessary consents and explains consents to the patient (does not explain procedure).

17. Records complete and accurate information for each admission and registration, obtaining copies of third-party payer information as necessary.

18. Obtains copies of insurance cards and insurance forms for charts.

19. Prepares patient charts.

20. Coordinates services of outpatient surgery department and business office under supervision of admitting supervisor and charge nurse/nurse manager of outpatient surgery.

21. Schedules special nursing procedures under supervision of charge/nurse manager.

22. Disasembles patient's charts for medical records after discharge.

23. Assists with counting, batching, charging, and delivery to data processing.

24. Performs other duties as assigned.

*P*REOPERATIVE PREPARATION

The nursing staff will prepare patients physically and emotionally for the impending surgery. Nursing personnel will shave and clean the operative area, regulate the patient's diet, administer enemas as necessary, and carry out any other **preoperative** doctor's orders.

You as the health unit coordinator will be responsible for seeing that certain clerical duties have been completed and for assembling the chart forms in the proper order.

Preoperative Checklist

The purpose of the preoperative checklist is to assure that all necessary tasks and information are complete before the patient goes to surgery. This checklist is sent to the operating room on the chart.

1. Tasks pertaining to the patient's chart forms and records, to be performed by the health unit coordinator.

2. Tasks pertaining to the preparation of the patient, performed by nursing personnel.

Nursing Responsibilities

The following procedures must be certified as having been completed by appropriate nursing personnel:

- Recording the time of the surgical prep of the operative area; when the enemas were completed, and by whom.
- Confirmation that the patient's TPR and BP were taken on the morning of surgery. If these values are not within the normal range, indicating possible disease, the surgery may have to be canceled. The health unit coordinator may be responsible for recording these values on the graphic chart.
- Noting the time, dosage, and name of the preoperative medications given. The anesthesiologist will then be able to coordinate the anesthesia with the medications given to achieve the optimum state of unconsciousness.
- Recording the time and amount of the patient's final voiding before transport to the operating room.
- Verifying the patient's identification number on the identification band on his or her wrist.
- Removal of the patient's dentures (sometimes not done until arrival in OR), jewelry, hairpins, nail polish, lipstick, and all prostheses prior to transport to the operating room.
- Having the patient properly dressed in hospital gown or other clothing, as required in your hospital.

Note: Special items may be required for patients with particular disease conditions or preoperative needs.

Health Unit Coordinator Responsibilities

The health unit coordinator must be sure that the following records are completed and included in the chart:

- The preoperative checklist (Fig. 17.11).
- The operative consent signed by the patient (or another person responsible for the patient according to the regulations of your hospital) (Fig. 17.12).
- A preanesthesia questionnaire and consent for anesthesia (Figs. 17.13 and 17.14).
- An anesthesia record (Fig. 17.15).
- A signed sterilization consent if the surgery will render the patient unable to reproduce (Fig. 17.16).
- History and physical records, completed and recorded by the physician responsible. These are required before surgery. Short forms are usually available for patients hospitalized under 24 to 48 hours.
- Preoperative laboratory results posted on the clinical pathology record. Preoperative patients routinely have a blood count and urinalysis done prior to surgery. There will be policies regarding the recency of CBC and UA tests. Usually they will be valid for no longer than 48 hours. If any patient has evidence of anemia or a bladder infection, these conditions must be corrected prior to surgery. If not, they could cause serious complications during or after surgery.
- Any other tests done preoperatively, such as ECGs and x-rays.

DATE	YES	NO	N/A	COMMENTS			UNIT RN INITIAL	HR RN INITIAL
Patient ID Band Checked								
Nickname								
Allergies				List:				
Allergy Band								
PATIENT CHART / CHART FORMS	YES	NO	N/A	COMMENTS			UNIT RN INITIAL	HR RN INITIAL
Face Sheet								
Conditions of Admission / Advance Directive Form								
History & Physical								
Surgical Consent								
Anesthesia Consent				☐ Dr. Orders ☐ Signed ☐ Witnessed				
Anesthesia Questionnaire								
Sterilization / Observation / Photo Consent								

LAB / CLINICAL REPORTS	YES	NO	N/A	ON CHART	ABNORMAL REPORT CALLED TO DR/OR	TIME	UNIT RN INITIAL	HR RN INITIAL
Tests Done								
Chest X-Ray								
EKG								
CBC								
LYTES								
UA								
Other: Nuclear Medicine Test within 24 hours				(If yes - contact Nuc. Med.)				

TYPE / X MATCH	AUTOLOGOUS DONATION		DESIGNATED DONATION	RED CROSS DONATION	TOTAL	UNIT RN INITIAL	HR RN INITIAL
No. Units Donated				N/A			
No. Units X Match							

BELONGINGS	YES	NO	N/A	COMMENTS	DISPOSITION	UNIT RN INITIAL	HR RN INITIAL
Dental Appliances				☐ Upper ☐ Lower			
Prosthesis				Type:			
Glasses / Contacts							
Jewelry				Type:			
Hearing Aids							
Other:				Type:			

MISCELLANEOUS

NPO SINCE	LAST VOID	PREOP TEACHING ☐ DONE	VISITORS WAITING

IV Started @_____ . Size #_____ gauge ☐ LR1000cc ☐D5W_____ cc. Site:_____

☐ Patent   ☐ Opsite   ☐ Pump Set   ☐ Secondary Set   ☐ Ext. Set   ☐ 1% Xylocaine_____ cc. infiltrate

☐ Alka Seltzer TT tabs in 30cc/H_2O po @_____   Versed_____ mg IVP @_____

Comments _____
_____
_____

NURSE SIGNATURE & TITLE	NURSE SIGNATURE & TITLE	TO O.R. @

PREOP CHECKLIST

FIGURE 17.11

AUTHORIZATION FOR AND CONSENT TO SURGERY OR SPECIAL DIAGNOSTIC OR THERAPEUTIC PROCEDURES

To _____
Name of Patient

Your admitting physician is _____, M.D.

Your surgeon is _____, M.D.

1. The hospital maintains personnel and facilities to assist your physicians and surgeons in their performance of various surgical operations and other special diagnostic and therapeutic procedures. These surgical operations and special diagnostic or therapeutic procedures all may involve calculated risks of complications, injury, or even death, from both known and unknown causes, and no warranty or guarantee has been made as to result or cure. Except in a case of emergency or exceptional circumstances, these operations and procedures are therefore not performed upon patients unless and until the patient has had an opportunity to discuss them with his physician. Each patient has the right to consent or refuse any proposed operation or special procedure (based upon the description or explanation received).

2. Your physicians and surgeons have determined that the operations or special procedures listed below may be beneficial in the diagnosis or treatment of your condition. Upon your authorization and consent, such operations or special procedures will be performed for you by your physicians and surgeons and/or by other physicians and surgeons selected by them. The persons in attendance for the purpose of administering anesthesia or performing other specialized professional services, such as radiology, pathology and the like, are not the agents, servants, or employees of the hospital or your physician or surgeon but are independent contractors performing specialized services on your behalf and, as such, are your agents, servants, or employees. Any tissue or member severed in any operation will be disposed of at the discretion of the pathologist, except _____

3. Your signature below the operations or special procedures listed below constitutes your acknowledgment (i) that you have read and agreed to the foregoing, (ii) that the operations or special procedures have been adequately explained to you by your attending physicians or surgeons and that you have all of the information that you desire, and (iii) that you authorize and consent to the performance of the operations or special procedures.

Operation or Procedure

_____

_____

_____

_____

SIGNATURE _____ DATE _____ TIME _____
Patient

SIGNATURE _____ DATE _____ TIME _____
Witness

(If patient is a minor or unable to sign, complete the following):

Patient is a minor, or is unable to sign, because _____

_____

_____

Father	Guardian
Mother	Other Person and Relationship

FIGURE 17.12

ANESTHESIA QUESTIONNAIRE   Name_____ Ht._____ Wt. _____

1. Please list all medications taken in last ten days (including aspirin):

    _____

    _____

    _____

2. Are you allergic to any medication, iodine, soap, latex, rubber products, or tape? What adverse reaction did you have?

    _____

    _____

    _____

3. Please check (✔) if you have had the following:

❑ High blood pressure	❑ Asthma or wheezing	❑ Nuclear medicine test within 24 hours
❑ Chest pains or angina	❑ Emphysema or chronic bronchitis	❑ Diabetes
❑ Heart attack	❑ Cough up phlegm daily	❑ Thyroid problems
❑ Palpitations	❑ Recent cold or flu	❑ Kidney problems
❑ Heart failure	❑ Polio	❑ Heavy bleeding
❑ Heart murmur	❑ Seizures or convulsions	❑ Prednisone or steroid in last 6 months
❑ Rheumatic fever	❑ Fainting spells	❑ Hepatitis
❑ Other heart disease	❑ Strokes	❑ Peptic ulcer disease
❑ Shortness of breath	❑ Weakness on one side of body	❑ Hiatal hernia or reflux
❑ Ankle swelling	❑ Temporary blindness, in an eye	❑ Other significant illness _____

4. Do you smoke? ❑ No ❑ How much_____ When did you quit? _____

5. What is your alcohol use? ❑ Never   ❑ Occasional   ❑ Few times a week   ❑ Daily

6. Is it possible that you are pregnant? ....❑ Yes ❑ No When was your last menstrual period? _____

7. Is your ability to exercise limited? ....❑ Yes ❑ No Explain _____

8. Has any relative had problems with anesthesia?....❑ Yes ❑ No

9. Do you have ....❑ Dentures ❑ Loose teeth ❑ Capped or bonded teeth ❑ Contact lenses

10. Do you have any problems with neck mobility or have you ever been told you have an abnormal airway? ❑ Yes ❑ No

11. Please list your previous operations:

Year	Operation	Type of Anesthesia (general, spinal, local)	Complications
_____	_____	_____	_____
_____	_____	_____	_____
_____	_____	_____	_____
_____	_____	_____	_____

12. This form has been filled out by _____

PREANESTHESIA QUESTIONNAIRE

FIGURE 17.13

CONSENT FOR ANESTHESIA

Although anesthesia is very safe, there are certain inherent risks every time anesthesia is administered. The medicines used for anesthesia may affect the cardiovascular system to lower blood pressure, may cause breathing problems, may cause allergic reations, and may directly cause injury to any of the organs of the body. There is the potential for very serious complications that even result in brain damage and/or death. Serious complications are very infrequent, and occur much less than 1% of the time in the general population.

Additional Risks Include the Following:

GENERAL ANESTHESIA:

Frequent (more than 1% occurrence): nausea and vomiting, sore throat, brief disorientation

Rare (less than 1% occurrence): damage to teeth, awareness under anesthesia, damage to peripheral nerves, damage to major organs (including brain, heart, lungs, liver, kidneys)

REGIONAL ANESTHESIA:

Frequent (more than 1% occurrence): bruising, minor pain and discomfort, residual sensation, need for general anesthesia, headache

Rare (less than 1% occurrence): damage to nerves and/or blood vessels, infection, convulsions, damage to major organs (including brain, heart, lungs, liver, kidneys)

I have read this and acknowledge that I understand that I am to have anesthesia to relieve pain during my surgical procedure and that this administration of anesthesia carries risk to life and limb. I understand that these risks stated above are not meant to be a complete list, and that other unexpected complications may occur. I have had the opportunity to have all of my questions answered by an anesthesiologist.

Date	Time	Patient/Parent/Guardian/Conservator
Date	Time	Witness

CONSENT FOR ANESTHESIA

FIGURE 17.14 Consent for anesthesia.

PREMED/EFFECT			ALLERGY	HCT	HT	WT	ASA 1 2 3 4 5 E	PG

AGENTS/FLUIDS	TIME	TOTALS
O₂		

MONITORS
- ☐ BP
- ☐ EKG
- ☐ TEMP
- ☐ PCS
- ☐ ES
- ☐ OXIMETER
- ☐ ETCO₂
- ☐ FIO₂
- ☐ CVP
- ☐ ART   ☐ PNS
- ☐ PA
- ☐ FOLEY
- ☐ DISCONNECT

200
190
180
170
160
150
140
130
120
110
100
90
80
70
60
50
40
30
20
10

PACU
BP
P
R
AIRWAY
LOC
O₂ SAT

☐ PT ID	☐ CHART REV	☐ CONSENT	**AIRWAY** ☐ OP ☐ NP ☐ OETT ☐ NETT ☐ MASK ☐ TRACH
☐ EQUIP CHECKED	☐ IV		

REMARKS   SIZE _____ DIFFICULTY _____

OPERATION	SURGEON
	ASSISTANT

ANES. START	SURG. START	SURG. END	ANES. END	DATE	ANESTHESIOLOGIST

ANESTHESIA RECORD

FIGURE 17.15

MEMORIAL HOSPITAL
STERILIZATION PERMIT

Datė _____ Hour _____.M.

I hereby authorize and direct Doctor _____
and assistants of his choice to perform the following operation upon me at the above
named hospital: _____ and to
do any other procedure that his (their) judgment may dictate during the above
operation. It has been explained to me that I may (or will probably) be sterile as a
result of this operation but no such result has been warranted. I understand that the
word "sterility" means that I may be unable to conceive or bear children and in giving
my consent to the operation have in mind the possibility (probability) of such a result.
I absolve said doctor, his assistants and the hospital from all responsibility for my
present condition or any condition that may result from said operation.

Signed _____

Signature Witnessed:

By _____   By _____

I have read the foregoing matter and, as the spouse of the above named patient, do
hereby join in authorizing the performance of the surgery under the terms set forth
and consented to above.

Signed _____

Signature Witnessed:

By _____   By _____

FIGURE 17.16

- Other preoperative forms (e.g., preanesthesia form) as required by your hospital.
- Blank chart forms to be used in the operating room and recovery room, such as the anesthesia record and intake and output sheets.
- The patient's imprinter plate for use on forms in the operating room and recovery room.

PREOPERATIVE ORDERS

TYPES OF PREOPERATIVE ORDERS

Orders for a patient prior to surgery vary not only according to the operation to be performed but also according to the preferences of each surgeon. Ordinarily, preoperative orders will include one order from each of the following categories (Fig. 17.17).

FIGURE 17.17

Enema

Many preoperative patients receive an enema. The type of enema ordered will depend on the operation to be performed. Cleaning out the bowel prior to surgery serves two purposes:

1. The patient is less likely to contaminate the operating field with feces when his rectal sphincter relaxes under anesthesia.

2. A bowel distended with feces will block the surgeon's view once he enters the abdominal cavity.

Prep

The area where the surgical incision will be made must be shaved and cleaned before surgery. The shave and scrub is called a surgical "prep" (Fig. 17.18).

The purpose of this preparation is to clean the skin and reduce the possibility of the spread of microorganisms from the skin into the operative incision.

Diet

If the patient does not have an empty stomach, he or she may vomit during and after surgery as a reaction to the anesthesia. Therefore, the patient is usually made NPO at midnight on the day of surgery (Fig. 17.19). If surgery is to be performed on the

DISPOSABLE PREP KIT

Plastic container used as a basin

Towels

Soap sponge

Disposable razor

FIGURE 17.18

FIGURE 17.19

lower GI system, the patient's diet may be modified for two to three days before the operation.

Consent

All patients must have an operative consent signed before the operation may take place. If the patient is underage or unable to sign, the person with power of attorney or as designated by hospital policy must do so.

The doctor may obtain the patient's written consent; if not, he or she writes an order to that effect and relies on the nursing staff to carry out the order. Surgical consents must be informed consents with many legal implications. Therefore, it is usually the doctor who explains the surgery and the nurse who obtains the consent.

Sleeping Medication (Sedatives and Hypnotics)

Most doctors order sleeping medications for their patients preoperatively, to reduce their anxiety and to help them sleep well the night before surgery.

Preoperative Medicine

Shortly before the patient is taken to the operating room, he or she is given injections to help the patient relax. In many hospitals, these medications are ordered by the anesthesiologist rather than the surgeon.

Blood Replacement

Most patients scheduled for major surgery should have blood reserved for them in the blood bank. Their blood must be typed and crossmatched with blood units available in the blood bank. This is usually done the evening before surgery, and the whole blood or packed cells are placed "on call" for the following day. Many patients bank their own blood for their surgery.

Other Preoperative Orders

The doctor may write an order for items that are to accompany the patient to the operating room. For example:

> To OR c̄ skull x-rays
> To OR c̄ 1 vial regular insulin

The doctor may also order that certain miscellaneous duties be performed the morning of surgery.

Figure 17.20 shows an example of preprinted preoperative anesthesia orders. The physician will check those that apply, and they are transcribed in the usual manner.

> Phone lab for results of CBC and UA. Include one chart.
> Start IV 500 cc 5% D/W prior to OR transport.
> Give one unit whole blood tonight.

*T*RANSCRIPTION

The following is a sample paper of preoperative orders. Transcribe these on a separate sheet of paper. Practice using the symbols and abbreviations you have been taught.

> Have operative consent signed.
> SS enema tonight and at 6 A.M.
> Abdominal-perineal prep c̄ 5 min antiseptic scrub.
> NPO p̄ midnight.
> Type and x-match 3 units whole blood. Give one tonight and place 2 on-call for 8 A.M.
> Sodium pentobarbital 200 mg po hs
> Catheterize pt prior to giving preop meds.
> Preop meds by order of Dr. Jones.
> Pt to OR c̄ pelvic x-rays.

1. **TESTS:**
   - ❏ EKG
   - ❏ CHEST X-RAY
   - ❏ PULMONARY FUNCTION SCREEN
   - ❏ OTHER_____
   - ❏ CBC
   - ❏ UA
   - ❏ SMA - 7
   - ❏ ELECTROLYTES

2. **DIET**
   - ❏ NPO p 2400
   - ❏ CLEAR LIQUIDS (NO JELLO, NO SOUP) UNTIL_____

3. **START IV**   ❏ OPS   ❏ HOLDING ROOM   ❏ FLOOR
   - ❏ Extension Set
   - ❏ 1000 D 5 ½ N.S. @ _____ cc/hr
   - ❏ 500 D 5 W @ _____ cc/hr
   - ❏ 1000 R L @ _____ cc/hr
   - ❏ 1000 D 5 Isolyte S @_____ cc/hr
   - ❏ OTHER_____
   - ❏ LIDOCAINE 1% plain intradermal infiltrate for IV start

4. **MEDICATIONS**
   - ❏ Daily meds c̄ sip of H_2O in a.m. pre-op

   SLEEP
   - ❏ NEMBUTAL 100 mgm p.o. H.S.   M.R. x _____ prn
   - ❏ DALMANE   15 mgm p.o. H.S.   M.R. x _____ prn
   - ❏ DALMANE   30 mgm p.o. H.S.   M.R. x _____ prn
   - ❏ HALCION .25 mgm p.o. H.S.   M.R. x _____ prn
   - ❏ OTHER_____

   PREOP
   - ❏ LEAVE DENTURES IN PLACE
   - ❏ NO PREOP MEDICATION
   - ❏ ALKA SELTZER COLD TABS II c̄ 30 cc H_2O ½ - 1 h. pre-op
   - ❏ VALIUM _____ mgm. ❏ IV ❏ P.O. @ _____
   - ❏ DROPERIDOL _____ mgm I.M. @ _____
   - ❏ MORPHINE _____ mgm I.M. @ _____
   - ❏ FENTANYL _____ mgm. ❏ IV ❏ I.M. @ _____
   - ❏ DEMEROL _____ mgm I.M. @ _____
   - ❏ VISTARIL _____ mgm ❏ p.o. ❏ I.M. @ _____
   - ❏ ATIVAN _____ mgm ❏ p.o. ❏ I.M. @ _____
   - ❏ ATROPINE _____ mgm I.M. @ _____
   - ❏ SCOPOLAMINE _____ mgm I.M. @ _____
   - ❏ ROBINUL _____ mgm I.M. @ _____
   - ❏ VERSED _____ mgm ❏ IV ❏ I.M. @ _____
   - ❏ OTHER_____

5. **ADDITIONAL PREOP ORDERS** _____

Nurse's Signature	Date	Time	Transcriber	M.D. Signature

PREOPERATIVE ANESTHESIA ORDERS

FIGURE 17.20

POSTOPERATIVE ORDERS

Most patients are taken to the recovery room (RR or PACU) immediately following surgery. They remain in the recovery room until they begin to recover from the effects of anesthesia. When it is felt that the patient may safely return to the floor (nursing unit), the recovery room staff will bring the patient, by gurney, back to his room.

TYPES OF POSTOPERATIVE ORDERS

Surgery usually affects a patient's hospitalization more than any other single event.

- Following surgery, the patient's diet and activity orders usually change.
- Treatments and medications given before the operation may no longer be necessary.
- The postoperative patient usually requires special care for a period of hours or days following surgery, and new orders for this care must be written.

Postoperative orders vary according to the operation performed. Following surgery, all preoperative orders written on a patient are automatically canceled. The postoperative orders must be rewritten by the time the patient is transferred to the recovery room so that the nurses there will know what must be done for the patient. You as health unit coordinator should be familiar with this type of order so that you will know if new orders were instituted in the recovery room. Figure 17.21 shows an example of postanesthesia orders for PACU and the floor. Postoperative orders usually include most of the following categories.

> *Postoperative Orders*
> - *Diet*   ■ *Medications*
> - *Activity*   ■ *Tubes and catheters*
> - *Intravenous feeding (IV)*   ■ *Intake and output*
> - *Vital signs*   ■ *Special equipment*
> - *Wound and dressing*

Diet

A diet order of some kind is generally indicated. A patient with minor surgery may have few, if any, restrictions. For example:

> *Diet as tolerated*
> *Regular diet; serve dinner*
> *Resume low Na diet as tolerated*

POSTANESTHESIA CARE UNIT

1. MEDICATIONS:

☐ **Fentanyl 25 mcg. IV q5 min. x _____doses prn pain**

☐ **Fentanyl 50 mcg. IV q5 min. x _____doses prn pain**

☐ **Morphine_____mgm. IV q5 min. x _____doses prn pain**

☐ **Demerol_____mgm. IV q5 min. x _____doses prn pain**

☐ **Droperidol_____mgm. IV prn nausea M.R. x _____**

☐ **Compazine ☐ 1.25 mgm. IV prn nausea M.R. x _____**

☐ **2.5 mgm. IV prn nausea M.R. x _____**

☐ **Atropine   mgm. IV prn pulse below_____and notify anesthesiologist**
   M.R. x _____prn

☐ **Narcan 0.1 mgm. IV prn respiratory depression M.R. x _____and notify**
   anesthesiologist.

2. ADDITIONAL ORDERS:
   OXYGEN

☐ **Mask   ☐ Nasal Prongs_____LPM   ☐ Mist_____%   ☐ Pulse Oximeter**

☐ **Warm Air Therapy for Temp ⏐ 96F.**

_____
_____
_____
_____

3. DISCHARGE FROM PACU TO: ☐ Ward ☐ DOU ☐ ICU ☐ Same day Surgery ☐ Extended Care

☐ **Time _____**

☐ **PACU Score of _____**

☐ **Block sensory level of _____**

☐ **Return of motor function _____**

☐ **DC EPIDURAL**

4. ☐ Discharge home in care of responsible party when V.S.S., awake, comfortable, takes P.O. fluids
   with minimal nausea/vomiting, voids, sits up and walks with assistance and instructed how
   to contact anesthesiologist if necessary through hospital operator.

☐ **DC I.V. BEFORE DISCHARGE**

Nurse's Signature	Date	Time

POSTANESTHESIA ORDER FOR FLOOR

_____
_____
_____
_____

Nurse's Signature	Date	Time	Transcriber	M.D. Signature

MEMORIAL HOSPITAL

POSTANESTHESIA ORDERS

FIGURE 17.21

A patient with major surgery usually is fed intravenously for a day or two. However, reference to diet may be made. For example:

> NPO
> Ice chips as tolerated
> Sips of tap water as pt desires

Activity

A patient's activity is almost always limited after surgery. Limitations may be insignificant in the case of minor surgery. For example:

> OOB ad lib p̄ pt awake.
> OOB tonight as tolerated.

When certain major surgery has been performed, far stricter regulations apply. The patient is often confined to bed entirely until the following morning, when orders for progressive ambulation are written. Some activity orders concern the surgical procedure performed. For example:

> Pt to be kept flat in bed for 24 hrs.
> Elevate right arm at all times.

IVs

An intravenous infusion is begun on almost every adult patient who has surgery. Moreover, some anesthetics are given intravenously; their administration is often simplified if an IV is running. Most physicians also consider it wise to have an IV running during surgery, in case of an emergency. The type of surgery and the patient's postoperative condition largely determine the type of IV order to be written. For example:

> Finish current IV; then discontinue.
> Hang 1 bottle 500 cc D/W after current IV finishes; then discontinue.
> Keep IV open with 1000 cc 5% D/W til 8 AM.
> 1000 cc 5% D/W follow c̄ 500 cc 5% D/S to run til morning.
> Finish blood, then hang 1000 cc NS c̄ 2 million U aqueous penicillin added.

As the last order shows, postoperative IV orders may contain orders for medication. Antibiotics to combat possible infection and vitamins to help rebuild the body after surgery are some of the most common medications given in connection with IVs.

Vital Signs

Accurate records of the blood pressure, pulse, and respirations are extremely important during the immediate postoperative period. A rising pulse, increased respirations, and falling blood pressure may indicate the onset of shock. Shock can occur after surgery from excessive or continuing blood loss or as a reaction to the anesthetic used. Since these two situations can occur in any postoperative patient, vital signs are generally taken every 15 minutes in the recovery room. The physician will usually write orders pertaining to the VS to be carried out after the patient has been returned to his or her own hospital unit. For example:

> VS q15min×4, q1h× q4h, then qd.
> VS q15min until stable.

Wound and Dressing

After surgery, there is often the possibility that the patient will bleed internally. Hemorrhage usually takes place near the wound site, so a frequent check of the dressing for blood may assist in early detection. Physicians often order continuous observation for signs of bleeding. For example:

> Check dressing q15min for bleeding.
> Call Dr. Green if bleeding excessive.

Medications

After all surgery, except the most minor, a physician will ordinarily write a prn order for the relief of pain. For treatment or prevention of postoperative nausea and vomiting, an order for an *antiemetic* drug might be written. In cases of potential infection, the doctor will usually order *antibiotics* postoperatively. Other medications may be ordered, but these types are ordered most often. Examples follow:

> Meperidine 75 mg IM q4h prn
> Codeine gr ⅱ (H) q3h prn.
> Prochlorperazine 5 mg IM q4h prn
> Streptomycin 0.5 Gm IM bid.

Tubes and Catheters

Many patients leave the operating room with tubes or a catheter in place. Observation and care of tubes or catheters require a written order, such as the following:

> *Foley catheter to gravity drainage. Irrigate q4h c̄ 10 cc NSS.*
> *Wound catheter to Hemovac.*
> *Levine tube to suction. Irrigate q4h.*

Intake and Output

Postoperative records of I&O are kept on almost every patient subjected to major surgery, primarily because fluid balance is easily upset by surgery. The doctor must know when to add fluids or withhold them to attain fluid balance. A record of out-put is also important, because urinary retention is a common complication fol-lowing certain types of surgery. Examples of orders associated with these difficulties follow:

> *Strict I & O for 3 days.*
> *Check voiding q8h.*
> *Cath pt q8h prn if unable to void.*
> *If pt has not voided by 4 AM, call Dr. White for cath order.*

Special Equipment

Sometimes patients require the postoperative use of special equipment. A patient with a spinal fusion may need a bedboard; a patient recovering from chest surgery may require chest tubes; a postoperative prostatectomy patient will sometimes require a special apparatus for irrigating the bladder with distilled water or a saline solution called a *Murphy drip*. Pneumatic and elastic stockings are ordered on patients following a variety of surgical procedures. Examples of orders of this type follow:

> *Bedboard.*
> *Murphy drip at gtts 10/min.*

TRANSCRIPTION

A group of typical postoperative orders follows. Transcribe them for practice in the manner indicated previously in the chapter.

> *NPO*
> *Complete bedrest*
> *VS q15 min until stable. Then q2h × 12 hrs.*
> *Check bleeding q15 min.*
> *Wound catheter to suction. Measure and empty q4h.*
> *I & O*
> *Cath pt. at 8 PM if unable to void.*
> *Elastic stockings toes to knees. Remove qd, wash and dry legs, then replace stockings.*
> *Meperidine 50 mg IM q3h prn.*
> *1000 cc 5% D/W c̄ 4,000,000 U aqueous penicillin to run until 12 Mn.; then keep open c̄ 500 cc 5% D/S.*

$\mathcal{T}$RANSFER OF PATIENTS

After patients have been admitted to a bed in a hospital unit, it may become necessary to **transfer** them elsewhere. Some transfers take place within the same nursing unit: the patient simply changes rooms. Other transfers may be between floors. The best time of day for a patient transfer is usually in the afternoon. This is because most patient care has been completed, patients have been discharged, and rooms are clean and ready to receive transfer patients. Whenever a doctor orders a patient transferred, the admitting office must be notified so that the census records can be corrected (Fig. 17.22). Another type of transfer is between hospitals, which will be discussed last.

NOTIFY FOLLOWING
DEPARTMENTS FOR
APPROPRIATE ACTION:

DIETARY KITCHEN   REROUTE MAIL   ADMITTING OFFICE

FIGURE 17.22

*T*RANSFERS TO OTHER ROOMS

Transfer of a patient to another room in the same nursing unit may be made for the following reasons (Fig. 17.23):

■ A patient may have been admitted to a ward room because there were no private rooms available. Once a private room becomes vacant, however, the patient may be transferred.

■ A patient may ask to transfer from a private room to a semiprivate room. This may be necessary for insurance purposes.

■ The age or condition of another patient in the room may warrant the transfer to a more appropriate room.

■ A patient may develop a postoperative wound infection or a contagious disease and require transfer to an isolation unit on the same floor.

Your duties in connection with transfers of patients to other rooms will be to make sure that the patient's records are kept in order and that their new locations are properly registered wherever necessary.

■ The change in the patient's room and bed number must be made:
  ■ On the chart holder
  ■ On the patient's Kardex, which must then be replaced in its holder in the newly designated place
  ■ On all of the patient's medicine tickets if used in your hospital.

FIGURE 17.23

- In the TPR book, if one is used in your hospital.
- On any other forms, such as the diet sheet that contains the patient's name and room number.
- Take care to redirect the patient's visitors and mail to the new location in the unit. It is very important that a visitor not enter the room and simply find the patient gone! (Fig. 17.24).

*T*RANSFERS TO OTHER UNITS

Patients are transferred to other nursing units because of a change in their condition and a change in the level of care that is required. For example, a patient's condition may worsen and the patient is transferred to the critical care unit, or it may improve and the patient is transferred to a less intensive level of care. When a patient is transferred, all orders cancel and must be reviewed and renewed.

Figure 17.25 shows a computer-generated patient transfer document. This document is often many pages long.

*R*ECEIVING TRANSFER PATIENTS

When a patient is transferred from another floor to your nursing unit, you will be responsible for many tasks similar to those carried out in connection with admission.

- When you expect a transfer patient, check with the responsible nursing personnel to make sure the new room is ready for the patient.
- When the patient arrives on the floor, you will be given the patient's medical records and new identification plate.
- Place the chart in the proper chart folder.
- Change all necessary information (floor number, room number, bed number) on the Kardex and file it properly.

FIGURE 17.24

```
********* PATIENT TRANSFER DOCUMENT *********
```

THIS IS A PERMANENT CHART DOCUMENT. PLEASE PLACE IN CHART. FAX TO PHARMACY

05/30/2XXX 16:49   Page: 1

```
4MS  00000  EXAMPLE, IMA      X
F  60    DOB: 111737                Pt. No: 100053677      Allergies:
64    150                           MR  No: 0000000000      PCN
Admit Date:  11/19/58 0000          Admit:  GOODDOCTOR JOHN  ASA
Isol:    Diab:                                               CODEINE
                                    Cons:   VERYFINE, MARY
```

```
    TRANSFER PATIENT:
                        _____  STAT
                        _____  WHEN BED AVAILABLE
                        _____  IN A.M.
                        _____  SPECIFY

                TO:
                        _____  CRITICAL CARE UNIT
                        _____  MEDICAL/SURGICAL UNIT
                        _____  TRANSITIONAL CARE UNIT
                        _____  BEHAVIORAL MEDICINE UNIT
                        _____  MATERNAL/CHILD HEALTH UNIT

ADMIT DX:    BRONCHITIS
CURRENT DX:  PNEUMONIA
             ARDS
UPDATE CURRENT DX AS FOLLOWS: _____

ATTENDING MD:  GOODDOCTOR, JOHN
UPDATE ATTENDING MD AS FOLLOWS:_____
```

       ALL PATIENT ORDERS HAVE BEEN REVIEWED BY THE PHYSICIAN SIGNED BELOW.
          ORDERS ARE TO BE REORDERED UNLESS INDICATED TO BE DISCONTINUED.

```
      ----- Laboratory ------------------------------    CONTINUE     D/C
 483 053097 URINE, CREATININE RANDOM

            COLLECT BY NURSE

                ROUTINE                                  _____   _____

 717 053097 TYPE & SCREEN

            COLLECT BY LAB

                ROUTINE                                  _____   _____
```

                                 CONT.

FIGURE 17.25

- Change the room and bed number on all the medication tickets if used and file them in the ticket holder according to the time of administration of the medication. You may need help from a nurse with this or other tasks; you should feel free to seek assistance if words or orders seem unfamiliar. Place MARs in the appropriate notebooks.
- Add the patient's name to your TPR book, diet sheet, and any other appropriate unit record.
- Make sure that the staff member responsible has oriented the patient to the new hospital environment (Fig. 17.26).

A patient who has been transferred, and the family, may be unnecessarily anxious about such a change because they do not fully understand the reasons for it. They may have become accustomed to the original hospital unit and may be apprehensive about the new one. In any direct meeting you may have with the patient or his visitors, be as reassuring and friendly as possible.

*T*RANSFER TO ANOTHER HOSPITAL

Sometimes a patient must be transferred from one hospital to another. This may be at the patient's request or it may be for another reason such as a change in level of nursing care required (from an acute-care hospital to a skilled nursing facility), because the patient needs specialized care (from the hospital to a burn unit in a specialized hospital), or because the patient's insurance contract requires that he or she may be in a certain hospital (such as one run by Kaiser Permanente). Figures 17.27 and 17.28 show examples of forms used for this purpose. The patient in other respects is treated as a discharge.

**PATIENT TRANSFER
(TO ANOTHER FLOOR)**

1. TELEPHONE TO BE SURE NEW ROOM IS READY.

2. GATHER PATIENT'S:

MEDICAL RECORDS

AND

DRUGS

3. RECORD TRANSFER ON CENSUS AND OTHER NECESSARY FORMS.

...TO BE TRANSFERED TO NEW UNIT

FIGURE 17.26

_____ **Patient Request for Transfer**
Initials

This is to certify that _____ ,
                              Name of Patient

a patient who has received services in this hospital, is being transferred at the request of the patient (or the patient's legal representative).

  I acknowledge that I have been informed of the risk and consequences potentially involved in the transfer, the possible benefits of continuing treatment at this hospital, and the alternatives (if any) to the transfer I am requesting. I hereby release the attending physician, any other physicians involved in the patient's care, the hospital and its agents and employees, from all responsibility for any ill effects which may result from the transfer.

_____ **Patient Transfer Acknowledgment**
Initials

I understand that I have a right to receive medical screening, examination, and evaluation by a physician, or appropriate personnel, without regard to my ability to pay, prior to any transfer from this hospital and that I have a right to be informed of the reasons for any transfer. I acknowledge that I have received medical screening examination and evaluation by a physician, or other appropriate personnel, and that I have been informed of the following reasons for my transfer.

_____ **Authorization to Release Medical Records**
Initials

Physician Certification

I _____ , the undersigned physician, have examined and evaluated
        Name of Physician

_____ . Based on this examination, the information available to me at the time, and the reasonable risks and benefits to the patient, I have concluded for the reasons which follow that the medical benefits reasonably expected from the provision of emergency treatment at another facility outweigh the increased risks to the patient's medical condition involved in the transfer process.

Please explain: _____

_____

_____ Date	_____ Time	X _____ E D Physician	X _____ Other Physician (if applicable)
_____ Date	_____ Time	X _____ Patient	_____ Relationship if signed by other than patient
_____ Date	_____ Time	X _____ Witness	

MEMORIAL HOSPITAL   ADDRESSOGRAPH

PATIENT TRANSFER

White – Receiving Facility   **Canary** – Medical Records   **Pink** – Nursing Unit

FIGURE 17.27

ACUTE INTERHOSPITAL PATIENT TRANSFER FORM

PATIENT:_____ DATE:_____

ADDRESS: _____ TIME OF DISCHARGE: _____

_____ D.O.B._____ AGE:_____

DIAGNOSIS:_____

PATIENT'S CONDITION AT TIME OF TRANSFER: ☐ Stable   ☐ Unstable   ☐ Critical   ☐ Serious

☐ Fair   ☐ Satisfactory   ☐ Other:_____

REASON FOR TRANSFER: _____

_____

ADDITIONAL COMMENTS: _____

PHYSICIAN ORDERING TRANSFER: _____

HOSPITAL ACCEPTING PATIENT: _____

PHYSICIAN ACCEPTING PATIENT: _____

DETAILS OF PHYSICIAN TO PHYSICIAN CONTACT:_____

NAME OF RESPONSIBLE PARTY/FAMILY: _____

TRANSPORT MODE: ☐ Ambulance   ☐ BLS   ☐ ALS   ☐ Paramedic   ☐ Taxi   ☐ Private

☐ Other:_____ Transport Service:_____
Accompanied by:_____

VITAL SIGNS ON TRANSFER: Time:_____:_____ P_____ R_____ BP_____ /_____

I.V. PATIENT: Solution_____ Amount Remaining_____ Amount Given_____

RECORDS ACCOMPANYING PATIENT: ☐ PATIENT TRANSFER FORM   ☐ WRITTEN TRANSFER

ORDERS (medication, fluids, etc.) ☐ X-RAYS (___originals___copies)   ☐ EKG   ☐ ED

HOSPITAL ADMIT FORM/CHART

LAB RESULTS _____

OTHER _____

PERSONAL EFFECTS _____

NAME AND SIGNATURE OF PHYSICIAN:_____

NAME AND SIGNATURE OF NURSE: _____

REPORT IS COMPLETE: (Signature)_____

MEMORIAL HOSPITAL
ACUTE INTERHOSPITAL PATIENT
TRANSFER FORM

Addressograph

FIGURE 17.28

DISCHARGE OF PATIENTS

Patients are normally discharged to their homes after correction of the medical condition for which they were admitted. Sometimes, however, additional care is needed, and the patient is discharged to another medical institution with special facilities such as a skilled nursing facility or nursing home (Fig. 17.29).

FIGURE 17.29

DISCHARGE PROCEDURES

The following outline of patient discharge procedures will give you an understanding of how your own duties fit into the entire patient discharge process.

- An order to discharge a patient must be written by the physician on the doctor's order sheet.
- In most hospitals, patients to be discharged must leave by a certain time in the morning so that their rooms can be cleaned and prepared for new patients.
- The patient may need a follow-up appointment with the patient's private physician or with the clinic if he or she is a service patient.
- The nurse performs all ordered treatments a final time before the patient is discharged and checks to see that the patient thoroughly understands the doctor's instructions about such matters as diet, medications, or further treatment. The nurse must also write a final discharge note on the nurses' notes.
- The patient/significant other should have received discharge education (Fig. 17.30), and the patient discharge record is completed (Fig. 17.31).
- Another department, such as social services or discharge planning, has seen the patient.

**PATIENT/SIGNIFICANT OTHER
EDUCATION LOG**

PRIMARY DX:					
OTHER MEDICAL PROBLEMS/DX:					
FAMILY/SIGNIFICANT OTHERS	**1 -**		**2 -**		
PHYSICAL/COGNITIVE DEFICIT/LIMITATION:					
SPECIAL LEARNING NEEDS/REQUESTS:					
DISCHARGE PLANNING FOLLOW-UP/RESOURCES:					

EDUCATION TOPIC	INSTRUCTION GIVEN	DEMONSTRATION GIVEN	VERBALIZES KNOWLEDGE	DEMONSTRATES SKILLS	NEEDS COMPLETE REINFORCEMENT	RESOURCES USED COMMENTS
Safe and effective use of medication.	PT/SO: DATE/INITIALS:	PT/SO: DATE/INITIALS:	PT/SO: DATE/INTITALS:	PT/SO: DATE/INITIALS:	PT/SO: DATE/INITIALS:	
Safe and effective use of medical equipment.	PT/SO: DATE/INITIALS:	PT/SO: DATE/INITIALS:	PT/SO: DATE/INITIALS:	PT/SO: DATE/INITIALS:	PT/SO: DATE/INITIALS:	
Potential drug/food interactions.	PT/SO: DATE/INITIALS:	PT/SO: DATE/INITIALS:	PT/SO: DATE/INITIALS:	PT/SO: DATE/INITIALS:	PT/SO: DATE/INITIALS:	
Dietary consult on modified diets.	PT/SO: DATE/INITIALS:	PT/SO: DATE/INITIALS:	PT/SO: DATE/INITIALS:	PT/SO: DATE/INITIALS:	PT/SO: DATE/INITIALS:	
Rehabilitation techniques to facilitate independence in ADL's.	PT/SO: DATE/INITIALS:	PT/SO: DATE/INITIALS:	PT/SO: DATE/INITIALS:	PT/SO: DATE/INITIALS:	PT/SO: DATE/INITIALS:	
	PT/SO: DATE/INITIALS:	PT/SO: DATE/INITIALS:	PT/SO: DATE/INITIALS:	PT/SO: DATE/INITIALS:	PT/SO: DATE/INITIALS:	
	PT/SO: DATE/INITIALS:	PT/SO: DATE/INITIALS:	PT/SO: DATE/INITIALS:	PT/SO: DATE/INITIALS:	PT/SO: DATE/INITIALS:	
	PT/SO: DATE/INITIALS:	PT/SO: DATE/INITIALS:	PT/SO: DATE/INITIALS:	PT/SO: DATE/INITIALS:	PT/SO: DATE/INITIALS:	
	PT/SO: DATE/INITIALS:	PT/SO: DATE/INITIALS:	PT/SO: DATE/INITIALS:	PT/SO: DATE/INITIALS:	PT/SO: DATE/INITIALS:	
	PT/SO: DATE/INITIALS:	PT/SO: DATE/INITIALS:	PT/SO: DATE/INITIALS:	PT/SO: DATE/INITIALS:	PT/SO: DATE/INITIALS:	

SIGNATURE:	INITIALS:	DISCIPLINE:	ADDRESSOGRAPH
_____ _____ _____ _____ **PT/SIGNIFICANT OTHER EDUCATION LOG**	_____ _____ _____ _____	_____ _____ _____ _____	

FIGURE 17.30

NURSING DISCHARGE SUMMARY

Dismissed by M.D. ☐ Yes ☐ No   ☐ Released   ☐ AMA Release Signed

☐ Ambulatory   ☐ Wheelchair   ☐ Ambulance Accompanied by _____

Discharge to: ☐ Home   ☐ SNF   ☐ Other _____

Vital Signs: T _____   P _____   R _____   B/P _____

Afebrile for 24 hrs. (< 99.6) _____   Temp. Above 99.6 _____   M.D. Notified _____

Mental Status: ☐ Alert   ☐ Oriented   ☐ Cooperative   ☐ Confused   ☐ Other _____

CONDITION OF SKIN	YES	NO	LOCATION/DESCRIPTION
Bruises			
Rashes			
Reddened Areas			
Pressure Ulcer			
Wound/Incision			

IMPAIRMENT	YES	NO	LOCATION/DESCRIPTION
Speech			
Hearing			
Vision			
Paralysis			
Contracture			

COMPLIANCE	YES	NO	COMMENTS
Understands physical condition			
Willing to comply with regimen			
States understanding of instructions			

SELF CARE:	INDEPEND	ASSIST	DEP	SELF CARE:	INDEPEND	ASSIST	DEP
Ambulatory				Dressing			
Turns self in bed				Transfer to W.C.			
Personal Hygiene				Other			

Bladder: ☐ Continent ☐ Incontinent ☐ Catheter Type: _____ ☐ Other _____

Bowel: ☐ Continent ☐ Incontinent ☐ Ostomy ☐ Other _____

Date _____/_____/_____   Time _____   Nurse Signature: _____

PATIENT DISCHARGE INSTRUCTIONS

DISCHARGE MEDICINES AND MEDICATION INSTRUCTIONS:

POST-DISCHARGE INSTRUCTIONS: (i.e. Diet, Activity, Equipment, Physical Therapy, Respiratory Therapy, Pharmacy, Support Group)

Office Appointment: Doctor _____ return to the office in ____ days / week. Please call _____ for an appointment.

DISCHARGE PLANNING

EQUIPMENT _____ COMPANY _____ Telephone (____) _____

HOME HEALTH CARE _____ Telephone (____) _____

OTHER _____ Telephone (____) _____

AUTHORIZATION: I acknowledge that the above information has been explained to me. I have had the opportunity to clarify any questions. I have received a copy of these instructions.

SIGNATURE

_____ _____ _____
PATIENT / FAMILY SIGNATURE   RELATIONSHIP   DATE

PATIENT DISCHARGE RECORD

SC W46 (2/94)

WHITE - CHART   Canary - Patient   Pink - Physician

FIGURE 17.31

■ Members of the nursing staff help the patient prepare for discharge by assembling the patient's belongings and, if necessary, helping him or her dress. Valuables are returned (Fig. 17.32).

■ When the patient is ready to leave, the patient must be accompanied by a friend or relative. Any exceptions require written permission from the doctor.

After the patient is discharged, the following procedure must be completed.

1. The diet kitchen must be notified so meals are not sent to the floor for that patient.

2. Other departments such as admitting and the laboratory may be notified. If medications that have been charged to the patient remain on the nursing unit, they must be returned to the pharmacy so the patient's account can be credited.

3. The physician must complete the discharge summary on the summary sheet.

4. The order of the chart forms must be rearranged when the patient is discharged, and the reassembled chart must be delivered to the medical records department, where it will be filed.

DISCHARGE AND HEALTH UNIT COORDINATOR RESPONSIBILITIES

Following is a list of instructions to guide you in discharging patients:

■ Make sure that a written order for discharge is included on the doctor's order sheet.

■ Check with the patient to make certain that he knows the time by which he must leave the hospital in order to avoid additional expense, that he has someone coming to accompany him home, and that he has a follow-up appointment.

■ If the patient does not have anyone to accompany him from the hospital, you may have to notify his doctor to write a taxi permission order.

FIGURE 17.32 The nurse helps the patient collect and pack personal possessions.

- If the person is a service patient, you will be responsible for calling the clinic by telephone for a follow-up appointment and writing up an appointment slip to give the patient.
- If the person is a private patient, you may need to call her doctor or the doctor's office to arrange for a follow-up appointment.
- If the patient needs special diet instructions, you may need to call the diet kitchen to arrange for a dietitian to come up to the floor and explain the instructions.
- If patients in your hospital do not routinely stop at the business office on their way out of the hospital, find out which patients must do so before leaving, according to the procedure in use at your hospital.
- Check to see what valuables are returned to the patient.
- If the patient is a "police case," permission for discharge home must be obtained from the local police department.
- Notify the diet kitchen of the patient's discharge.
- Add the patient's name to your daily census records as a discharge.
- Record the discharge of the patient in the discharge and transfer book if one is used.
- Rearrange the chart forms in proper sequence for discharge. Remove and discard all blank forms, and send the chart to the medical records department.
- In many hospitals, a written notice of discharge must be sent to other departments, such as the admitting and business offices. The instructor will explain the regulations in use in your hospital.

When you have completed your training course, you will also be responsible for transcribing the discharge orders written by the doctor and returning medications to the pharmacy for credit, as necessary (Fig. 17.33).

DISCHARGE TO ANOTHER FACILITY

Patients are not always discharged directly to their homes. The Joint Commission or Accreditation of Health Care Organizations (JCAHO) requires that accredited hospitals that accept Medicare patients review the condition of all patients who remain in the hospital longer than a certain prescribed amount of time. A JCAHO-accredited hospital must have a Utilization Review Committee for this purpose.

When the committee deems that a patient no longer requires "acute nursing care," the doctor is asked to transfer the patient to an extended care facility (ECF). An ECF is also called a convalescent or nursing home.

The discharge of a patient to an ECF is similar to a routine discharge except that

- The bed patient will likely require transportation to the new facility by ambulance.
- A special form for interhospital transfer will be required. This form will often be partially completed by the health unit coordinator and partially by nursing. Photocopies of the patient's chart are made by medical records and placed in an envelope to be sent with the ambulance attendant or with the family to the new facility.

The procedure for routine discharge is then completed by the health unit coordinator.

HEALTH UNIT COORDINATOR RESPONSIBILITIES

FIGURE 17.33

$\mathcal{D}$ISCHARGE AGAINST MEDICAL ADVICE (AMA)

On occasion, a patient will decide that he does not want to remain in the hospital, even though his doctor feels that he is not yet well enough to go home. The patient may believe that the doctors and nurses are not helping him to get better. He may think he is well enough to go home despite the doctor's opinion, or he may simply be tired and depressed by a lengthy hospitalization. Whatever his reasons, you can encourage him to stay, but you cannot prevent him from leaving if he wants to go.

If this situation should arise, steps must be taken to protect the hospital and its personnel from liability in case serious medical consequences arise from premature discharge. As a health unit coordinator you have certain responsibilities to the patient who insists on leaving the hospital against the advice of his doctor.

■ First, notify the nurse in charge, who will ask you to call the patient's attending physician, or the chief resident, if the person is a service patient. In most hospitals, you would also notify the nursing administration office.

- The patient must sign a special release form. The signature must be witnessed.
- Once this release is signed and the patient and/or family are fully aware of the possible consequences of premature discharge, your responsibilities and duties are the same as for any routine discharge.

DISCHARGE ORDERS

TYPES OF DISCHARGE ORDERS

If the patient has fully recovered and needs little or no follow-up care or detailed home instruction, the doctor may write simple discharge orders on the day of discharge, for example:

> *Discharge home in PM.*
> *Make 6-week follow-up clinic appointment.*

Ordinarily, discharge orders are written prior to the actual day of discharge and include more details. Orders from the following categories are usually included.

Discharge

The doctor must always state in writing that the patient is to be discharged and must include the date and time of day. The order may also specify where the patient is to be discharged and by what means (e.g., may be discharged to home or to a nursing home; may be leaving by ambulance or by taxi).

Medications

In some hospitals, the pharmacy provides the patient with medications he or she must continue to take at home. If this is the case, the doctor will write an order for the medications, and they must be requisitioned from the pharmacy.

Follow-up Appointments

Many patients are discharged from the hospital to convalesce at home. Ordinarily, every patient who has been hospitalized is advised to continue under a doctor's care until recovery is complete. Most doctors will write discharge orders for follow-up appointments that include the date or time the patient is expected to see him or her or visit the clinic.

Special Instructions

Many patients and their family must be taught to perform care related to their illnesses that they will carry out at home. Some patients will be taught to change dressings on draining wounds. Others may require special diet instructions. Diabetics must often learn to test their own urine and blood for glucose and to give their own insulin injections. This instruction is the responsibility of the patient educator, who is usually a nurse.

Other Discharge Orders

Discharge orders that do not fall into any of the categories already discussed may include the following:

> *Disposable-type enema on AM discharge, if pt has not defecated during previous 24 hours.*
>
> *Change dressing before discharge.*
>
> *Notify brother of impending discharge.*
>
> *Sent pt home c̄ elastic stockings in place.*

*T*RANSCRIPTION

Transcribe the following group of discharge orders:

> *Discharge home Tuesday AM.*
>
> *Teach urine testing prior to discharge.*
>
> *Have dietician discuss diabetic diet c̄ pt and wife.*
>
> *To diabetic follow-up clinic in 4 weeks.*
>
> *Instruct pt in care of leg ulcer.*
>
> *Order Colace tab ī po qd hs*
>
> *Order multivitamins tabs īī po AM*

*P*ATIENT DEATHS

Some patients who enter a health care institution are terminally ill, that is, dying. Sometimes death is sudden or unexpected. More often it is not. Nursing's first responsibility is to help make the patient as comfortable as possible. Their second responsibility is to assist in meeting the emotional needs of the patient and his family.

The most important single fact to remember about the dying patient is that he or she is just as important as the patient who is going to recover. It is the goal of the health care team to help a human being end his or her life in peace, comfort, and dignity. Everyone must die. Surely we would all prefer to die in reassuring and comfortable surroundings (Fig. 17.34).

A great deal of research was done on death and dying by Elisabeth Kübler-Ross. She interviewed many dying patients over a period of years and developed what has been called the stages of dying. These are not always experienced by all patients in the same way, and not all patients pass through all the stages. Briefly they are:

- Denial
- Anger

FIGURE 17.34

- Bargaining
- Depression
- Acceptance

In the presence of death, there are certain attitudes your hospital expects of you—toward yourself, the dying patient, and the family. Try to adopt these attitudes with sympathy and tact.

- First, try hard to avoid becoming emotionally involved in deaths and medical tragedies. To show sympathy and quiet understanding for the misfortunes of others at such a time is praiseworthy, but to identify yourself with a dying patient will prevent you from extending the warmth and understanding necessary at such times and may keep you from being able to perform your job and helping other patients who also need you.

- Second, you must never forget that most people fear the uncertainty of death. You must learn to accept the patient regardless of his or her reactions or possible unreasonableness to you or other members of the staff. Never categorize patients as "good" or "bad." Simply try to appreciate the difficulties they face and learn to accept their behavior.

- Finally, you must respect the feelings of the patient's family and friends when they come to visit the patient. Under the pressure of helplessness and anxiety, these visitors may not always act reasonably. Accept their behavior and try to help them through a difficult period.

- Realize that for some patients their family consists of people other than traditional family members. The people closest to them may not be actual "family" and their significant other may be a person of the same sex.

When it is known that death is approaching, the people closest to the dying patient's family and close friends may want to spend a lot of time with the patient. This is usually permitted as much as possible. Be as helpful to them as you can. You might suggest that they have a cup of coffee or tea. Tell them where the coffee shop is. Also learn the policy in your institution of serving meals to visitors. You may be able to arrange for trays to be delivered to the patient's family at mealtimes. If this is not a

FIGURE 17.35 Supporting the family of the terminally ill patient is very important.

lowed, tell the visitors where they can find the cafeteria or a nearby restaurant. Make sure the visitors know the location of the restrooms, lounge, telephones, and chapel (Fig. 17.35).

SIGNS OF APPROACHING DEATH

Death comes in different ways. It may come quite suddenly after a patient has seemed to be recovering; or it may come after a long period during which there has been a steady decline of body functions. Death also may result from complications during convalescence. The following are some signs showing that death may be near:

- Blood circulation slows down. The patient's hands and feet are cold to the touch.
- If the patient is conscious, the patient may complain that he or she is cold.
- The patient's face may become pale because of decreased circulation.
- The patient's eyes may be staring blankly into space. There may be no eye movement when the nurse's hand moves across the patient's line of vision.
- The patient may perspire heavily, even though his or her body is cold.
- The patient loses muscle tone, and the body becomes limp. The patient's jaw may drop, and the mouth may stay partly open.
- Respirations may become slower and more difficult.
- Mucus collects in the patient's throat and bronchial tubes and may cause a sound that is sometimes called the "death rattle."
- The pulse often is rapid, but it becomes weak and irregular.
- Just before death, respiration stops and the pulse gets very faint. The nurse may not able to feel the patient's pulse at all.
- Contrary to popular belief, a dying person is rarely in great pain. As the patient's condition gets worse, less blood may be flowing to the brain. Therefore, the patient may feel little or no pain.

In some health care institutions, the head nurse or team leader confirms that a patient has no pulse or has stopped breathing and the nurse can call a "code." Code Blue, Cardiac Arrest, or whatever name is used for the code in your institution, is an emergency announcement to the entire staff. As previously discussed, a preassigned team will come to help the patient. Only when the team fails to keep the patient alive is the patient declared to be dead by a physician. If because of the patient's Advance Directive and terminal condition, an order for No Code, do not resuscitate (DNR), or do not attempt resuscitation (DNAR) has been written by the doctor, no Code Blue will be called and no resuscitation will be attempted.

After a patient's death, his or her body still is treated with respect and is given gentle care. If family members are present, they usually wait outside the room until the doctor has finished his or her examination. The patient's family will probably be allowed to view the body if they wish.

Sometimes the family is not present when the patient dies. In this case, the nurse calls the doctor and tells him or her that the family is not there. Either the doctor or the nurse then notifies the family and finds out whether they wish to view the body before it is sent to the morgue. If so, the body stays in the room until the family arrives.

When the family is present, they may be given the patient's personal belongings, which they sign for. These items are checked against the clothing list to be sure that everything is accounted for. You will learn the procedure in your health care institution for taking care of the deceased patient's clothes. If the members of the family do not wish to view the body, the nurse will then proceed with the postmortem care.

𝒫OSTMORTEM PROCEDURE

Although as a health unit coordinator you will have no direct responsibility for postmortem procedures, it will help you to be familiar with them. After the patient has been pronounced dead, nursing personnel carry out postmortem (after death) care.

■ The body must be cleaned, the eyes and jaw closed, and the limbs positioned in good body alignment. If members of the family are present, they are often allowed to view the body at this time.
■ Following this, the limbs are carefully tied together and the body is wrapped in a large sheet, called a shroud. Policies will differ somewhat on this procedure.

The body is then placed on a special stretcher. It is covered with a sheet and removed to the morgue. It is stored in a large refrigerator there until the family has made funeral arrangements with a mortician. The mortician, having obtained proper authorization, removes the body from the hospital premises.

𝒫ATIENT DEATHS AND HEALTH UNIT COORDINATOR RESPONSIBILITIES

As a health unit coordinator, your duties at the time of a patient's death will be primarily clerical, although you may often be asked to make necessary telephone calls. The following are some of the responsibilities you may be assigned.

- You may be asked to locate, by paging or by telephone, the patient's doctor for certification of death.
- You may be expected to notify the nursing administration office, the reception or information desk, and the business office and admitting office. This may be done by telephone, computer, or in writing.
- For situations in which the deceased patient's family cannot be reached by telephone by the doctor or nurse, your hospital will have regulations specifying who should be notified to contact the family. In small communities, this responsibility is often given to the police department.
- The death certificate is usually processed for the physician's completion and signature by the admitting office or the medical records department. You may be asked to expedite this form by taking a copy from the file on request.
- You must have a stamped autopsy consent form ready if it is to be used.
- You may be required to requisition a shroud pack for use in wrapping the body.
- You may be asked to prepare identifications tags to be used on the body in several places and in the morgue.
- You may be responsible for collecting and identifying the patient's personal belongs and sending them to a designated hospital area, if the family is not at hand.
- You must add the patient's name to the daily census record as a death and record the proper information in summary records, such as a discharge and transfer book.
- Finally, you will be required to assemble the patient's chart records in discharge sequence and send them to the medical records department. Delete the patient's name from all current hospital records in use on the unit. Carry out any other procedures associated with a routine discharge, such as returning medications to the pharmacy for credit, if they apply to the deceased patient's situation.

CERTIFICATION OF DEATH

Certification of death can take place only after examination by a physician. The death certificate is signed by the doctor, and permission to perform an autopsy is usually requested from the family.

Autopsies

Autopsies are dissections of the corpse. They are performed to determine the extent of disease and the cause of death. They cannot be done routinely without the permission of the family. The signed permission of the next of kin is given in a special chart form called the autopsy consent (Figs. 17.36 and 17.37).

Coroner's Cases

In corner's cases, hospital personnel are not allowed to approach the family for autopsy authorization; the responsibility for conducting the autopsy lies with the coroner. Usually, the local, county, or state government will have regulations defining coroner's cases. For example, cases of deaths occurring within 24 hours after hospitalization, or of victims of suspected poisoning, or of apparently accidental deaths may be considered coroner's cases in your locality.

AUTHORIZATION FOR AUTOPSY

TO: PATHOLOGIST, MEMORIAL HOSPITAL   DATED: _____ 19 ____

I certify that I am the _____
                                                        (Relationship)

of _____ deceased, and have the right to control the disposition of the remains of said decedent. I hereby authorize you, together with your assistants, to perform an autopsy and complete postmortem examination on the body of such deceased, including the taking of photographs, and the removal of such structures or organs as you may deem necessary for special study or for therapeutic or scientific uses as provided in the health and safety code.

I also authorize the pathologist to have present at the examination such person or persons as he may deem proper.

I also authorize any cemetery authority, licensed funeral director or licensed hospital, having custody of such remains, through its authorized personnel, to permit or assist in such autopsy and examination including the transportation of the remains by any such cemetery authority or funeral director to and from the hospital or other place as may be arranged by you for such autopsy and examination.

WITNESS: _____ SIGNED _____

WITNESS: _____ SIGNED _____

The nurse is instructed to list the names of the physicians to whom reports are to be sent. These are physicians who have attended the patient on present or previous admission.

ATTENDING PHYSICIAN _____ M.D.

SURGICAL CONSULTANT _____ M.D.

MEDICAL CONSULTANT _____ M.D.

UROLOGIC CONSULTANT _____ M.D.

OTHER PHYSICIANS WHO ATTENDED THE DECEASED _____ M.D.

_____ M.D.

INSTRUCTIONS:

1. The autopsy permission is to be completed in duplicate and witnessed.

2. Send both copies of autopsy premission, with hospital chart, to the pathologist's office.

3. Notify the pathologist, who will arrange the time of the postmortem examination.

4. When the postmortem exam is completed, the pathology office will notify nursing supervisor when the remains may be released to the mortician.

FIGURE 17.36

(Complete this in duplicate—one for the mortician)

AUTHORITY FOR RELEASE OF REMAINS

PART I: MEMORIAL HOSPITAL

Release Remains of _____

To Mortician _____ Address _____

_____

Date _____ Signed _____

Relationship _____

PART II: RECEIVED FROM MEMORIAL HOSPITAL THE PERSONAL EFFECTS LISTED BELOW:

_____   _____

_____   _____

_____   _____

_____   _____

_____   _____

_____   _____

Date _____ Signed _____

Witness _____

PART III: REMAINS RECEIVED:

Date _____ Mortuary _____

Signed _____

INFORMATION FOR MORTICIAN

Date of Death _____ Hour _____

Attending Physician _____

Address _____

Telephone Number _____

FIGURE 17.37

*L*EARNING ACTIVITIES

Complete the following.

1. Explain how you would greet a patient being admitted to your unit.

   _____

   _____

   _____

   _____

   _____

2. List the two types of patient admissions.
   (a) _____
   (b) _____

3. What is the MSSU? _____

4. List the forms or items that will come to the unit from the admitting department when a patient is admitted.
   (a) _____
   (b) _____
   (c) _____

5. In your words, explain how you would admit a patient to a nursing unit.

   _____

   _____

   _____

   _____

   _____

   _____

   _____

   _____

   _____

   _____

   _____

6. List the categories of orders that are usually included for new admissions.
   (a) _____
   (b) _____
   (c) _____
   (d) _____
   (e) _____

7. List the two most commonly ordered diagnostic tests.
   (a) _____
   (b) _____

8. Define *routine orders*. _____

   _____

9. Surgery may be _____ or _____ in nature

10. List three groups into which surgical patients can be divided.
    (a) _____
    (b) _____
    (c) _____

11. List the two categories of activities that generally will require checking preoperatively.

(a) _____

(b) _____

12. List the records that may be included in the preoperative chart.

(a) _____

(b) _____

(c) _____

(d) _____

(e) _____

(f) _____

(g) _____

(h) _____

13. List orders frequently included preoperatively.

(a) _____

(b) _____

(c) _____

(d) _____

(e) _____

(f) _____

(g) _____

14. Before surgery an _____ must be signed.

15. List the two laboratory tests that must be current preoperatively according to hospital policy.

(a) _____

(b) _____

16. List four reasons why a patient might be transferred to another room.

(a) _____

(b) _____

(c) _____

(d) _____

17. Why might a patient be transferred to another unit?

_____

_____

_____

_____

18. Explain your duties when a patient is transferred to another room.

_____

_____

_____

To another unit. _____

_____

_____

_____

19. Describe your responsibilities when a patient is discharged.

_____

_____

_____
_____
_____
_____
_____
_____
_____

20. What does it mean when a patient leaves the hospital AMA?

_____
_____

21. In the presence of death, there are certain attitudes the hospital expects of you. List at least three.

(a) _____
_____
_____

(b) _____
_____
_____

(c) _____
_____
_____

22. List the five stages of dying according to Elisabeth Kübler-Ross.

(a) _____
(b) _____
(c) _____
(d) _____
(e) _____

23. List some of your clerical and communication duties at the time of a patient's death.

(a) _____
(b) _____
(c) _____
(d) _____
(e) _____
(f) _____
(g) _____
(h) _____
(i) _____

24. Admitting calls and tells you they need a female bed stat. You have two semi-private rooms, both of which contain male patients. One male is 19 years old and is recovering from a fractured leg. The other is an 80-year-old terminally ill patient. The only other empty bed (which is ready) on the floor is in a semi-private room with a noisy, confused, elderly woman. What should you do? What criteria will you use in deciding what to do?

_____
_____
_____
_____

_____

_____

25. What do you think a patient worries about when he or she is admitted to the hospital for surgery? _____

_____

26. What could happen if a new patient is brought to a room by wheelchair and no one on your nursing unit knows the patient is there? _____

_____

27. Mr. Jacobs in Room 213 comes to the nurses' station. He insists he is going to be discharged today. His doctor has just been on the floor and has written new orders on other patients' charts, but now you no longer see the doctor. What should you do? _____

_____

28. A patient that the staff has become very fond of was supposed to go home today. Early this morning she suddenly died. How would you feel? What kinds of questions do you think would go through your mind? How do you think you and the staff would manage to keep working on a bad day like this? What would you say to the family? What should you not say to the family?

_____

_____

_____

_____

_____

_____

29. Sometimes patients have DNR (do not resuscitate) orders. How do you feel about this? How do you feel about the fact that sometimes patients are kept on life support or given life-sustaining fluids and medications when there appears to be no hope at all?

_____

_____

_____

_____

_____

30. Mr. Swansen was taken to the operating room at 8:00 AM, and his wife was told he should be back in his room by noon. It is 1:30 PM and she has asked you to call the OR every half-hour since 11:00 . Now she wants you to call again. How should you handle this? Is there anything else you can do to help Mrs. Swansen?

_____

_____

_____

_____

_____

_____

31. When a patient is transferred from one place to another on the nursing unit, what records must be changed? Why is this important?

_____

_____

_____

32. Why is it important that all required departments such as laboratory, dietary, and admitting be notified when a patient moves to another room or nursing unit?

_____

_____

_____

_____

_____

*S*AMPLE HEALTH UNIT COORDINATOR PROCEDURES

1. ADMITTING
Use the information and the forms provided by your instructor to admit the following patients.
(a) Joseph P. Anyone
Rm. 123
Admitting M.D.—James Stevens, M.D.
Diagnosis—congestive heart failure
Age—78
Unit #—68754
(b) Clara Fied
Rm. 765
Admitting M.D.—Laila Morgan, M.D.
Diagnosis—COPD
Age—82
Unit #—98123

2. SURGICAL PATIENTS
Using the forms and procedures required by your hospital, set up the following patients for surgery:
(a) Ryan A. Cox
Rm. 794
Diagnosis—acute appendicitis
Surgery—appendectomy
Date of surgery—use tomorrow's date
Age—22
Surgeon—Velma Blade, M.D.
Allergies—penicillin
(b) Kathleen Doyle
Rm. 8921
Diagnosis—uterine fibroids
Surgery—hysterectomy
Date of surgery—use tomorrow's date

Age—39
Surgeon—Calvin Cutter, M.D.
Allergies—none

3. TRANSFER
Use the following information and the forms provided by your instructor to transfer the following patients.
(a)   Transfer Mr. Anyone to Rm. 124 on the same floor.
      Transfer Mr. Anyone to ICU.
(b)   Transfer Mrs. Fied to Riversweet Convalescent Hospital today.

4. DISCHARGE
Use your hospital's forms and procedures to discharge Mr. Anyone. (Following ICU he returned to your floor, Room 124. He has improved and is going home today.)

5. DEATHS
Use the forms and procedures required by your hospital and complete this exercise.

Mr. John C. Over was admitted to your floor three days ago. His condition became worse, and this morning he expired. He was pronounced dead by his physician, Tod Matthew, M.D., at 8.03 A.M. His diagnosis was acute myocardial infarction and he was in Room 888. His wife was with him at the time of his death and has taken home all of his belongings. He is not a coroner's case. He is to go to Drake's Mortuary. There is no autopsy.

Kardexing

Use the Kardexes provided in Figure 17.38, or ones given to you by your instructor.

DATE

X-RAY AND OTHER

LAB

DATE

DAILY LAB

RESPIRATORY

HEIGHT: WEIGHT:

CODE STATUS:

DISCHARGE PLANNING/REHAB:

SURGICAL OR SPECIAL PROCEDURES

DATE

DIET

FORCE FLUIDS

TUBE FEEDING

TEST DIET

ALLERGIES:

I & O

ACTIVITY

DATE LAST BM

RELATIVE PHONE #

FIGURE 17.38

DATE	MEDS - ROUTINE	DOSE	RT	FREQ	RO	DATE	FREQ	BOTTLES	IVs	DO
								MEDS		DO

DATE	MEDS - PRN	DOSE	RT.	FREQ.	RO

TREATMENTS

DATE

DATE	MEDS - ONE TIME	DOSE	RT.	FREQ.	RO

SURGICAL PROCEDURE DATE:

DIAGNOSIS:

ROOM # NAME:	AGE	SEX	CONSULTING M.D.
			ADMITTING M.D.
	ADMIT DATE		TRANSFER DATE

FIGURE 17.38b (*Continued*)

DATE

X-RAY AND OTHER

LAB

DATE

DAILY LAB

DATE

SURGICAL OR SPECIAL PROCEDURES

RESPIRATORY

HEIGHT: WEIGHT:

CODE STATUS:

DISCHARGE PLANNING/REHAB:

DIET

FORCE FLUIDS

TUBE FEEDING

TEST DIET

ALLERGIES:

I & O

ACTIVITY

DATE LAST BM

RELATIVE PHONE #

FIGURE 17.38c (*Continued*)

DATE	MEDS - ROUTINE	DOSE	RT	FREQ	RO	DATE	FREQ	BOTTLES	IV'S	DO

DATE	MEDS - PRN	DOSE	RT.	FREQ.	RO	DATE	FREQ	MEDS		DO

DATE	MEDS - ONE TIME	DOSE	RT.	FREQ.	RO	DATE	TREATMENTS

SURGICAL PROCEDURE DATE:

DIAGNOSIS:

ROOM #	NAME:	AGE	SEX	CONSULTING M.D.
				ADMITTING M.D.
	ADMIT DATE			TRANSFER DATE

FIGURE 17.38d (*Continued*)

LAB

DATE

X-RAY AND OTHER

DAILY LAB

RESPIRATORY

DATE

SURGICAL OR SPECIAL PROCEDURES

HEIGHT: WEIGHT:

CODE STATUS:

DISCHARGE PLANNING/REHAB:

DIET

FORCE FLUIDS

TUBE FEEDING

TEST DIET

ALLERGIES:

I & O

ACTIVITY

DATE LAST BM

RELATIVE PHONE #

FIGURE 17.38e (Continued)

DATE	MEDS - ROUTINE	DOSE	RT	FREQ	RO	DATE	FREQ	BOTTLES	IV'S	DO

DATE	MEDS - PRN	DOSE	RT.	FREQ.	RO	DATE	FREQ	MEDS	DO

DATE	TREATMENTS

DATE	MEDS - ONE TIME	DOSE	RT.	FREQ.	RO

| | AGE | SEX | CONSULTING M.D. |

SURGICAL
PROCEDURE DATE:

DIAGNOSIS:

ADMITTING M.D.

ROOM # NAME:

ADMIT DATE TRANSFER DATE

FIGURE 17.38f (*Continued*)

This is a rotated (landscape) Kardex-style patient care form. The form contains the following labeled fields and column headers:

Top row headers (left to right):
- DATE | X-RAY AND OTHER | DATE | LAB | DAILY LAB
- DATE | SURGICAL OR SPECIAL PROCEDURES

Left-side field labels (rows):
- RESPIRATORY
- HEIGHT: | WEIGHT:
- CODE STATUS:
- DIET | DISCHARGE PLANNING/REHAB:
- FORCE FLUIDS
- TUBE FEEDING
- TEST DIET
- ALLERGIES:
- I & O
- ACTIVITY
- DATE LAST BM | RELATIVE PHONE #

FIGURE 17.38g (*Continued*)

DATE	MEDS - ROUTINE	DOSE	RT.	FREQ	RO	DATE	FREQ	BOTTLES	IV'S	DO

DATE	MEDS - PRN	DOSE	RT.	FREQ.	RO	DATE	FREQ	MEDS		DO

DATE	MEDS - ONE TIME	DOSE	RT.	FREQ.	RO	DATE	TREATMENTS			

SURGICAL PROCEDURE DATE:

DIAGNOSIS:

		AGE	SEX	CONSULTING M.D.

ROOM #   NAME:

		ADMITTING M.D.

ADMIT DATE		TRANSFER DATE

FIGURE 17.38h (*Continued*)

Review

Now that you have completed your health unit coordinator training course, consider all that you have accomplished. Throughout this program you have been taught skills, attitudes, and information necessary to perform your duties.

- You have learned to answer the telephone and intercom, and how to receive and give instructions to patients and visitors; and you have learned the proper attitudes you should have toward all the people you meet in your work.
- You have studied the routine of the hospital, the duties of its staff, and the variety of services offered by its departments. You have recognized the important role you play in helping the hospital run efficiently to give each patient the best of care.
- You have learned how to handle charts and have become familiar with patient care records.
- You have learned how to transcribe doctors' orders so that the patients receive the treatments and care that have been prescribed for them at the correct time and exactly as the doctor intended.
- You have learned the importance of accuracy, promptness, and attention to detail in carrying out your tasks.

You must keep these points in mind, then, as you assume your full responsibilities as a health unit coordinator.

REVIEWING FOR YOUR EXAMINATION

To effectively and meaningfully review your course work, you will find it helpful to follow a few simple recommendations.

GETTING READY

- Choose a time when you are not likely to be disturbed. It is difficult to organize your thoughts when you are subject to constant interruptions.
- Find a quiet place for study. Be sure that you have a good light and a flat surface (a table, desk, or countertop) on which you can spread your materials.
- Assemble all the equipment you will need. This will include your health unit coordinator manual, pencils, and some scratch paper.
- Sit up straight. Bad posture causes fatigue. Your mind will be more alert and your attention span longer if your body is not too relaxed.

ℋOW TO REVIEW

Your review should have three primary objectives:

1. To refresh your memory about all the material you have studied during the course.

2. To help you relate the specific tasks you have learned to your total job.

3. To identify any subject areas about which you may still be confused or unsure of yourself.

Everyone has his or her own method of reviewing, and what works well for one person may not work at all for another. Here are some further suggestions that may be helpful.

■ Begin by jotting down the titles of each of the chapters in your manual. Look over the list and try to recall the main points of each chapter.

■ Turn to the first chapter and scan it quickly, noting especially the main headings. If you have already underlined the most important points, read them over. Also, reread any notes you may have taken in class.

■ Proceed in this way through the remaining chapters. Copy out any lists of detailed procedures (such as chart order) as an aid in your review.

■ Write down any points about which you are still unsure so that you can discuss them with your instructor before the examination.

■ There are certain things, such as the following, that you absolutely *must know*. If you have not already memorized them, start now.
  ■ Abbreviations for times of administration for medications and your hospital's time schedule.
  ■ The hospital's regulations regarding visitors, patients, and personnel.
  ■ Correct chart order.
  ■ The appropriate hospital department to which you must send each requisition.
  ■ The seven steps of the transcription procedure and their application.

■ There are many other abbreviations and symbols with which you are expected to be familiar. These include, for example, abbreviations for treatments, diet, diagnostic examinations, dosages, and routes of administration. Review these lists carefully.

As you prepare for your final examination prepare yourself for the NAHUC national certification examination. If you will not be taking this until after your final, be sure to save your notes and plan to review again before the examination.

The NAHUC national certification examination is offered at testing sites nationwide. It is a comprehensive examination designed to test your skills as a health unit coordinator and give you recognition as an educated member of the health team in this important health occupation. For information on the NAHUC examination, contact NAHUC.

Your final examination will cover all the material you have studied in this course. The examination will give you an opportunity to demonstrate the knowledge you have acquired, the skills you have learned, and your readiness to assume the full responsibilities of a health unit coordinator.

$\mathcal{H}$EALTH UNIT COORDINATOR CERTIFICATION EXAMINATION CONTENT OUTLINE

Students should note that this is a *sample* content outline and should request the most current information before sitting for the examination. The new examination content outline is based on the results of a 1996 health unit coordinator job analysis conducted by NAHUC. The percentages of questions in each area were statistically determined by the number of knowledge statements associated with those areas.

Clinical Training Plan: Health Unit Coordinator (pp. 520–524) contains a list of skills a health unit coordinator should possess. If you are a student, your instructor may wish you to use this training plan to document your learning during your externship.

If you are already employed as a health unit coordinator, you may wish to use this skill list to review what you already know and that which you need to learn.

$\mathcal{N}$AHUC OUTLINE
(BASED ON 1996 JOB ANALYSIS)

	Percentage
I. Coordination of the Health Unit	48%
A. Operations	
1. Supplies and services management	
2. Information management: patient record, unit staff, organization	
B. Communications	
1. Equipment	
2. Skills	
C. Orientation and training personnel	
D. Safety	
II. Confidentiality and Patient Rights	10%
III. Critical Thinking	6%
A. Problem identification and resources	
B. Prioritization and decision making	
IV. Order Transcription	31%
A. Process	
B. Classifications: Diagnostics, Dietary, Nursing, Pharmacy, Therapy, Misc.	
C. Medical terms, abbreviations, and symbols	
V. Professional Development	5%

(Courtesy of NAHUC.)
Note: Content and percentage of emphasis may change.

$\mathcal{C}$LINICAL TRAINING PLAN: HEALTH UNIT COORDINATOR
STUDENT: _____   **SEMESTER:** _____

*Tasks	Est. Time Needed	On-Site Trainer Signature	Date of Competency	Actual Time
ORIENTATION				
Shows knowledge of:				
Hospital environment				
Nursing Service Dept.				
Working environment				
Daily routine				
COMMUNICATIONS				
Uses computer				
Uses the telephone				
Pages				
Records and delivers messages				
Operates the intercom				

(continued)

*C*LINICAL TRAINING PLAN: HEALTH UNIT COORDINATOR (CONTINUED)
STUDENT: _____   **SEMESTER:** _____

*Tasks	Est. Time Needed	On-Site Trainer Signature	Date of Competency	Actual Time
PATIENTS AND VISITORS				
Greets new patients				
Handles patient requests				
Delivers patients' gifts, mail, etc.				
Receives and directs visitors				
EMERGENCIES				
Shows knowledge of emergency procedures				
Knows locations of fire alarms and extinguishers				
Shows knowledge of safety procedures				
Knows emergency telephone numbers and codes (e.g., cardiac arrest)				
Reports hazards				
Reports fires				
Shows knowledge of incident report forms				
Reports medical emergencies				
Shows ability to carry out HUC responsibilities by keeping telephone lines free and remaining alert and responsive to supervisor's directions				
CLERICAL RESPONSIBILITIES— General				
Keeps the nurses' station neat				
Handles mail				
Maintains files and supplies				
Posts bulletin board notices				
Helps fill out routine forms				
THE PATIENT'S CHART				
Is able to assemble patients' charts				
Shows knowledge of routine and supplemental chart forms				
Keeps track of charts: records, removals, and replacements				
Does routine chart checks				
Demonstrates understanding of chart as legal document that must be in ink, legible, current, and signed as prescribed by hospital				
CHARTING RESPONSIBILITIES				
Enters information on graphic sheet as applicable to hospital				
Keeps chart forms in standard sequential order				
PATIENT-CENTERED ACTIVITIES *Admitting Patients:*				
Makes up new chart				
Enters name on all records				
Notifies nurse of admission				
Checks for signature on release of liability				
Makes note of allergies				
Adds proper supplemental chart forms				
Shows knowledge of all prescribed HUC admitting procedures				
Makes patient appointments for treatments and examinations				
Makes appointments for consultations				

(continued)

CLINICAL TRAINING PLAN: HEALTH UNIT COORDINATOR (CONTINUED)

STUDENT: _____   SEMESTER: _____

*Tasks	Est. Time Needed	On-Site Trainer Signature	Date of Competency	Actual Time
Surgery Patients:				
Prepares preoperative chart forms and checklists				
Checks for current CBC & Ua				
Makes sure all ordered tests are on chart				
Checks for history and physical				
Checks for allergies				
Checks chart for completeness				
Shows ability to follow all prescribed HUC preop procedures				
Transferring Patients:				
Redirects patients' mail and visitors				
Records patient transfers				
Notifies appropriate departments				
Redirects all incoming test results				
Notifies housekeeping				
Receiving Transfer Patients:				
Receives patients' medical records and identification plates				
Makes changes on all necessary records				
Notifies all appropriate departments				
Discharging Patients:				
Checks discharge orders				
Makes follow-up appointments				
Checks with business office				
Returns valuables to patients				
Notifies diet kitchen and other depts. as prescribed				
Records discharges in daily census records				
Notifies housekeeping				
Rearranges chart forms				
Records discharges on all records as prescribed				
Returns medications to pharmacy				
Discharging Patients against Medical Advice				
Notifies attending physician at nurse's direction				
Notifies patient's family at nurse's direction				
Uses appropriate forms and procedures				
Patient Deaths				
Locates patient's doctor for certification if applicable				
Notifies nursing service office, reception desk, business office, and/ or admitting office, and any other dept. as prescribed by hospital				
Procures autopsy consent form				
Requisitions shroud pack				
Prepares identification tags				
Collects patient's personal belongings and/or knows procedure for placement in hospital until claimed by family				
Adds patient's name to daily census record as an expiration				
Assembles patient's chart records in proper sequence				
Sends patient's chart records to medical records department				
Shows knowledge of all forms utilized				
Maintains professional and helpful attitude				

(*continued*

CLINICAL TRAINING PLAN: HEALTH UNIT COORDINATOR (CONTINUED)

STUDENT: _____   SEMESTER: _____

*Tasks	Est. Time Needed	On-Site Trainer Signature	Date of Competency	Actual Time
WORKING WITH THE DIETARY DEPARTMENT				
Notifies dietary department of number and kinds of meals needed on the unit by utilizing prescribed procedures				
Checks and orders stocks of supplemental nourishments				
Requisitions meals				
Notifies diet department of changes				
Requisitions individual patient nourishments				
Requisitions guest trays				
WORKING WITH THE LABORATORIES				
Prepares requisition forms for laboratory tests/orders by computer				
Transcribes orders directly from doctor's order sheet				
Notifies the laboratory of emergency tests or appointments to be made				
Cancels patient meals				
Compiles lists of patients scheduled for tests				
Compiles lists of patients needing special preparations				
WORKING WITH OTHER HOSPITAL DEPARTMENTS				
(e.g., X-ray, Inhalation Therapy, Cardiopulmonary, Physical Therapy, Housekeeping, Environmental Services, Engineering)				
Prepares requisitions/orders by computer				
Makes appointments				
Telephones stat orders				
Contacts departments for repairs or supplies				
Sends requisitions to blood bank				
Sends requisitions to business office				
TRANSCRIPTION OF ORDERS				
Recognizes that a doctor's order needs transcription.				
After doctor's order sheet is stamped with identification plates, sends copies to appropriate departments				
Requisitions all equipment and services needed				
Transfers orders to special records and forms; shows understanding of Kardex				
Writes transcription symbols to show that the order is being processed				
Has transcribed orders checked and initialed by nurse				
Transcribing Medication Orders				
Recognizes that a doctor's order needs transcription				
After doctor's order sheet is stamped with identification plates, sends copies to appropriate departments				

(continued)

CLINICAL TRAINING PLAN: HEALTH UNIT COORDINATOR (CONTINUED)
STUDENT: _____   SEMESTER: _____

*Tasks	Est. Time Needed	On-Site Trainer Signature	Date of Competency	Actual Time
Requisitions equipment and services				
Transfers orders to special forms; shows understanding of Kardex				
Writes transcription symbols to indicate order is in process				
Checks transcribed order with nurse				
Cancels medication orders				
Transcribes renewal orders				
Transcribes single-dose and stat orders				
Transcribing Treatment Orders				
Transcribes standing orders				
Transcribes stat and single-time orders				
Transcribes cancellations and changes in orders				
Transcribing Miscellaneous Orders				
Can properly transcribe:				
Diet orders				
Activity orders				
Diagnostic test orders				
Permission, restrictions				
Consultations				
Critical condition list				
Other orders: transfers, deaths, blood bank, isolation				
Common Order Groups				
Can demonstrate ability to transcribe:				
Admission orders				
Preoperative orders				
Postoperative orders				
Discharge orders				

Note: Utilization of medical terminology to be integrated into practical experience.

This is to certify that _____ has successfully performed the skills listed under the direct supervision of the designated on-site trainer and/or the instructor of record.

Date of completion of complete training plan: _____

Comments:

_____   _____
On-Site Trainer   Student

_____   _____
Instructor   Date

Student: In the following spaces list additional tasks included in this occupation in your hospital but not listed in the preceding pages. This page will be especially useful when you are assigned to special areas of the hospital such as ICU, Mental Health, or Obstetrics. Please show number of hours spent on additional tasks performed.

Additional Tasks Performed	Hours	Date

CHAPTER 19

Order Transcription Practice

There are 48 sets of authentic physician's orders in this section. Sets 1 to 11 are examples of preprinted doctor's orders. Practice transcribing these first, and you will build your skills using orders that are easy to read.

Sets 12 to 17 are real handwritten orders. An answer key is included below each set.

Sets 18 to 48 offer a variety of actual orders to give you further practice with different writing styles.

Transcribe the following orders for Sets 1 through 48. Use the computer or your hospital's Kardexes and requisitions if possible. A sample Kardex is included at the end of Chapter 17.

PHYSICIAN'S ORDER SHEET

DATE & TIME				ORDERS	PATIENT NAME
				1. Admit.	
				2. Bedrest—May feed self, read.	
				3. Bedside commode prn BM c̄ full assistance 1–2x/day.	
				4. TPR & BP/qid.	
				5. I & O	
				6. Low salt diet.	
				7. Maalox 30 cc q 2h while awake.	
				8. Valium 5 mg p.o. q 8 hrs.	
				9. Valium 5–10 mg p.o. additional h.s. prn sleep.	

APPROVED EQUIVALENTS MAY BE DISPENSED UNLESS CHECKED HERE

	TIME NOTED	NURSE'S SIGNATURE	DOCTOR'S SIGNATURE	☐ TO BE DISCHARGED

		DATE & TIME		
			10. Surfak i̇ daily.	
			11. MOM 30 cc prn constipation.	
			12. Demerol 75 mg–100 mg IM q 2–4 hrs. PRN chest pain.	
			13. O$_2$ 6L/min, Nasal prn chest pain or dyspnea.	
			14. EKG, CPK, SGOT, HBD, SGPT tomorrow.	
			15. Bilirubin, alk ptase, ceph floc tomorrow.	
			16. IV keep open c̄ D5W.	

UNLESS CHECKED HERE

t 1

			ORDERS
			1. Pentobarb 100 mg. IM (or PO) hs.
			2. Oil retention enema followed by ss enema for impaction.
			3. Vital signs & temp q.i.d.
			4. I & O
			5. Up to bathroom c̄ help PRN.
			6. Demerol 25–50 mgm IM q 3h prn.
			7. CBC, Ua, Na, K, BUN now.
			8. IV's 5% D/1/2 N saline (add K$^+$ 30 mEq/1000) 100 cc's/hr.
			9. NPO

Set 2

DATE & TIME				ORDERS	PATIENT NAME
				1. Transfer to the Rehabilitation Unit.	
☐				2. Rehabilitation Evaluation: P.T., O.T., Speech Therapy	
				and Social Worker.	
				3. B.I.D. P.T., gait and exercise.	
				4. B.I.D. O.T., ADL, ROM, strengthening and coordination exercises.	
				5. Vital signs q. shift.	
				6. May have shampoo.	
				7. Diet as follows: *1000 mg Na — 1800 cal.*	
				8. See medication orders on separate Physician's Order Sheet.	

APPROVED EQUIVALENTS MAY BE DISPENSED UNLESS CHECKED HERE

Set 3

DATE & TIME	ORDERS	PATIENT NAME

ROUTINE BED REST ORDERS

1. Foot board attached to bed.

2. Knee length antiembolism stockings.

3. Push feet against foot board ten times hourly.

4. Ascriptin 2 B.I.D. if not allergic to aspirin.

5. Vitamin C 500 MGS Q.I.D.

6. Bathroom privileges or bedside commode for bowel movements.

7. Overhead frame with trapeze.

8. Semi-Fowler's for position of comfort.

TIME NOTED	NURSE'S SIGNATURE	DOCTOR'S SIGNATURE	☐ TO BE DISCHARGED

DATE & TIME

9. Sheepskin or air mattress.

10. Bran cereal daily.

11. Metamucil 1 oz. daily in juice.

12. Surfak 1 cap. T.I.D.

13. Enema, Laxative, or suppository of choice PRN.

14. 4000 CC'S oral fluid each 24 hrs.

15. Shampoo PRN.

TIME NOTED	NURSE'S SIGNATURE	DOCTOR'S SIGNATURE	☐ TO BE DISCHARGED

DATE & TIME

16. Incentive spirometry hourly while awake, 10 breaths,

VT ten times patients' body weight to be supervised by

respiratory therapist twice daily.

TIME NOTED	NURSE'S SIGNATURE	DOCTOR'S SIGNATURE	☐ TO BE DISCHARGED

APPROVED EQUIVALENTS MAY BE DISPENSED UNLESS CHECKED HERE

PHYSICIAN'S ORDER SHEET

		DATE & TIME	ORDERS	PATIENT NAME

APPROVED EQUIVALENTS MAY BE DISPENSED UNLESS CHECKED HERE ☐

1. T & C 3 UPC for surgery.

2. Transfuse 3 UWB—each over 3 period.

3. DSW @ 100 cc/h.

4. Consent: Reconstruction ® carotid artery.

5. Prep neck.

6. Dalmane 30 mgm po HS prn sleep.

7. Teds

8. Ampicillin 250 mgm po QID.

9. Preop Meds.

TIME NOTED	NURSE'S SIGNATURE	DOCTOR'S SIGNATURE	☐ TO BE DISCHARGED

APPROVED EQUIVALENTS MAY BE DISPENSED UNLESS CHECKED HERE ☐

DATE & TIME

Demerol 50 mgm IM i̇ preop or on call.

Vistaril 25 mgm IM i̇ preop or on call.

Valium 5 mgm po i̇ preop or on call.

10. Pt to void immediately before leaving for surgery.

11. NPO p̄ midnight.

TIME NOTED	NURSE'S SIGNATURE	DOCTOR'S SIGNATURE	☐ TO BE DISCHARGED

APPROVED EQUIVALENTS MAY BE DISPENSED UNLESS CHECKED HERE ☐

DATE & TIME

TIME NOTED	NURSE'S SIGNATURE	DOCTOR'S SIGNATURE	☐ TO BE DISCHARGED

Set 5

1. TESTS:

☐ EKG
☐ CHEST X–RAY
☐ PULMONARY FUNCTION SCREEN
☐ OTHER _____

☐ CBC
☐ UA
☐ SMA – 7
☐ ELECTROLYTES

2. DIET

☑ NPO p 2400
☐ CLEAR LIQUIDS UNTIL _____

3. START IV   ☑OPS   ☐HOLDING ROOM   ☐FLOOR

☐ Extension Set
☐ 1000 D 5 ½ N.S. @ _____ cc/hr
☐ 500 D 5 W @ _____ cc/hr
☑ 1000 R L @ _TKO_ cc/hr
☐ 1000 D 5 Isolyte S @ _____ cc/hr
☐ OTHER _____

4. MEDICATIONS

☐ Daily meds c̄ sip of H$_2$O in a.m. preop

SLEEP

☐ NEMBUTAL 100 mgm p.o. H.S.   M.R. x _____ prn
☐ DALMANE   15 mgm p.o. H.S.   M.R. x _____ prn
☐ DALMANE   30 mgm p.o. H.S.   M.R. x _____ prn
☐ HALCION   .25 mgm p.o. H.S.   M.R. x _____ prn
☐ OTHER _____

PRE – OP

☐ LEAVE DENTURES IN PLACE
☐ NO PREOP MEDICATION
☑ ALKA SELTZER GOLD TABS ii c̄ 30 cc H20 ½ - 1 h. preop
☐ VALIUM _____ mgm. ☐IV ☐P.O. @ _____
☐ DROPERIDOL _____ mgm I.M. @ _____
☐ MORPHINE _____ mgm I.M. @ _____
☐ FENTANYL _____ mgm. ☐IV ☐I.M.@ _____
☐ DEMEROL _____ mgm I.M. @ _____
☐ VISTARIL _____ mgm ☐p.o. ☐I.M. @ _____
☐ ATIVAN _____ mgm ☐p.o. ☐I.M. @ _____
☐ ATROPINE _____ mgm I.M. @ _____
☐ SCOPOLAMINE _____ mgm I.M. @ _____
☐ ROBINUL _____ mgm I.M. @ _____
☒ VERSED _2-4_ mgm ☒IV ☐IM@ ____ on call
☐ OTHER _____

5. ADDITIONAL PREOP ORDERS ———————————————

Nurse's Signature	Date	Time	Transcriber	

**PREOPERATIVE ANESTHESIA
ORDERS**

Set 6

PHYSICIAN'S ORDER SHEET

DATE & TIME	ORDERS	PATIENT NAME
	PREOPERATIVE ORDERS FOR COLOSTOMY CLOSURE:	
	1. Laboratory: CBC, U/A, Lytes, Creatinine, Glucose.	
	2. Chest X-Ray.	
	3. Plain abdominal film.	
	4. EKG—to be read by patient's internist.	
	5. Dulcolax, two (2) tabs on admission; repeat in the A.M.	
	6. Fleet enemas through both colostomy stomas on admission.	
TIME NOTED	NURSE'S SIGNATURE DOCTOR'S SIGNATURE	☐ TO BE DISCHARGED
DATE & TIME	7. Cleansing enemas rectally the night of admission.	
	8. Fleet enema at bedside for physicians to administer.	
	9. Minimum residue diet on admission.	
	10. Change to clear liquid diet the morning after admission.	
	11. Ambulate prn.	
	12. Consent for colostomy closure.	
	13. Prep for possible laparotomy.	
	14. Dalmane, 30 mg, p.o., @ hs, prn sleep.	
	15. D.S.S., 250 mg, p.o., bid.	
TIME NOTED	NURSE'S SIGNATURE DOCTOR'S SIGNATURE	☐ TO BE DISCHARGED
DATE & TIME	16. Petrogalar, one (1) ounce, p.o., bid.	
	17. Routine colostomy care.	
	18. Other medications:	
TIME NOTED	NURSE'S SIGNATURE DOCTOR'S SIGNATURE	☐ TO BE DISCHARGED

APPROVED EQUIVALENTS MAY BE DISPENSED UNLESS CHECKED HERE

Set 7

PHYSICIAN'S ORDER SHEET

			DATE & TIME	ORDERS	PATIENT NAME

PREOPERATIVE ORDERS

Patient Name: Date:

1. Type of surgery:

   Date:

   Time:

2. Anesthesia:

3. Operation permit to be obtained.

4. Notify O.R. & Anesthesia Department.

5. NPO after midnight.

(left margin: APPROVED EQUIVALENTS MAY BE DISPENSED UNLESS CHECKED HERE)

TIME NOTED	NURSE'S SIGNATURE	DOCTOR'S SIGNATURE	☐ TO BE DISCHARGED

DATE & TIME

6. Upon rising in the morning of surgery, patient must wash face

   with Phisohex, void urine, and have a bowel movement.

7. Chloroptic Ophthalmic Solution

   1 drop to _____ q 1 hr. upon rising in the morning of

   surgery.

8. Preoperative Medication

   _____ mgm Demerol I.M. 1 hr. preoperative (time _____)

   _____ mgm Valium P.O. 1 hr. preoperative (time _____)

9. Preoperative Antibiotics

(left margin: APPROVED EQUIVALENTS MAY BE DISPENSED UNLESS CHECKED HERE)

TIME NOTED	NURSE'S SIGNATURE	DOCTOR'S SIGNATURE	☐ TO BE DISCHARGED

DATE & TIME

   _____ mgm Ampicillin I.M. 1 hr. preoperative (time _____)

10. Void urine immediately before patient leaves for O.R.

11. Diamox 250 mgm _____ tab P.O. 1 hr. preoperative (time _____)

12. Special Medications:

(left margin: APPROVED EQUIVALENTS MAY BE DISPENSED UNLESS CHECKED HERE)

TIME NOTED	NURSE'S SIGNATURE	DOCTOR'S SIGNATURE	☐ TO BE DISCHARGED

et 8

PHYSICIAN'S ORDER SHEET

			DATE & TIME	ORDERS	PATIENT NAME

	ADMITTING ORDERS: PREOP COLON SURGERY

☐ APPROVED EQUIVALENTS MAY BE DISPENSED UNLESS CHECKED HERE

1. Clear liquid diet with gum drops.

2. Dulcolax tabs ii on admission, repeat in A.M.

3. D.S.S. 250 mg po BID.

4. Petrogalar 1 oz. po q hs.

5. CBC, Lytes, Creatinine, Glucose, U/A.

6. EKG—to be read by patient's internist.

7. CXR.

TIME NOTED	NURSE'S SIGNATURE	DOCTOR'S SIGNATURE	☐ TO BE DISCHARGED

☐ APPROVED EQUIVALENTS MAY BE DISPENSED UNLESS CHECKED HERE

DATE & TIME

8. SMA-12 in A.M.

9. T & C _____ u. pc. for surgery.

10. May shower.

11. Ambulatory.

12. Routine vital signs.

13. Abdominal prep.

14. Cleansing enema on eve. prior to surgery.

15. Consent for:

TIME NOTED	NURSE'S SIGNATURE	DOCTOR'S SIGNATURE	☐ TO BE DISCHARGED

☐ APPROVED EQUIVALENTS MAY BE DISPENSED UNLESS CHECKED HERE

DATE & TIME

16. Dalmane 30 mg po @ hs PRN.

TIME NOTED	NURSE'S SIGNATURE	DOCTOR'S SIGNATURE	☐ TO BE DISCHARGED

Set 9

PHYSICIAN'S ORDER SHEET

DATE & TIME	ORDERS	PATIENT NAME

POSTOPERATIVE ORDERS FOR:

1. Vital signs until stable.

2. Bed rest. head up.

3. May be up to bathroom with assist only.

4. Progress to regular diet as tolerated.

5. Chloral hydrate 0.5 gm h.s. PRN for sleep

   repeat × 1 PRN.

6. Compazine 5 mgm I.M. q 4 hr. PRN for nausea.

TIME NOTED	NURSE'S SIGNATURE	DOCTOR'S SIGNATURE	☐ TO BE DISCHARGED

DATE & TIME

7. Milk of Magnesia 30cc PRN for laxative.

8. Empirin with codeine #3 tabs ii q 4 hr.

   PRN for pain.

9. Place eye medications at bedside tray, especially note

   those from O.R.

10. Continue previous medications as follows:

TIME NOTED	NURSE'S SIGNATURE	DOCTOR'S SIGNATURE	☐ TO BE DISCHARGED

DATE & TIME

TIME NOTED	NURSE'S SIGNATURE	DOCTOR'S SIGNATURE	☐ TO BE DISCHARGED

POSTOP PACU ORDERS

1. MEDICATIONS:

☒ Fentanyl 25 mcg. IV q5 min. x ___4___ doses prn pain
☐ Fentanyl 50 mcg. IV q5 min. x _____ doses prn pain
☐ Morphine _____ mgm IV q 5 min x _____ doses prn pain
☐ Compazine ☒ 1.25 mgm. IV prn nausea M.R.X.- _Ø_____
☒ Inapsine ☐ 2.5 mgm. IV prn nausea M.R.X. _____
☐ Atropine 0.2 mgm. IV prn pulse below _____ and notify anesthesiologist
M.R. x _____ prn
☒ OTHER _____Pulse Oximetry_____
                    ABG's 1200 *✗*

2. ADDITIONAL ORDERS:
OXYGEN
☐ Mask   ☐ Nasal Prongs _____ LPM ☒ Mist ___40___ %

Verapamil 2.5mg IV } in PAR stat
Digoxin 0.25 mg IV }
Call Dr. ████████ for ICU orders

3. DISCHARGE:

To ☐ Ward   ☐ DOU   ☒ ICU   ☐ Home
☒ Time 1300
☐ PACU Score of _____
☐ Block sensory level of _____
☐ Return of motor function

4. POST – OP ANESTHESIA ORDERS FOR FLOOR

O₂ mist 40%   ABGs in AM
Suction airway q 2 hr + prn poor cough
CXR in AM
Pulse Oximetry

[Handwritten physician's orders]

Admit: DOU.

Dx: R/O R Hip Fx

S/P ⓁHip replace

Cond: guarded

Vit sh q 2-4, q 4°

Diet Regular

Ensure prn tid 240 cc

Act immobility Ⓡ hip. Bedrest

Date	Time	R.N.	Date	Time	M.D.

Allergy ∅

Medications

Tylenol ᵢᵢ po q 4°

Ascriptin ᵢᵢ po q 6°

Demerol 25 ᵐᵍ

Vistaril 25 ᵐᵍ   IV q 3° prn pain

MVI ᵢᵢ po q am.

IV D5½ NS @ 50 cc/hr

c̄ 20 KCl

Date	Time	R.N.	Date	Time	M.D.

Deep breathing & foot flexion q 1 hr.

Eggcrate Mattress

Admit—Definitive Observation Unit

Diagnosis—Rule out right hip fracture
    Slipped left hip replacement

Condition—Guarded

Vitals—every 2–4 hrs to every 4 hrs

Diet—Regular
    Ensure when necessary three times a day—240 cc

Activity—Immobility right hip. Bedrest.

Allergy—None

Medications—Tylenol $\bar{ii}$ po q 4 hrs

    Ascriptin $\bar{ii}$ po q 6 hrs

    Demerol 25 mg ⎫
    Vistaril 25 mg ⎭ IV q 3° prn pain

    MVI $\bar{ii}$ po q AM

IV D5½ NS at 50 cc/hr c̄ 20 KCl

Deep breathing & foot flexion q 1 hr

Eggcrate mattress

Set 12

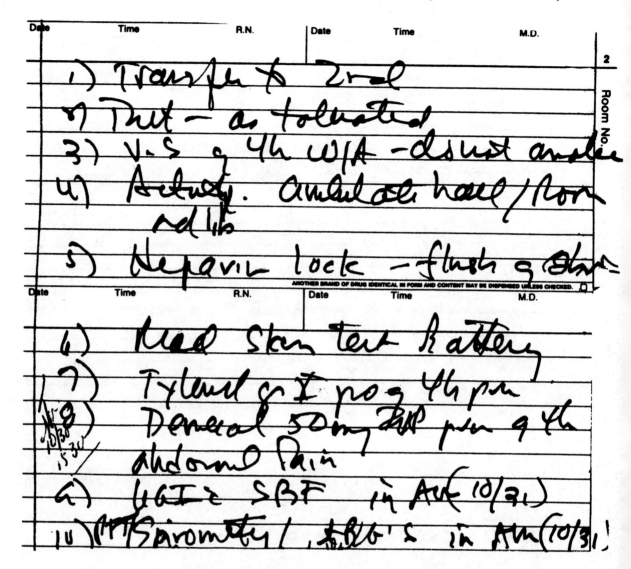

1) Transfer to 2nd (floor)
2) Diet as tolerated
3) Vital signs every 4 hrs while awake—do not awake
4) Activity—ambulate hall/room ad lib
5) Heparin lock—flush every 8 hrs
6) Read skin test battery
7) Tylenol grain 10 po every 4 hrs prn
8) Demerol 50 mg prn every 4 hrs abdominal pain
9) Upper gastrointestinal series, small bowel film in AM
10) Pulmonary function tests/spirometry/arterial blood gases in AM

Set 13

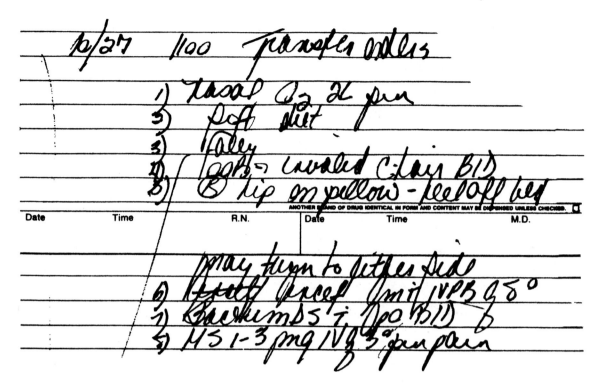

1) Nasal oxygen 2 L prn
2) Soft diet
3) Foley
4) Out of bed invalid chair twice a day
5) Right hip on pillows—heel off bed. May turn to either side.
6) Ancef Gm ⅰ intravenous piggyback every 8 hrs
7) Bactrim DS ⅰ po BID
8) Morphine sulfate 1–3 mg IV q3° prn pain

Set 14

Change IV orders:
    Continue current L DSW c̄ 40 KCl/L at 85 cc/hr
    Next L D5NS c̄ 40 KCl @ 85/hr
    Then D5½ c̄ 40 KCl/L at 85/hr continuous
    Lytes in AM

Set 15

Date	Time	R.N.	Date	Time	M.D.
ANOTHER BRAND OF DRUG IDENTICAL IN FORM AND CONTENT MAY BE DISPENSED UNLESS CHECKED. □					

Tagamet 300 mg IM q 6h
NPO
Chart I&O
Sodium luminal gr ⅱ Ⓗ prn sleep
Hematocrit & hemoglobin at 6 AM
Continuous gastric suction

Set 16

Physical therapy consult with patient with ruptured disc lumbar 5–sacral 1 with nerve root S_1

Sponge baths and shampoo

Continue bedside commode

Zantac 150 mg po BID

Discontinue IV

Increase Percocet to 2 tablets po every 3 hrs prn pain

K-pad to left buttock and low back

Set 17

Set 18

1. Sign Consent → exploratory laparotomy c̄ appendectomy

2. Mefoxin ī gm IV now

Date	Time	R.N.	Date	Time	M.D.
11/3/8	1300				

3. Demerol 75 mg IM now –

Set 19

Post op appendectomy

1. PR → 2nd
2. VS q̄ 8h

Date	Time	R.N.	Date	Time	M.D.

3. NPO
4. IV D5½ NS + 20 mEq KCl/l @ 150 cc/h.
5. Mefoxin ī gm IV q̄ 6h disc @ 1900
6. TCDB q̄ 2h while awake
7. Leg exercises

Date	Time	R.N.	Date	Time	M.D.

8. Ambulate tid
9. St. cath. q̄ 8h prn –

Set 20

Date	Time	R.N.	Date	Time	M.D.

ANOTHER BRAND OF DRUG IDENTICAL IN FORM AND CONTENT MAY BE DISPENSED UNLESS CHECKED. ☐

Set 21

Dx: Severe back pain c̄ sciatica + slipped lumbar disc.
1. Reg diet
2. Exercise mattress
3. BR strict – BSC for BM only
4. Pelvic Tx 20#
5. Hep lock

Time	R.N.		Date	Time	M.D.

ANOTHER BRAND OF DRUG IDENTICAL IN FORM AND CONTENT MAY BE DISPENSED UNLESS CHECKED. ☐

6. Robaxin 500mg IVPB q8° for 3× then
7. Oral Robaxin 750 po q10
8. Percocet ī tab q3° prn pain
9. CT scan of back in AM. LS spine
10. Colace 200mg po q12°
11. Naprosyn 500mg BID c̄ meals

Set 22

---

① UGI today
② Triple lumen cath c̄ bedside
③ Sign consent → insertion triple lumen catheter
④ Hold KCl in IV for

Date	Time	R.N.	Date

ANOTHER BRAND OF DRUG IDE...

CHART ⑤ SmA-14 today

Set 23

① IV - D5½NS c̄ 20mEq KCl at 125cc/hr.

② Digoxin 0.25mg 2 hrs p̄ dose given in d.R.

③ Verapamil 5mg IVP q̄ 4° prn SVT > 150/min
     Maximum of 4 doses in 24°

       Call Dr. ████████ if rate remains > 150
       p̄ one dose of Verapamil

④ M.S. 1-3mg IV q̄ 3° prn pain

⑤ H+H at 1500

⑥ CPK X3 per ICU protocol - starting now

<table>
<tr><th>Date</th><th>Time</th><th>R.N.</th><th>Date</th><th>Time</th><th>M.D.</th></tr>
</table>

⑦ K at 1800°

⑧ CBC° and SMA 7° in AM

⑨ EKG° in AM

Set 24

CBC°
UA
SMA 14
ABG
EKG
Chest X-ray
T + C 2 units

STAT

Set 25

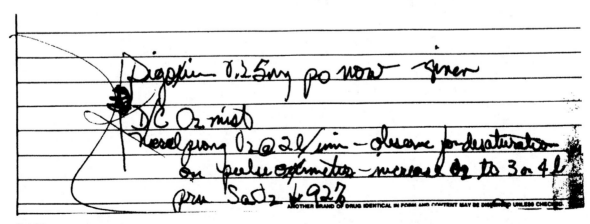

Digoxin 0.25mg po now given

DC O₂ mist

Nasal prong O₂ @ 2L/min - observe for desaturation
on pulse oximeter - increase O₂ to 3 or 4L
prn SaO₂ < 92%

Set 26

Type & X match for 2 units of
blood

Give one unit blood now &
repeat H&H @ 4PM & 7AM

Time	R.N.	Date	Time

digoxin .25 mg ⊙ q day

5% D/W c̄ 40 KCl c̄ 85cc/hour

Set 27

Darvocet N-100 ī q4h prn pain

ORUDIS 75 mg ī bid

D/C digoxin

I.V. 5% glucose in Ringer's lactate
at 85/hour.

Date	Time	R.N.	Date	Time	M.D.

H&H in AM

Give 2nd unit of blood today

O₂ prn

Set 28

Zantac 150 y bid

K⁺ N   m̄   ATY / Buffer / hypo also

.40 g dehomedrol 1 cc   ⎤   1. d
40 u ACTH   1 cc   ⎦

Qué davoulte, N — 100   ī q 6 h
        pm pain

Use IV M. S only if absolutely necessary

Compazine 5 mg   ī q 4 h prn
        nausea

Set 29

1) Halcion 0.5mg po q HS prn

2) MOM 30cc po QD prn

3) Lomotil 2 q 6h prn diarrhea

4) Ambulate tid
   BRP č Amb prn

5) D/C Cefoxitin after 1 post
   Biopsy dose

Set 31

1) Abdominal CT scan and chest CT today, STAT

2) CBC daily   NO EZ CATH

3) ~~Amy Ca~~ ~~~~ PRN

Date   **Time**   **R.N.**   **Date**   **Time**   **M.D.**

ANOTHER BRAND OF DRUG IDENTICAL IN FORM AND CONTENT MAY BE DISPENSED UNLESS CHECKED.

4) ESR in AM 10/29

5) EKG in AM (10/29)

6) Obtain old charts STAT on floor

7) CEA titer ~~today~~ STAT

8) Skin test Battery: PPD, Candida, mumps today

Set 32

1) Obtain consent for colonoscopy c per Dr. ~~~~ for 8:30 AM

Set 33

For Colonoscopy in am
Begin go-lytely colonic lavage 4L as
prepped NG tube over 2-3 hrs.

Set 34

2) Diet. — Regular
No Caffeine. No Alcohol
3) V.S. q 4w w/A
4) IV — D5NS at 100 cc/hr
5) Ambulate BR c̄ Asst ās needed

Date	Time	R.N.	Date	Time	M.D.

6) Nystatin Oral Suspension — 5 cc swish & swallow QID — pt may use own — pt has his own
7) Hycodan 5 mg T̄T̄ tab po q HS
— may repeat T̄ q 4h prn cough
8) Ativan 2 mg po q HS

Date	Time	R.N.	Date	Time	M.D.

9) Pepcid 20 mg po BID
10) Digoxin 0.25 mg po QD
11) Tylenol gr X̄ po q 4h prn pain
12) Imodium 2 mg po q 4h prn diarrhea
13) IPPB c̄ NS q 4h w/A°C
14) ABG on Room Air Now
15) Urinalysis — Now

Date	Time	R.N.	Date	Time	M.D.

16) NPO after Midnight tonight
17) Septra DS T̄ tab po BID
18) Blood Culture X3 — 5 min apart

Set 35

4) Diuretion to recopt today

5) Ensure Plus ↑ can TID

6) Obtain copy of pt's EKG for outpatient record of 11/4
dor

Date	Time	R.N.	Date	Time	M.D.

7) Demerol 75 mg ⎫ IM on
   Vistaril 50 mg ⎭
   Call to Radiology to
   Thoracenesis — may repeat
   q 4h prn chest pain

Date	Time	R.N.	Date	Time	M.D.

8) Chest x-ray in am (11/6)

9) ~~May DIC RO if labs~~

5) May DIC RO after Thoracen
   if pt stable

incision care to abd + axilla incisions
as done at home, BID — clean
incisions c̄ hydrogen peroxide +
apply new bandaide
send culture tubes to radiology c̄
pt + have thoracentesis fluid sent
to lab for aerobic + anaerobic
organisms

Set 37

NPH insulin 70 units SQ
        now

Call me c̄ AM glucose
when available — notified
Glucose at 1600 STAT

Time	R.N.	Date	Time	M.D.

Call me c̄ results

Sit OOB for meals + prn
en cough — assist prn
P.T. eval in _____ today

EKG in AM (11/3)
H/H _____ in AM (11/3)
SMA-7

Increase Heparin to 1000 u/min

Time	R.N.	Date	Time	M.D.

Daily PTT in AM's

Set 38

① D/C Robaxin
② Soma 350 mg po qid
③ Prednisone 60mg po today
   40 mg po 11/8
   20 mg po 11/9
   10 mg po. 11/10 & 11/11 then D/C
④ For acute severe back pain or spasm give
   Demerol 50 c̄ Vistaril 50 mg I.M. q3 hrs prn.

Set 39

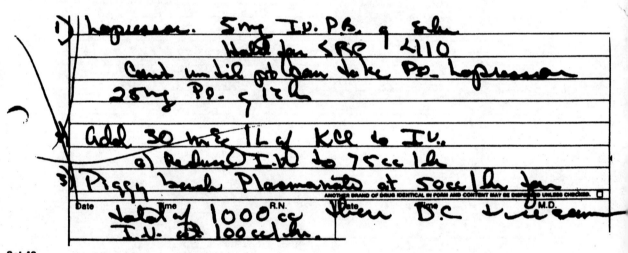

1) Lopressor 5mg IV. PB. q 5hr
   Hold for SBP ∠110
   Cont until pt can take PO. Lopressor
   25mg PO. q 12h
2) Add 30 mEq/L of KCl to IV.
   a) Reduce IV to 75cc/hr
3) Piggy back Plasmanate at 50cc/hr then
   total of 1000 cc then D/C
   IV at 100cc/hr.

Set 40

1) DC Compazine
2) Torecan 10mg PO or IM q4h prn N/V
3) Valium 2-10mg IV q 2h prn acute
   agitation
4) Increase IV to 125cc/hr
5) Temperg - called

Set 41

Room No. 3

I.S., Q4H W/A

St. cath if no void by midnight
→ Q10H prn thereafter.

P.T.: isometrics & bed mobility

Set 42

↑ ↓C wife's 1 unit of whole
blood & transfuse today

Set 43

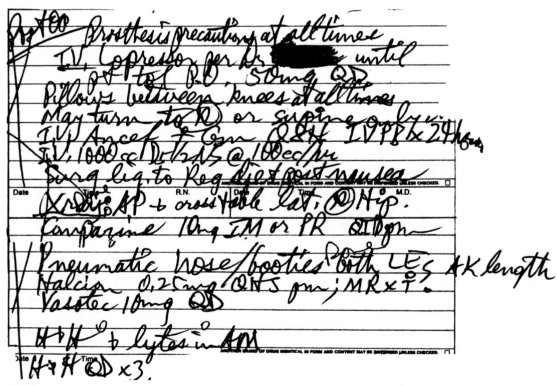

Prosthesis precaution at all times
I.V. Lopressor per Dr. ___ until
___ to P.O. 50mg QD
Pillows between knees at all times
May turn to ® or supine only
I.V. Ancef 1 Gm Q8H IVPB x 24 hours
I.V. 1000cc D5½NS @ 100cc/hr
Sling leg. to Reg diet post nausea
X-ray ® AP & cross-table lat. ® Hip.
Compazine 10mg I.M. or PR Q4H prn
Pneumatic hose/booties both LE's AK length
Halcion 0.25mg QHS prn; MR x 1.
Vasotec 10mg QD

H & H & lytes in AM
H & H QD x 3.

Set 44

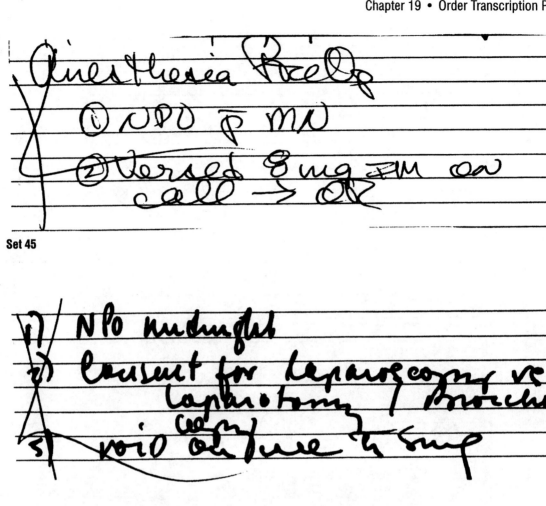

Set 45

Set 46

1) ICU → floor
2) V.S. Q15min til stable then Q 2hrs x 4 then Q 8hrs.
3) NPO
4) IV's D5½NS + 50meq KCl/L✓ at 100cc QH
5) Collect all post bronch sputum for Cytology. ∅

Date	Time	R.N.	Date	Time	M.D.

ANOTHER BRAND OF DRUG IDENTICAL IN FORM AND CONTENT MAY BE DISPENSED UNLESS CHECKED. ☐

6) Pneumatic boots Done
7) EKG in ICU ✓ done
8) Demerol 50-75mg IM Q 2 hrs pr pain.
9) Restoril 100mg IM HS ✓ pr sleep
10) Torecan 10mg IM Q 6 hrs ✓ IV meds, pr nausea.

Set 47

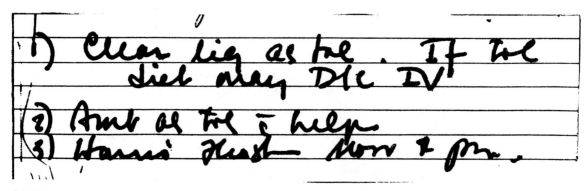

1) Clear liq as tol. If tol diet may D/C IV
2) Amb as tol c̄ help
3) Harris Flush now & prn.

Set 48

Bibliography

BADASCH, SHIRLEY, and CHESEBRO, DOREEN, *Introduction to Health Occupations* (4th ed.). Upper Saddle River, NJ: Brady, 1997.

BARBER, LINDA, *Being a Medical Admissions Clerk.* Upper Saddle River, N.J.: Brady, 1994.

BENTLY McDANIEL, JAN; and ORANGE COUNTY APIC. *New Guidelines for Isolation Precautions in Hospitals,* 1996.

BLACKBURN, ELSA, *Health Unit Coordinator.* Upper Saddle River, N.J.: Brady, 1991.

BORTON, DOROTHY, *Isolation Precautions. Nursing 1997,* January, pp. 49–51.

BROOKS-LA FLEUR, MYRNA, *Health Unit Coordinating* (4th ed.). St. Louis MO: Mosby, 1999.

BRUST, DONNA, and FOSTER, JOYCE, *From Nursing Assistant to Patient Care Technician.* Philadelphia: W. B. Saunders Co., 1997.

BURTON, GWENDOLYN, and ENGELKIRK, PAUL, *Microbiology for the Health Sciences* (6th ed). Philadelphia: Lippinott Williams Wilkins, 2000.

CHABNER, DAVI-ELLEN, *The Language of Medicine* (5th ed.). Philadelphia: W. B. Saunders Co., 1996.

CLARK, MADELINE, and MAZZA, VIRGINIA, *Health Unit Coordinating: Expanding the Scope of Practice.* Philadelphia: W. B. Saunders, 1999.

DAMJANOV, IVAN, *Pathology for the Health-Related Professions.* Philadelphia: W. B Saunders Co., 1996.

EDGE, RAYMOND, and KRIEGER, JOHN, *Legal and Ethical Perspectives in Health Care.* Albany, N.Y.: Del Mar, 1998.

FREMGEN, BONNIE F., *Essentials of Medical Assisting.* Upper Saddle River, N.J. Prentice-Hall, 1998.

GARBER, DEBRA, *Introduction to Clinical Allied Healthcare* (2d ed.). Orange, Calif. Career, 1998.

GARBER, DEBRA, *Introduction to Clinical Allied Healthcare.* Orange, Calif.: Caree Publishing, Inc., 1996.

HARTSHORN, JEANETTE, SOLE, MARY LOU, and LAMBORN, MARILYN, *Introduction to Critical Care Nursing* (2d ed.). Philadelphia: W. B. Saunders Co., 1997.

HODGSON, BARBARA, and KIZIOR, ROBERT, *Saunders Nursing Drug Handbook 2000,* Philadelphia: W. B. Saunders Co., 2000.

HODGSON, BARBARA, KIZIOR, ROBERT, and KINGDON, RUTH, *Nurse's Drug Handbook 1997.* Philadelphia: W. B. Saunders Co., 1997.

KARCH, AMY, *1997 Lippincott's Nursing Drug Guide.* Philadelphia: Lippincott, 1997

LAFLEUR-BROOKS, MYRNA, *Health Unit Coordinating* (3d ed.). Philadelphia: W. F Saunders Co., 1993.

LUCKMANN, JOAN, *Transcultural Communication in Nursing.* Albany, N.Y.: Del Mar 1999.

MARSHALL, JACQUELYN, *The Clinical Laboratory Assistant/Phlebotomist,* Orange, Calif.: Career, 2000.

MARTINI, FREDERIC, *Fundamentals of Anatomy and Physiology.* Upper Saddle River, N.J.: Prentice Hall, 1989.

McCAFFERY, MARGO, and PASERO, CHRIS, *Pain Control. Nurseweek,* September 2000, pp. 18–19.

McMILLER, KATHRYN, *Being a Medical Records Clerk.* Upper Saddle River, N.J.: Brady, 1992.

Miller-Keane Encyclopedia and Dictionary of Medicine, Nursing, and Allied Health (6th ed.). Philadelphia: W. B. Saunders Co., 1997.

Mosby's Nursing Drug Reference 2001. St. Louis, MO.: Mosby, 2001.

PAGANA, KATHLEEN, and PAGANA, TIMOTHY, *Mosby's Diagnostic and Laboratory Test Reference* (4th ed.). St. Louis MO.: Mosby, 1999.

POZGAR, GEORGE, *Legal Aspects of Health Care Administration* (6th ed.). Gaithersburg. Md.: Aspen Publishers, Inc., 1996.

RICE, JANE, *Principles of Pharmacology for Medical Assisting* (3rd ed.). Albany, N.Y.: Del Mar, 1999.

Taber's Cyclopedic Medical Dictionary, (18th ed.). Philadelphia: F. A. Davis Co., 1997.

WOLGIN, FRANCIE, *Being a Nurse Assistant* (8th ed.). Upper Saddle River, N.J.: Prentice Hall, 2000.

WOLGIN, FRANCIE, *Being a Nursing Assistant* (7th ed.). Upper Saddle River, N.J.: Brady, 1997.

Index